C WILCOX, MD
DEPT OF RADIOLOGY

C WILCOX, MD
DEPT OF RADIOLOGY

AIDS IMAGING

A Practical Clinical Approach

To my wife Nienke, my children Loes and Puck, and to my mother and
in memory of my father for all their love and support.

To my wife Jane, my children Julia, Ian, David and Fiona,
and to my parents, Jack and Gloria for all their love and support.

AIDS IMAGING
A Practical Clinical Approach

Edited by

Jacques W.A.J. Reeders, MD, PhD

Head, Division of Gastrointestinal Radiology and Hepato-pancreato and Biliary Imaging,
Academic Medical Center, Amsterdam,
The Netherlands

John R. Mathieson, MD, FRCPC

Head, Section of Radiology, Medical Imaging Services, Capital Health Region,
Victoria, BC,
Canada

Formerly: Head of Gastrointestinal and Interventional Radiology,
St Paul's Hospital, University of British Columbia, Vancouver, BC,
Canada

W.B. Saunders Company Ltd
London Philadelphia Toronto Sydney Tokyo

W. B. Saunders Company Ltd   24–28 Oval Road
London NW1 7DX

The Curtis Center
Independence Square West
Philadelphia, PA 19106-3399, USA

Harcourt Brace & Company
55 Horner Avenue
Toronto, Ontario M8Z 4X6, Canada

Harcourt Brace & Company, Australia
30–52 Smidmore Street
Marrickville, NSW 2204, Australia

Harcourt Brace & Company, Japan
Ichibancho Central Building, 22-1 Ichibancho
Chiyoda-ku, Tokyo 102, Japan

A catalogue record for this book is available from the British Library

ISBN 0-7020-1904-6

Typeset by Florencetype Ltd, Stoodleigh, Devon
Printed by Jarrold Book Printing Ltd, Norfolk

CONTENTS

Part III   Quick Reference Tables

CONTRIBUTORS

Michael M. Ambrosino, MD
Department of Radiology,
New York University Medical Center,
New York,
USA

Joep F.W.M. Bartelsman, MD
Department of Gastroenterology
Academic Medical Center,
University of Amsterdam,
Amsterdam,
The Netherlands

Patrick J.E. Bindels, MD, PhD
Municipal Health Service,
Amsterdam,
The Netherlands

Kees Boer, MD, PhD
Department of Gynecology,
Academic Medical Center,
University of Amsterdam,
Amsterdam,
The Netherlands

Charles A.B. Boucher, MD
Department of Microbiology,
Academic Medical Center,
Human Retrovirus Laboratory,
Amsterdam,
The Netherlands

Anne-Elizabeth Cabée, MD
Centre d'Imagerie,
Paris-Nord 95,
200 Sarcelles,
France

Norman H. Chan, MD
Department of Laboratory Medicine,
St Paul's Hospital,
University of British Columbia,
Vancouver, BC,
Canada

Esther C.J. Consten, MD, PhD
Department of Surgery,
Academic Medical Center,
Amsterdam,
The Netherlands

Roel A. Coutinho, MD, PhD
Department of Public Health,
Municipal Health Service,
Amsterdam,
The Netherlands

Sven A. Danner, MD, PhD
AIDS Clinics,
Division of Infectious Diseases,
Academic Medical Center,
Amsterdam,
The Netherlands

Muriel Eliaszewicz, MD
Service de Maladies Infectieuses,
Hôpital de l'Institut Pasteur,
Paris,
France

Roelien H. Enting, MD
Department of Neurology,
Academic Medical Center,
University of Amsterdam,
Amsterdam,
The Netherlands

Nancy B. Genieser, MD
Department of Radiology,
NYU Medical Center,
New York,
USA

Mieke H. Godfried, MD, PhD
Department of Internal Medicine,
Academic Medical Center,
Amsterdam,
The Netherlands

Richard M. Gore, MD
Department of Gastrointestinal Radiology,
Evanston Hospital–McGaw Medical Center of
    Northwestern University,
Evanston,
Illinois,
USA

Jaap Goudsmit, MD, PhD
Human Retrovirus Laboratory,
Academic Medical Center,
University of Amsterdam,
Amsterdam,
The Netherlands

Philip B. Harrison, MD
Department of Radiology,
St Paul's Hospital,
University of British Columbia,
Vancouver, BC,
Canada

Hendrik J. Hulsebosch, MD, PhD
Department of Dermatology,
Academic Medical Center,
University of Amsterdam,
Amsterdam,
The Netherlands

Marla C. Kiess, MD
Echocardiography Laboratory,
St Paul's Hospital,
University of British Columbia,
Vancouver, BC,
Canada

Keith Krasinski, MD
Department of Pediatrics,
New York University Medical Center,
New York,
USA

Jan J.B. van Lanschot, MD, PhD
Department of Surgery,
Academic Medical Center,
Amsterdam,
The Netherlands

Robert L. Lavayssière, MD
Centre d'Imagerie,
Paris-Nord 95,
200 Sarcelles,
France

Donna Magid, MD
Department of Radiology,
Johns Hopkins University,
Baltimore,
USA

John R. Mathieson, MD, FRCPC
Section of Radiology,
Medical Imaging Services,
Capital Health Region,
Victoria, BC,
Canada

Frank H. Miller, MD
Department of Gastrointestinal Radiology,
Northwestern Memorial Hospital
Chicago, Illinois,
USA

Julio S.G. Montaner, MD, FRCPC, FCCP
Infectious Disease Clinic,
St Paul's Hospital,
AIDS Research Program,
University of British Columbia,
Vancouver, BC,
Canada

Nestor L. Müller, MD
Department of Chest Radiology,
Vancouver General Hospital,
Vancouver, BC,
Canada

Peter Phillips, MD
Infectious Disease Clinic,
St Paul's Hospital,
AIDS Research Program,
University of British Columbia,
Vancouver, BC,
Canada

Peter Portegies, MD, PhD
Department of Neurology,
Academic Medical Center,
Amsterdam,
The Netherlands

D. Randall Radin, MD
Professor of Radiology,
University of Southern California,
School of Medicine,
Los Angeles, California,
USA

Jacques W.A.J. Reeders, MD, PhD
Division of GI-Radiology and
Hepato-pancreato and Biliary Imaging,
Academic Medical Center,
University of Amsterdam,
Amsterdam
The Netherlands

Kevin J. Roche, MD
Department of Radiology,
New York University Medical Center,
New York,
USA

Eric A. van Royen, MD, PhD
Department of Nuclear Medicine,
Academic Medical Center
University of Amsterdam,
Amsterdam,
The Netherlands

Marguerite E. I. Schipper, MD, PhD
Department of Pathology,
University Hospital Utrecht,
Utrecht,
The Netherlands

Frederick J. Smith, MD
Department of Diagnostic Imaging,
Oakville-Trafalgar Memorial Hospital,
Oakville, Ontario,
Canada

Eric van Sonnenberg, MD
Department of Radiology,
University Hospital Clinic,
Galveston, TX
USA

Catherine A. Staples, MD
Department of Radiology,
Kelowna General Hospital,
Kelowna, BC,
Canada

Christopher R. Thompson, MD
Echocardiography Laboratory,
St Paul's Hospital,
Vancouver, BC,
Canada

Pierre M. Trotot, MD
Service de Radiologie,
Hôpital de l'Institut Pasteur,
Paris,
France

Jan G. van den Tweel, MD, PhD
Department of Pathology,
University Hospital Utrecht,
Utrecht,
The Netherlands

Susan D. Wall, MD
Department of Interventional Radiology,
University of California,
San Francisco, CA
USA

Judy Yee, MD
Department of Radiology,
University of California,
Veterans Administration Medical Center,
San Francisco, CA,
USA

FOREWORDS

Foreword by Peter L. Cooperberg

The spread of AIDS in the last 15 years has been alarming and devastating. However, research into the cause and effects of AIDS has been equally rapid and, in some ways, gratifyingly successful. Much has been learned about the causative organism, the complicating infections, and the treatment of both. The disease is tending to become chronic rather than acute as before. Furthermore, there has been a tendency for the disease to spread from parts of the world and districts of large cities, where it is endemic, to a much more wide-spread distribution within and surrounding cities, as well as to all countries around the world. Therefore, the incidence of AIDS is still increasing and, since patients are now living longer, the prevalence is also on the rise.

This book is edited by two radiology experts from two different continents, but from hospitals that have similar downtown, endemic-type populations with HIV disease. These and other hospitals have been the source of much of the case material as well as research and investigation into HIV diseases. As illustrated in this book, the editors and the other contributors have a wealth of experience based on referral patterns, particularly from their local areas.

As the disease is now tending to spread out to more peripheral communities, it is important for all radiologists to be aware, not only of the typical radiographic presentation of all the manifestations of this disease and its complications, but even of the more subtle and variable findings.

The book is divided into three parts. The first gives a general overview of the history, epidemiology, and pathology of the AIDS phenomenon. This provides interesting reading and a solid background of information regarding the disease. The second part consists of a review of each organ system. The typical, as well as the occasional, clinical and imaging findings in each organ system are presented. There are excellent chapters within the organ systems section discussing different imaging modalities.

Perhaps the most useful part of this book is Part III. This consists of tables summarizing the different imaging findings seen with the most common infections and tumors in each organ system. It is a very extensive index and allows the practicing radiologist an easy way to quickly review the widespread and myriad aspects of this disease.

It is rare for a text to be both encyclopedic and a good reference source, as well as easy to read. However, this is an example of such a book. It will certainly make an impact on the way we investigate, treat, and teach this disease.

Peter L. Cooperberg
Professor and Vice-Chairman,
Department of Radiology,
University of British Columbia;
Chairman of Radiology,
St Paul's Hospital,
Vancouver, Canada, BC

Foreword by Guido N. J. Tytgat

The discovery of HIV infection and its recognition as one of the most important pathogens of humankind have granted a variety of scientists – from clinicians to molecular geneticists, from epidemiologists to experimental pharmacologists – membership of a new club of unprecedented variety. This is reflected in this well-conceived multiauthored book which places great emphasis on this indispensable multidisciplinary character of the research on AIDS. This book details, in a clear and concise manner, the techniques available for investigation of patients with HIV infection. First, a general introduction is given covering the state of affairs of HIV infection and AIDS in humans by world-renowned experts. Then a systematic discussion follows of the imaging modalities of the various organ systems, comprising the neurological, cardiopulmonary, abdominal, hepatopancreatic, retroperitoneal, dermatological, and musculoskeletal system. Special sections are devoted to the special problems of women and children with AIDS.

The last few years have witnessed a pandemic of books devoted to the pathology of the gastrointestinal tract in AIDS. How can clinicians and researchers make an informed decision about their next purchase? Price is hardly a consideration. The clarity of writing, the comprehensiveness, the timely nature, and the abundance and the excellence of figures and tables should be primary considerations in choosing a book of this kind. Readers want to know and see how organs and tissues affected by this tragic infection look and behave.

Throughout this book, a lavish selection of well-focused color and black and white photomicrographs gratify the eyes and the mind. The text is well written, and contains a wealth of well-referenced basic and practical information.

The chief editors and all the contributors are to be congratulated on a masterly AIDS imaging 'classic' which will be used as a major reference book for many years to come.

Guido N.J. Tytgat
Professor and Chairman,
Department of Gastroenterology,
Academic Medical Center,
University of Amsterdam

PREFACE

In less than two decades AIDS has become one of the most devastating illnesses in human history. Not long ago the concept of a retroviral infection rewriting the genetic code and causing destruction of the immune system was in the realm of science fiction. The AIDS epidemic differs from most other diseases in many ways, has challenged conventional medical thinking, and has broadened the boundaries of knowledge of human biology and medicine. The patterns of disease and pathological changes seen in AIDS patients can be perplexing and challenging, particularly in the Medical Imaging department.

As the epidemic continues to spread, AIDS patients are no longer confined to a few specialized AIDS hospitals, and are now seen in general hospitals and clinics everywhere. We feel there is a need for an AIDS Imaging textbook that is not only comprehensive, but also practical and easy to apply to daily clinical problem solving.

In this book we present a review of the current knowledge about the wide range of manifestations in AIDS and how the role of modern Medical Imaging techniques in diagnosis and treatment can be applied. Each chapter is written by leading experts from major AIDS hospitals in a variety of centres throughout North America and Europe. The book is organized in three parts. *Part I* consists of a review of basic medical sciences as they apply to AIDS. In *Part II*, the clinical and imaging features of AIDS (organized by body system) are presented, central nervous system, cardiopulmonary system, lumenal gastrointestinal tract, hepato-pancreatobiliary system, retroperitoneum, urinary tract, reproductive system, skin and musculoskeletal system. AIDS in children has evolved from a clinical syndrome meeting with scepticism regarding its relationship to immunosuppresive disease in adults, to a well-characterized disease process, becoming the ninth leading cause of death in children. Therefore, a special chapter has been devoted to pediatric AIDS radiology. *Part III* comprises Quick Reference Tables, summarizing the radiological abnormalities and imaging findings in AIDS-related disease of each body system.

We have structured the book so that each chapter can be read on its own, without requiring referral to other material, so that clinical problems can be solved as they arise. The textbook should be most useful as a guide in the encounter with AIDS patients in daily clinical practice. We hope that the reader will forgive the repetition of material needed to allow the chapters to be read out of sequence.

We hope that the coming years will see light shed upon our current state of ignorance of this baffling affliction.

J.W.A.J. Reeders
J.R. Mathieson

Part I General Overview

1 HISTORY OF AIDS

Jacques W.A.J. Reeders

Acquired immune deficiency syndrome (AIDS), the most severe clinical expression of immunosuppression following infection with human immune deficiency virus (HIV), was first diagnosed as a clinical entity in 1981 [1–4]. At the Centers of Disease Control and Prevention (CDC) in Atlanta, Georgia, USA, the first indications of the impending AIDS epidemic became evident. Upon retrospective review of clinical cases and blood and tissue samples, the disease was found to have already existed at least as early as 1978 in the USA [5]. In 1981, Gottlieb et al. (at three different hospitals in Los Angeles, California) became intrigued by a cluster of five young patients whose ages ranged from 29 to 36 years [2]. Two of the patients died and the remaining three were seriously ill. All of these patients had evidence of having been infected with *Pneumocystis carinii*, thrush and a cytomegalovirus (CMV), which was similarly common in immuno-suppressed patients. All pointed to an association with a homosexual lifestyle and a sexually transmitted disease [6].

The first report of these observations appeared in the *Morbidity and Mortality Weekly Report* of the CDC on 5 June 1981 [2,5]. A month later, there were similar reports of 26 homosexual men, 20 from New York and 6 from California, with a very uncommon tumor known as Kaposi's sarcoma (named after the nineteenth-century Hungarian dermatologist Moritz Kaposi, who first described this skin tumor). Kaposi's sarcoma had previously only been observed in elderly men, often of Mediterranean and Jewish extraction, and also in tropical Africa, mainly in children and young adults. These patients also had evidence of infections such as thrush and CMV.

It was at the beginning of the 1980s that the relatively few cases of homosexual male patients with unusual infections and tumors heralded the onset of one of the most devastating epidemics in

Table 1.1. CDC Clinical Classification System of HIV Infections.

Group I	Acute HIV infection (mononucleosis-like syndrome)
Group II	Asymptomatic HIV infection
Group III	Persistent generalized lymphadenopathy
Group IV	

    A   ARC (AIDS-related complex) (weight loss more than 10%, diarrhea and fever for more than one month)

    B   Primary neurological disease (dementia, myelopathy, peripheral neuropathy)

    C   Secondary infectious disease

        C1 Specified secondary infectious disease listed in the CDC surveillance definition for AIDS: *Pneumocystis carinii* pneumonia; chronic cryptosporidiosis; toxoplasmosis; extraintestinal strongyloidiasis; isosporiasis; candidiasis – esophageal, bronchial or pulmonary; cryptococcosis; mycobacterial infections; cytomegalovirus infections; chronic mucocutaneous; disseminated herpes simplex infection; pulmonary tuberculosis or recurrent bacterial pneumonia

        C2 Other specified secondary infectious diseases: oral hairy leukoplakia; herpes zoster; *Salmonella* sepsis; nocardiosis; tuberculosis; oral candidiasis

    D   Secondary cancers: Kaposi's sarcoma; non-Hodgkin lymphoma; primary lymphoma in central nervous system (CNS); invasive cervical cancer

    E   Other conditions, e.g. HIV-associated thrombocytopenia

N.B.   Patients are diagnosed with AIDS if classified IVB to IVE.

Table 1.2. Major developments in AIDS biomedical research in chronological order [10].

1981–1985

- Acquired immunodeficiency syndrome is first described in young homosexual men [2–4], intravenous drug users [12], hemophiliacs [13], blood transfusion in recipients [14], infants [15], and immigrants from certain countries [7]
- AIDS infectious agent is transmitted by sexual means, by blood products, and from mothers to infants [16]
- A non-transforming retrovirus isolated independently from a number of individuals with AIDS or related syndromes [17–20].
- Antibodies to this retrovirus (HIV-I) are detected in the majority of individuals with AIDS or pre-AIDS using a variety of serological techniques [21–23]
- Cell lines are developed to allow continuous propagation of HIV-I [19,24,25]
- The major receptor for the virus is identified as the CD4 molecule [26,27]
- Isolates of HIV-I are obtained from semen [28,29]

1986–1990

- Isolates of HIV-I are obtained from the CNS [30–32]
- The spectrum of disease associated with the virus is expanded to range from asymptomatic virus carriers, to primary HIV syndromes [33,34], to advanced dementia
- The HIV-I external glycoprotein, gp±120, is identified [35,36]
- HIV-I is molecularly cloned [37,38]
- The nucleotide sequence is established [39–42]
- Reliable antibody screening assays are developed and implemented for HIV-I blood screening [22,23]
- Techniques are developed to inactivate HIV-I in certain blood products such as factor VII for hemophiliacs [43,44]
- A Simian immune deficiency retrovirus (SIV) is shown to induce an AIDS-like illness in macaque monkeys [45–47]
- HIV-2 is isolated in west Africa and is related to SIV [48]
- Successful demonstration that zidovudine (ZDV, AZT) prolongs life and reduces opportunistic infections in persons with advanced HIV-I disease [49]
- Successful prophylaxis against *Pneumocystis carinii* pneumonia is also shown in patients with advanced HIV-I infection, utilizing oral trimethoprim-sulfamethoxazole [50]
- Spread of HIV-I infection occurs throughout most of the world
- Different patterns of transmission are described in different areas [51] with sexual transmission remaining the major vehicle for global spread
- Individuals are found to harbor swarms of genetically polymorphic viruses with varied tropisms [52,53] defined as quasi-species [54]
- Monocyte-macrophages infected with HIV-I are found in blood, lungs, and brain [55–60]
- Monocytes are found to be infectible *in vitro* [55]. Host immune responses to HIV-I proteins are well characterized, including neutralizing antibodies [61–64] and cytotoxic T-lymphocytes [65,66]. The major structural and regularity genes of HIV-I are defined [67–71] and molecular mechanisms of HIV-I replication are elucidated [72,73]

1991–present

- Early ZDV therapy in individuals with ⩽500 CD4 lymphocytes/mm³ delays progression of disease [74,75]
- Other nucleoside derivatives, such as didanosine and zalcitabine, also demonstrate potential clinical benefit in HIV-I infection, either as monotherapy [76–80] or in combination with zidovudine [81]
- Kaposi's sarcoma (KS)-associated herpesvirus (KSHV), a newly discovered human gamma herpesvirus, is found in the majority of KS lesions from patients with and without AIDS [82–87]

medical history, with a profound impact on all aspects of medical practice [7]. Because the new disease was mainly seen in homosexuals with frequently changing sexual contact, the name gay-related immunodeficiency disease (GRID) was given.

After the initial reports of AIDS, the CDC set up a task force to detect the syndrome in the population and identify those at risk. Criteria for the definition of AIDS were drawn up based primarily on diagnosis of opportunistic infections and rare tumors in individuals with no evidence of immune suppression. The CDC formulated the first case definition in 1981, which was revised in 1985 and 1987 [8,9]. In 1993, the definition was altered again. Besides three additional clinical conditions, one laboratory parameter was included as indicative for AIDS: a peripheral blood CD4-lymphocyte count (T-cell in a HIV-infected patient) [10]. Contrary to the USA, the latter criterion is not accepted as the sole definition of AIDS in Europe. The stages of HIV disease according to the

CDC Clinical Classification System are presented in Table 1 [8–10].

Major developments in AIDS biomedical research are summarized in Table 1.2 in chronological order and according to Hersch and Kaplan [10].

Since the early 1990s many clinical trials have been conducted. Intense societal pressure and the urgency of the AIDS epidemic have also greatly reduced regulatory roadblocks to the approval of new and promising drugs, and changed the position of regulators from extreme caution to active participation, resulting in a number of approvals of new antiviral compounds in record speed [11].

Many clinical trials are now cooperative efforts among pharmaceutical companies, academic investigators, government regulators and community participants [11].

Undoubtedly the HIV epidemic will continue to grow this century. The harvest of new biomedical knowledge from expanded research efforts will hopefully continue. Strides will be incremental and cures are not on the horizon yet. The knowledge gained may eventually prolong useful lives and may change AIDS from a rapidly fatal disease to a controlled chronic illness [11].

References

1 CDC. Update: Acquired immunodeficiency syndrome – United States. *MMWR* 1986; **35**: 17–21.

2 Gottlieb MS, Schroff R, Schanker HM et al. *Pneumocystis carinii* pneumonia and mucosal candidiasis in previously healthy homosexual men: evidence of a new acquired cellular immunodeficiency. *N Engl J Med* 1981; **305**: 1425–1431.

3 Masur H, Michelis MA, Greene JB et al. An outbreak of community-acquired *Pneumocystis carinii* pneumonia. *N Engl J Med* 1981; **305**: 1431–1438.

4 Siegal FP, Lopez C, Hammer GS et al. Severe acquired immunodeficiency in male homosexuals, manifested by chronic perianal ulcerative herpes simplex lesions. *N Engl J Med* 1981; **305**: 1439–1444.

5 CDC. Kaposi's sarcoma and *Pneumocystis* pneumonia among homosexual men in New York City and California. *MMWR* 1981; **25**: 305–308.

6 Schoub BD. *AIDS and HIV in Perspective.* Cambridge University Press, Cambridge, 1994.

7 CDC. Revision of the case definition of acquired immune deficiency syndrome for national reporting. *MMWR* 1985; **34**: 373.

8 CDC. Revision of the CDC surveillance case definition for acquired immune deficiency syndrome. *MMWR* 1987; **36** (1S): 1.

9 CDC. Revised classification for HIV infection and expanded surveillance case definition for acquired immune deficiency syndrome among adolescents and adults. *MMWR* 1993; **41**: 1–19.

10 Hirsch MS, Kaplan JC. The biomedical impact of the AIDS epidemic. In: Broder S, Merigan TC, Bolognesi D (eds) *Textbook of AIDS Medicine.* Baltimore: Williams & Wilkins, 1994: 3–12.

11 CDC. Update on acquired immune deficiency syndrome (AIDS) – United States. *MMWR* 1982; **31**: 504–514.

12 CDC. *Pneumocystis carinii* pneumonia among persons with hemophilia A. *MMWR* 1982; **31**: 365–367.

13 CDC. Possible transfusion-associated acquired immune deficiency syndrome (AIDS). *MMWR* 1982; **31**: 652–654.

14 CDC. Unexplained immunodeficiency and opportunistic infection in infants – New York, New Jersey, California. *MMWR* 1982; **31**: 665–667.

15 CDC. Acquired immune deficiency syndrome (AIDS): precautions for clinical and laboratory staff. *MMWR* 1982; **31**: 577–580.

16 Barre-Sinoussi F, Chermann JC, Rey F et al. Isolation of a T-lymphotropic retrovirus from a patient at risk for acquired immune deficiency syndrome (AIDS). *Science*, 1983; **220**: 868–871.

17 Gallo RC, Salahuddin SZ, Popovic M et al. Frequent detection and isolation of cytopathic retroviruses (HTLV-III) from patients with AIDS and at risk for AIDS. *Science*, 1984; **224**: 500–502.

18 Popovic M, Sarngadharan MG, Read E, Gallo RC. Detection, isolation and continuous production of cytopathic retroviruses (HTLV-III) from patients with AIDS and pre-AIDS. *Science* 1984; **224**: 497–500.

19 Levy JA, Hoffman AD, Kramer SM, Landis JA, Shimabukuro JM, Oshiro LS. Isolation of lymphocytopathic retroviruses from San Francisco patients with AIDS. *Science* 1984; **225**: 840–842.

20 Brun-Vezinet F, Rouzioux C, Barre-Sinoussi F et al. Detection of IgG antibodies to lymphadenopathy-associated virus in patients with lymphadenopathy syndrome. *Lancet* 1984; **1**: 1253–1256.

21 Schupbach J, Popovic M, Gilden RV, Gonda MA, Sarngadharan MG, Gallo RC. Serological analysis of a sub group of human T-lymphotropic retroviruses (HTLV-II) associated with AIDS. *Science* 1984; **224**: 503–505.

22 Sarngadharan MG, Popovic M, Bruch L, Schupbach J, Gallo RC. Antibodies reactive with human T-lymphotropic retro-

viruses (HTLV-III) in the serum of patients with AIDS. *Science* 1984; **224**: 506–508.

23 Montagnier L, Gruest J, Chamaret S et al. Adaptation of lymphadenopathy associated virus (LAV) to replication in EBV-transformed B lymphoblastoid cell lines. *Science* 1984; **225**: 63–66.

24 Popovic M, Reda-Connole E, Gall RC. T4 positive human neoplastic cell lines susceptible to and permissive for HTLV-III. *Lancet* 1984; **2**: 1472–1473.

25 Dalgleish AG, Beverley PCL, Clapham PR, Brawford DH, Greaves MF, Weiss RA. The CD4 (T4) antigen is an essential component of the receptor for the AIDS retrovirus. *Nature* 1984; **312**: 763–767.

26 Klatzmann D, Barre-Sinoussi F, Nugeyre MT et al. Selective tropism of lymphadenopathy associated virus (LAV) for helper-inducer T lymphocytes. *Science* 1984; **225**: 59–63.

27 Zagury D, Bernard J. Leibowitch J et al. HTL-III in cells cultured from semen of two patients with AIDS. *Science* 1984; **226**: 449–451.

28 Ho DD, Schooley RT, Rota TR, et al. HTLV-III in the semen and blood for a healthy homosexual man. *Science* 1984; **226**: 451–453.

29 Ho DD, Rota TR, Schooley RT et al. Isolation of HTLV-III from cerebrospinal fluid and neural tissues of patients with neurologic syndromes related to the acquired immunodeficiency syndrome. *N Engl J Med* 1985; **313**: 1493–1497.

30 Levy JA, Shimabukuro J, Hollander H, Mills J, Kaminsky L. Isolation of AIDS-associated retroviruses from cerebrospinal fluid and brain of patients with neurological symptoms. *Lancet* 1985; **2**: 586–588.

31 Shaw GH, Harper ME, Hahn BH et al. HTLV-III infection in brains of children and adults with AIDS encephalopathy. *Science* 1985; **227**: 177–181.

32 Cooper DA, Gold J, Maclean P et al. Acute AIDS retrovirus infection. Definition of a clinical illness associated with seroconversion. *Lancet* 1985; **1**: 537–540.

33 Ho DD, Sarngadharan MG, Resnick L, Dimarzo-Veronese F, Rota TR, Hirsch MS. Primary human T-lymphocytic virus type III infection. *Ann Intern Med* 1985; **103**: 880–883.

34 Kitchen LW, Barin F, Sullivan JL, et al. Aetiology of AIDS-antibodies to human T-cell leukemia virus (type III) in haemophiliacs. *Nature* 1984; **312**: 367–369.

35 Allan J, Coligan JE, Barin F et al. Major glycoprotein antigens that induce antibodies in AIDS patients are encoded by HTLV-III. *Science* 1985; **228**: 1091–1094.

36 Alizon M, Sonigo P, Barre-Sinoussi F et al. Molecular cloning of lymphadenopathy-associated virus. *Nature* 1984; **312**: 757–760.

37 Hahn BH, Shaw GM, Arya SK, Popovic M, Gallo RC, Wong-Staal F. Molecular cloning and characterization of the HTLV-III virus associated with AIDS. *Nature* 1984; **312**: 166–169.

38 Meusing MA, Smith DH, Cabradilla CD, Benton CV, Lasky LA, Capon DJ. Nucleic acid structure and expression of the human AIDS/lymphadenopathy retrovirus. *Nature* 1985; **313**: 450–458.

39 Ratner L, Haseltine W, Patarca R et al. Complete nucleotide sequence of the AIDS virus, HTL-III. *Nature* 1985; **313**: 277–284.

40 Sanchez-Pescador R, Power MD, Barr PJ et al. Nucleotide sequence and expression of an AIDS-associated retrovirus (ARV-2). *Science* 1985; **227**: 484–492.

41 Wain-Hobson S, Sonigo P, Danos O, Cole S, Alizon M. Nucleotide sequence of the AIDS virus, LAV. *Cell* 1985; **40**: 9–17.

42 CDC. Update: acquired immunodeficiency syndrome (AIDS) in persons with hemophilia. *MMWR* 1984; **33**: 589–592.

43 Levy JA, Mitra G, Mozen MM. Recovery and inactivation of infectious retroviruses from factor VIII concentrates. *Lancet* 1984; **2**: 722–723.

44 Kanki PJ, McLane MF, King NWJ et al. Serologic identification and characterization of a macaque T-lymphotropic retrovirus closely related to HTLV-III. *Science* 1985; **228**: 1199–1201.

45 Daniel MD, Letvin NL, King NW et al. Isolation of T-cell tropic HTLV-III-like retrovirus from macaques. *Science* 1985; **228**: 1201–1204.

46 Letvin NL, Daniel MD, Sehgal PK et al. Induction of AIDS-like disease in macaque monkeys with T-cell tropic retrovirus STLV-III. *Science* 1985; **230**: 71–73.

47 Clavel F, Guetard D, Brun-Vezinet F et al. Isolation of a new human retrovirus from West African patients with AIDS. *Science* 1986; **233**: 343–346.

48 Fischl MA, Richman DD, Grieco MH et al. The efficacy of 3′-azido-3′deoxythymidine (azidothymidine) in the treatment of patients with AIDS and AIDS-related complex: a double-blind, placebo-controlled trial. *N Engl J Med* 1987; **317**: 185–191.

49 Fischl MA, Dickinson GM, La Voie L. Safety and efficacy of sulfamethoxazole and trimethoprim chemoprophylaxis for *Pneumocystis carinii* in AIDS. *JAMA* 1988; **259**: 1185–1189.

50 Mann JM, Chin J, Piot P, Quinn T. The international epidemiology of AIDS. *Sci Am* 1988; **259**: 82–89.

51 Tersmette M, de Goede REY, Al BJM et al. Differential syncytium-inducing capacity of human immunodeficiency virus isolates: frequent detection of syncytium-inducing isolates in patients with acquired immunodeficiency syndrome (AIDS) and AIDS-related complex. *J Virol* 1988; **62**: 2026–2032.

52 Cheng-Mayer C, Seto D, Tateno M, Levy JA. Biologic features of HIV-I that correlate with virulence in the host. *Science* 1988; **240**: 80–82.

53 Goodenow M, Huet T, Saurin W, Kwok S, Sninsky J, Wain-Hobson S. HIV-I isolates are rapidly evolving quasispecies: evidence for viral mixtures and preferred nucleotide substitutions. *J Acquir Immune Defic Syndr* 1989; **2**: 344–352.

54 Ho DD, Rota TR, Hirsch MS. Infection of monocyte–macrophages by human T-lymphotropic virus type III. *J Clin Invest* 1986; **77**: 1712–1715.

55 Popovic M, Gartner S. Isolation of HIV-I from monocytes but not from T lymphocytes. *Lancet* 1987; **2**: 916.

56 Salahuddin SZ, Rose RM, Groopman JE, Markham PD, Gallo RC. Human lymphotropic virus type III infection of human alveolar macrophages. *Blood* 1986; **68**: 281–284.

57 Gartner S, Markovits P, Markovitz DM, Kaplan MH, Gallo RC, Popovic M. The role of mononuclear phagocytes in HTLV-III/LAV infection. *Science* 1986; **233**: 215–219.

58 Koenig S, Gendelman HE, Orentsein JM et al. Detection of AIDS virus in macrophages in brain tissue from AIDS patients with venecephalopathy. *Science* 1986; **233**: 1089–1093.

59 Wiley CA, Schrier RD, Nelson JA, Lampert PW, Oldstone MBA. Cellular localization of human immunodeficiency syndrome patients. *Proc Natl Acad Sci USA* 1986; **83**: 7089–7093.

60 Weiss RA, Clapham PR, Cheinsong-Popov R et al. Neutralization of human T-lymphotropic virus type III by sera of AIDS and AIDS-risk patients. *Nature* 1985; **316**: 69–72.

61 Robert-Guroff M, Brown M, Gallo RC. HTLV-III neutralizing antibodies in patients with AIDS and AIDS-related complex. *Nature* 1985; **316**: 72–74.

62 Ho DD, Sarngadharan MG, Hirsch MS et al. Human immunodeficiency virus neutralizing antibodies recognize several conserved domains on the envelope glycoproteins. *J Virol* 1987; **61**: 2024–2028.

63 Nara PL, Robey WG, Pyle SW et al. Purified envelope glycoproteins from human immunodeficiency virus type I variants induce individual, type-specific neutralizing antibodies. *J Virol* 1988; **62**: 2622–2628.

64 Walker BD, Chakrabarti S, Moss B et al. HIV-specific cytotoxic T lymphocytes in seropositive individuals. *Nature* 1987; **328**: 345–348.

65 Plata F, Autran B, Martins LP et al. AIDS virus-specific cytotoxic T lymphocytes in lung disorders. *Nature* 1987; **328**: 348–351.

66 Arya SK, Guo C, Josephs SF, Wong-Staal F. Trans-activator gene of human T-lymphotropic virus type III (HTLV-III). *Science* 1985; **229**: 69–73.

67 Sodroski J, Patarca R, Rosen C, Wong-Staal F, Haseltine WA. Location of the trans-activating region of the genome of human T-cell lymphotropic virus type III. *Science* 1985; **229**: 74–77.

68 Sodroski J, Goh WC, Rosen C, Dayton A, Terwilliger E, Haseltine WA. A second post-transcriptional trans-activator gene required for HTLV-III replication. *Nature* 1986; **321**: 412–417.

69 Feinberg MB, Jarret RF, Aldovini A, Gallo RC, Wong-Staal F. HTLV-III expression and production involve complex regulation at the levels of splicing and translation of viral RNA. *Cell* 1986; **46**: 807–817.

70 Cullen BR, Greene WC. Functions of the auxiliary gene products of the u/human immunodeficiency virus type I. *Virol* 1990; **178**: 1–5.

71 Cullen BR, Greene WC. Regulatory pathways governing HIV-I replication. *Cell* 1989; **58**: 423–426.

72 Haseltine WA. The molecular biology of HIV-I. In: Devita VT, Hellman S, Rosenberg SA (eds) *AIDS: Etiology Diagnosis, Treatment and Prevention*, 3rd edn. Philadelphia: Lippincott 1992: 39–59.

73 Fischl MA, Richman DD, Hansen N et al. The safety and efficacy of zidovudine (ZVT) in the treatment of subjects with mildly symptomatic human immunodeficiency virus type I (HIV) infection. *Ann Intern Med* 1990; **112**: 727–737.

74 Volberding PA, Lagakos SW, Koch MA et al. Zidovudine in asymptomatic human immunodeficiency virus infection. A controlled trial in persons with fewer than 500 CD$_4$-positive cells per cubic millimeter. The AIDS Clinical Trials Group of the National Institute of Allergy and Infectious Diseases. *N Engl J Med* 1990; **322**: 941–949.

75 Lambert JS, Seidlin M, Reichman RC et al. 2′3′-dideoxyinosine (ddI) in patients with the acquired immunodeficiency syndrome or AIDS-related complex. *N Engl J Med* 1990; **322**: 1333–1340.

76 Cooley TP, Kunches LM, Saunders CA et al. Once-daily administrations of 2′3′-dideoxyinosine (ddI) in patients with the acquired immunodeficiency syndrome or AIDS-related complex. Results of a Phase I trial. *N Engl J Med* 1990; **322**: 1340–1345.

77 Kahn JO, Lagakos SW, Richman DD et al. A controlled trial comparing continued zidovudine with didanosine in human immunodeficiency virus infection. *N Engl J Med* 1992; **327**: 581–587.

78 Merigan TC, Skowron G, Bozzette SA et al. Circulating p24 antigen levels and responses to dideoxycytidine in human immunodeficiency virus (HIV) infections. *Ann Intern Med* 1989; **110**: 189–194.

79 Merigan TC, Skowron G. Safety and tolerance of dideoxycytidine as a single agent: results of early-phase studies in patients with acquired immunodeficiency syndrome (AIDS or advanced AID-related complex). *Am J Med* 1990; **88**(Suppl 5B): 11S–15S.

80 Meng TC, Fischl MA, Boota AM et al. Combination therapy with zidovudine and dideoxycytidine in patients with advanced human immunodeficiency virus infection. A phase I/II study. *Ann Intern Med* 1992; **116**: 13–20.

81 Chang Y, Cesarman E, Pessin MS et al. Indentification of herpesvirus-like DNA sequences in AIDS-associated Kaposi's sarcoma. *Science* 1994; **265**: 1865–1869.

82 Chang Y, Ziegler JL, Wabinga H et al. Kaposi's sarcoma-associated herpesvirus DNA sequences are present in African endemic and AIDS-associated Kaposi's sarcoma. *Arch Intern Med* 1996; **156**: 202–204.

83 Moore PS, Chang Y. Detection of herpesvirus-like DNA sequences in Kaposi's sarcoma lesions from persons with and without HIV infection. *N Engl J Med* 1995; **332**: 1181–1185.

84 Boshoff C, Whitby D, Hatziionnou T et al. Kaposi's sarcoma-associated herpesvirus in HIV-negative Kaposi's sarcoma. *Lancet* 1995; **345**: 1043–1044.

85 Su I-J, Hsu Y-S, Chang Y-C, Wang I-W. Herpesvirus-like DNA sequence in Kaposi's sarcoma from AIDS and non-AIDS patients in Taiwan. *Lancet* 1995; **345**: 722–723.

86 Dupin N, Grandadam M, Calcez V et al. Herpesvirus-like DNA in patients with Mediterranean Kaposi's sarcoma. *Lancet* 1995; **345**: 761–762.

87 Moore PS, Kingsley LA, Holmberg SD et al. Kaposi's sarcoma-associated herpesvirus infection prior to onset of Kaposi's sarcoma. *AIDS* 1996; **10**: 175–180.

2 AIDS: A RETROVIRUS INFECTION IN HUMANS

Jaap Goudsmit
Charles A.B. Boucher

Introduction

The acquired immune deficiency syndrome (AIDS) is characterized by the appearance of opportunistic infections and tumors. Generally, AIDS does not emerge until years after the infection with the human immunodeficiency virus (HIV) has actually occurred. However, it has to be realized that HIV may cause AIDS in a few years. This is as rare as AIDS failing to appear within a period of 20 years following sero-conversion.

This chapter discusses the course and diagnostics of the infection, the structure and replication of HIV, and the pathogenesis and treatment of HIV infections.

The course of an HIV infection

The case history of a 58-year-old woman illustrates the full extent of the average course of an HIV infection (Figure 2.1). In January 1985, she was admitted to the hospital with a serious form of the Guillain–Barré syndrome. The decision was made to treat her with plasmapheresis, and for 2 weeks her plasma was replaced by a total of 16 litres of plasma derived from 82 different plasma donors. Two and half years after the plasmapheresis, a Kaposi's sarcoma and a *Candida* esophagitis were diagnosed. Also at that time, HIV antibodies could be demonstrated. In her case, the plasmapheresis procedure was the most probable source of HIV infection.

Retrospective analysis of the plasma samples with which she had been treated revealed that one plasma sample contained HIV antibodies. On the basis of stored serum samples from the patient, the development of serologic parameters could be investigated.

Using the HIV antigen test, proteins originating from the core of the virus can be detected in serum. Two weeks after infection, HIV antigen was found in her serum for a period of 1 week. The presence of these viral core proteins in her serum indicates that viral replication was occurring in the patient's cells. This was followed by the detection of HIV antibodies in her serum.

Some of the HIV antibodies are directed against the viral core, and these antibodies can bind with the viral core proteins and form complexes with them. If an excess of core-protein antibodies is produced, all antibodies will be trapped in complexes and the antigen test will become negative. At a certain point during the infection, the production of antigen is activated, resulting in an excess of antigen; thus the antigen test becomes positive again.

A prospective study of large groups of infected homosexual men has shown that the reappearance of HIV antigen in the serum of an asymptomatic individual is the precursor to the development of AIDS. A similar pattern could be seen in the patient discussed above. She was symptom-free for 2.5 years and no HIV antigen could be demonstrated. HIV antigen only reappeared when AIDS was diagnosed. With antiviral therapy (zidovudine), viral production could be reduced, as is apparent from the drop in serum level of HIV antigen following the initiation of therapy. Recently it has been discovered that the majority of virus detectable in the peripheral blood is produced by cells of lymph nodes and other lymphoreticular organs. The turnover of the virus population is extremely high, therefore, HIV infection can best be characterized as a persisting acute infection. The virus particles detected at any given time in the blood is produced in the last few days prior to detection.

Despite this high virus turnover, the steady-state level of HIV genomic RNA is relatively stable in the course of HIV infection. Figure 2.2 shows the distribution of AIDS patients related to the individual course of infection. From our own studies it was clear that virus load is a major determinant of the clinical

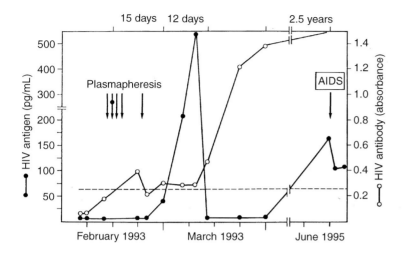

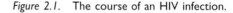

Figure 2.1. The course of an HIV infection.

progression rate. The course of infection in the patient shown in Figure 2.1 is representative of a rapid progressor. As can be seen, HIV-1 RNA levels do not decrease as dramatically after acute HIV infection as HIV-1 p24 levels. Progression rates in HIV-1 infection are directly related to HIV-1 RNA copy numbers in serum of plasma. *Rapid progressors* show persistent RNA levels and rapid CD4 cell decline; *average progressors* show an intermediate decline and a subsequent rise of HIV RNA levels following acute infection, in *slow progressors* the same kinetics are seen but somewhat retarded. *Non-progressors* show only the decline in HIV RNA levels and do not rebound.

Recognizing acute or chronic HIV infection

An acute HIV infection can present symptomatically, but this is not necessarily the case. Sometimes an infection is accompanied by a flu-like syndrome. Skin abnormalities can occur and retrosternal pain combined with swallowing problems have been described as a result of *Candida* esophagitis. Encephalopathy, meningitis and neuropathies can also occur in an acute infection. The incubation time for the flu-like syndrome varies from 1 to 4 weeks; the incubation time for the neurologic symptoms is 2–6 weeks. Because the complaints or symptoms are not specific, the case history makes an important contribution to establishing whether there is an acute HIV infection; in particular, details of recent events which could have resulted in the transmission of the HIV (sexual contact, blood transfusion, intravenous drug abuse) can lead to the diagnosis.

As shown in Figure 2.1, the serologic diagnostics in the early phase can be helpful. HIV antigen can be

demonstrated over a period of a few weeks in about 10–40% of those primarily infected, then antibodies develop. It is not possible in all cases to demonstrate antibodies following the antigen peak, and thus a 'window' phase can occur in which neither antibody or antigen is demonstrable. IgM antibodies to HIV can only be demonstrated in about 50% of all primary infections, but no earlier than IgG antibodies, and thus they do not play a role in routine diagnosis.

It is obvious that occasionally an individual will experience an acute HIV infection without any precious serologic indications. This is why it is recommended that the antigen test and the antibody test be repeated in follow-up sera taken at intervals of several weeks in those cases in which infection is strongly suspected. If no antibodies can be demonstrated after 3 months in the third-generation HIV enzyme-linked immunosorbent assay (ELISA), which can also detect HIV-2 antibodies, the patient can be regarded as not being infected. Once the HIV antibody test is positive, then it will remain positive for the rest of the patient's life.

The structure and replication of HIV

In order to be able to discuss the pathogenesis of HIV infections, it is essential to be aware of the structure and replication cycle of the virus.

Structure

The outside of an HIV particle is an envelope, consisting of a membrane derived from a cell, into

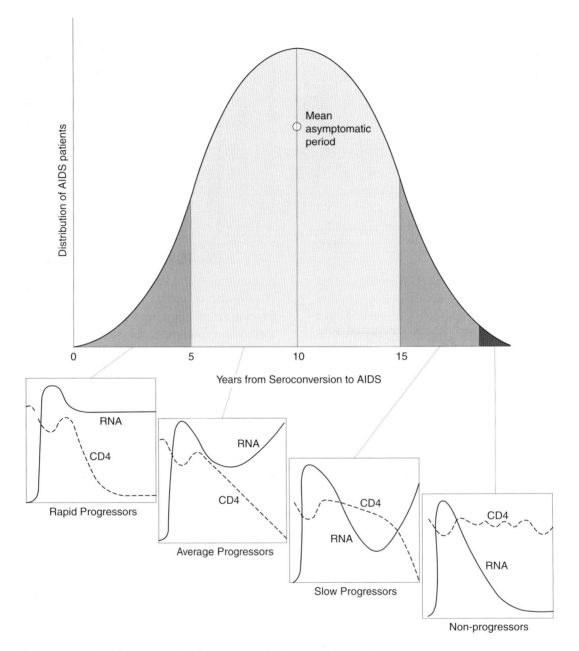

Figure 2.2. Distribution of AIDS patients related to the individual course of HIV infection.

which thumbtack-shaped objects have been inserted; these are encoded by the viral genome (Figure 2.3). This thumbtack (composed of proteins coupled to sugar groups/carbohydrate groups) consists of a head, glycoprotein 120, and a point, glycoprotein 41. This envelope contains the core proteins p17 (situated on the outside) and p24 (the innermost core protein). In the nucleus of the particle are two identical molecules of single-stranded RNA (the viral genome) and several copies of the enzyme, reverse transcriptase.

Replication

The *retro*viruses, to which the HIV belongs, derive their name from the enzyme reverse transcriptase. These enzymes have the unique property of being able to transcribe RNA into DNA. Converting RNA into DNA is an essential step in the replication cycle of a retrovirus (Figure 2.4). Once a cell has become infected, the viral RNA is transcribed into DNA by the reverse transcriptase which was brought into the

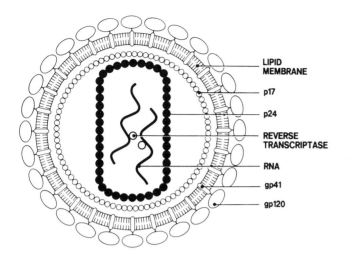

Figure 2.3. Schematic representation of a virus particle.

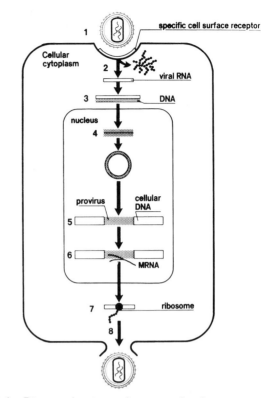

Figure 2.4. Diagram showing replication cycle of virus.

cell by the virus. The DNA is then integrated into the host cell genome; this is a 'provirus'. It can exist for a long time (years) before messenger RNA is produced; this is the latent phase. If the cell is 'activated', the provirus will also be activated via largely unknown mechanisms, resulting in the manufacture of viral messenger RNA (mRNA), which in turn stimulates the cell to procedure viral proteins. Genomic RNA is also produced. The viral proteins, together with the genomic RNA and the modified cell membrane derived from the host cell, form a new virus particle (Figures 2.5 and 2.6).

Analysis of the viral genome of HIV has revealed that, in addition to the genes that encode for structural proteins (of which the virus is composed, such as gp120, gp41, p17 and p24), other genes are also present. These code for enzymes which regulate the amount of virus produced (tat, nef, rev, protease) or the infectivity of the virus particle. Furthermore, there are genes which code for viral proteins whose function has not yet been elucidated.

Pathogenesis

HIV uses the CD4 receptor to penetrate cells. The most important host cell is the CD4 receptor-bearing T-lymphocyte, the T-helper cell (Figure 2.7).

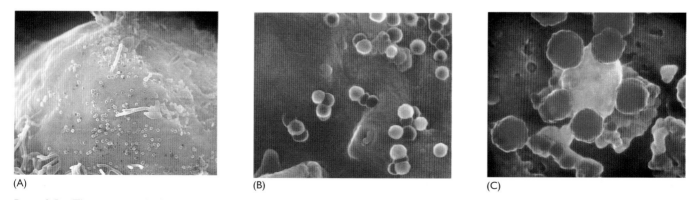

(A) (B) (C)

Figure 2.5. The process which a cell uses to produce new viral particles involves budding. The particles free themselves *en masse* from the cell surface. Virus particles often develop on the finger-shaped protrusions. Young (red) and more mature buds (blue) are visible. In (B), scarring can also be seen. (Enlargements of Figure 2.7; © Boehringer Ingelheim International GmbH; photography by L. Nilsson.)

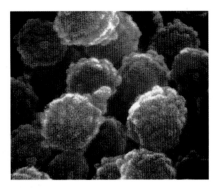

Figure 2.6. A few mature HIV particles, enlarged almost 1 000 000 times. The glycoprotein projections can even be seen. This electron microscopic technique does not allow further enlargement. The virus particles are not yet complete, but undergo a maturational process which also gives them a definitive inner structure. (© Boehringer Ingelheim International GmbH; photography by L. Nilsson.)

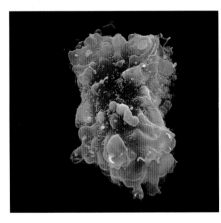

Figure 2.7. A major component of the immune system, a helper T-cell, can be seen to be under attack by the AIDS virus (blue). Multiple bladder- and finger-shaped protrusions of the cell can be seen. (© Boehringer Ingelheim International GmbH; photography by L. Nilsson.)

However, other CD4-positive cells, such as macrophages, B-cells, dendritic (antigen-presenting), and microglia cells can also become infected *in vivo*. The T-helper cell fulfils a central role in the regulation of the immune response. In the course of an HIV infection, functional disorders of the T-helper cell can already be established in the laboratory during the asymptomatic phase of the infection. These disorders are independent of the number of helper cells. Moreover, the number of T-helper cells gradually decreases during the infection (Figure 2.2). Ultimately, in the final stage of the illness, the existence of an

immune disorder can be directly deduced from the nature of the syndrome, i.e. the occurrence of opportunistic infections.

The T-helper cells are probably the most important reservoir and the most important site of production of the virus. The drop in the number of T-helper cells is possibly due to a direct lethal effect of intracellular virus production. *In vitro* studies have shown that signals which are a physiological stimulus for the T-helper cell also activate the integrated provirus, with the result that the production of viral particles starts.

Although at a cellular level the HIV can remain latent, it would appear to be incorrect to talk in general about a latent infection, because at each phase of the HIV infection, cell-free virus can be demonstrated in serum (Figure 2.2). This illustrates that continual replication proceeds at a low level. However, in the phase of disease progression, the continual drop in the number of T-helper cells seems to be associated with either a persistently high or a rising level of virus replication. This suggests that, at a certain time, there is a transition from a steady-state, low level of virus production to increased virus production in the average progressor.

Several mechanisms which operate during the infection cycle could contribute to the course described above. These mechanisms can be subdivided into viral immunologic factors. Investigation of viruses isolated during the course of HIV infections has shown that the biological properties of the virus in a person can change in the sense that viruses acquire properties that allow them to grow in several laboratory cell lines and that cause T-helper cells to fuse. Furthermore, during the course of an infection, the virus gradually changes the composition of the membrane protein at sites aimed at by the immune response. The most important site (epitope) is situated on gp120. Early in the infection, antibodies to this gp are manufactured which retard penetration of the virus into the cells, and thus neutralize it. These neutralizing antibodies could play a role *in vivo* to counteract massive viral spread. By altering this epitope precisely, the virus could eventually escape the neutralizing antibodies. Even in the asymptomatic phase, functional disorders can be demonstrated at several levels of the immune apparatus (T-helper cell, B-cell response, chemotaxis of the macrophage, cytotoxic T-cell response). The extent to which certain factors are the cause or the result of the advancing immunodeficiency, and what the effects are of interaction between viral and immunologic processes, is the subject of intense investigation.

Treatment of HIV infection

In the ideal situation, curing a person infected with HIV requires the complete abolition of all viruses from the body. This means that all proviruses should also be eliminated. In the absence of such a method, the prevention of virus production is an alternative. The first medicine to be successfully applied for this purpose on a large scale is zidovudine. The action of zidovudine, or AZT, lies in a specific interaction between the medicine and the enzyme reverse transcriptase. This enzyme incorporates the zidovudine into the growing DNA of the new provirus. Once incorporated, the zidovudine prevents further extension of the DNA molecule, so that a complete virus cannot be produced. The effect is that no further spread of the virus can occur, but the virus does remain in previously infected cells. Treatment of AIDS patients with zidovudine results in a drop in the amount of virus, an increase in the amount of T-helper cells and an extension of the life expectancy by a few years. Thus, zidovudine only yields a few extra years of life. It has been established in the laboratory that, during the course of treatment with zidovudine, HIV strains develop which are insensitive to zidovudine levels attainable *in vivo*. It is not inconceivable that the development of resistant strains is partially to blame for the fact that zidovudine is only effective for a limited time.

Several substances have been developed whose antiviral effect is based on the same mechanism as that of zidovudine. However, their application on a large scale is prevented by serious side effects. Recently it has been shown that the most promising therapy is combination therapy, in particular AZT combined with 3TC (lamivudine), which is a novel reverse transcriptase inhibitor that rapidly induces viral resistance. However, the RT mutation (codon 184) conferring 3TC resistance reverses AZT resistance in viruses carrying RT genes with both AZT and 3TC resistance mutation.

In the search for new medicines, one looks to other viral enzymes such as protease. Recent results with a combination of two RT inhibitors and a protease inhibitor are very encouraging.

Conclusion

It appears that the majority of all individuals with HIV eventually die from an acquired immunodeficiency. The length of the period from the moment of infection to the actual development of AIDS can, however, vary considerably (from a few months to 9 years). From the above, one can deduce that the human immune system does not (yet) have a satisfactory solution to suppressing or eliminating the infection. The cytotoxic T-cell response and neutralizing antibodies, two important pillars on which the fight against other infections rests, do not appear to be capable of successfully combating an HIV infection. Two properties of the virus are partially responsible for this: the ability to remain latent in some cells and the ability to continually change those components at which the human immune response aims. Because the virus infection has direct effects on different compartments of the immune system, for many disorders it is difficult to indicate whether they are the cause or result of disease progression. An important question remains: does reactivation of virus infection occur because of the appearance of certain immunologic disorder, or do immune disorders develop because of reactivation, or are both hypotheses correct? Answers to these questions can be obtained by studying the regulation of viral replication and the role of the viral variation which occurs in relation to the immunologic parameters.

Intervention via administration of antiviral substances (zidovudine), neutralizing antibodies, and immune modulators (interferon, interleukines) can help to provide insights into the importance of the different processes in retarding or preventing progression of disease. Until a strategy has been developed which can eliminate host cells with (latent) provirus, it is impossible actually to cure the infection.

Much research in the next few years will be aimed at developing methods to eliminate HIV and at developing an effective vaccine. Until this has been achieved, the medical profession can help AIDS patients by establishing diagnosis rapidly, so that adequate treatment can be initiated early on. Furthermore, there are indications that one should examine the effect of treatment with virostatic substances of individuals in the asymptomatic stages of HIV infection, with a view to determining the extent to which progression to AIDS can be delayed or even prevented.

Further reading

Fauci AS. The human immunodeficiency virus: infectivity and mechanisms of pathogenesis. *Science* 1988; **239**: 617–22.

Gottlieb MS, Groopman JE. *Acquired Immune Deficiency Syndrome (UCLA Symposia on Molecular and Cellular Biology)*. New York: Alan R. Liss, 1984.

Groopman JE, Chen ISY, Essex M, Weiss RA. *Human Retroviruses (UCLA Symposium on Human Retroviruses)*. New York: Wiley-Liss, 1989.

Ho DD, Pomerantz RJ, Kaplan JC. Pathogenesis of infection with human immunodeficiency virus. *N Engl J Med* 1987; **317**: 278–286.

Hogervorst E, Hurriaans S, De Wolf et al. Predictors for non- and slow progression in human immunodeficiency virus type 1 infection: low viral RNA copy numbers in serum and maintenance of high HIV-1 p24-specific but not V3-specific antibody levels. *J Infect Dis* 1995; **171**: 811–821.

Jurriaans S, Gemen van B, Weverling GJ et al. The natural history of HIV-1 infection: virus load and virus phenotype independent determinants of clinical course. *Virology* 1994; **204**: 223–233.

Levy JA. Mysteries of HIV: challenges for therapy and prevention. *Nature* 1988; **333**: 519–522.

Rosenblum ML, Levy RM, Bredesen DE. *AIDS and the Nervous System*. New York: Raven Press, 1988.

Schuurman R, Nijhuis M, Van Leeuwen R et al. Rapid changes in human immunodeficiency virus (HIV)-1 RNA load and appearance of drug resistant virus population in individuals treated with 3TC (Lamivudine). *J Infect Dis* 1995; 411–419.

Varmus H. Retroviruses. *Science* 1988; **240**: 1427–1435.

3 THE CLINICAL SPECTRUM OF HIV INFECTION

Sven A. Danner

The clinical spectrum

The prevalence of human immune deficiency virus (HIV) infection and its clinical end stage acquired immune deficiency syndrome (AIDS) has continued to increase world-wide during the last few years, as will be described elsewhere (see page 26). The clinical spectrum has not changed profoundly. Some infections with microorganisms which were previously hardly known have been added to the list of opportunistic infections, and additional information has been achieved on the many atypical clinical presentations of infections and malignancies in advanced HIV infection. The incidence of the different complications has changed as a result of a somewhat longer survival, changes in the size of the different risk groups, and increasing use of primary prophylaxis against infectious complications. For example, generalized atypical mycobacteriosis and retinitis caused by cytomegalovirus are seen more frequently. These are really end-stage complications, occurring usually in individuals with less than $100/mm^3$ $CD4^+$ lymphocytes. On the other hand, the incidence of Kaposi's sarcoma is decreasing. This is the result of the decreasing contribution of homosexual/bisexual men to the total number of AIDS patients. For reasons still to be elucidated, Kaposi's sarcoma is mainly seen in this group and far less in other groups such as intravenous drug abusers or heterosexual individuals.

Pneumocystis carinii pneumonia as an AIDS indicator is declining owing to the widespread use of primary prophylaxis with cotrimoxazole in HIV-infected people with $<200/mm^3$ $CD4^+$ lymphocytes. Because cotrimoxazole is also active against toxoplasmosis, the incidence of encephalitis by *Toxoplasma gondii*, a late stage complication, is also declining.

Since the widespread use of zidovudine, the incidence of the AIDS dementia complex has declined sharply. Zidovudine, which penetrates relatively well in the cerebrospinal fluid (CSF), apparently protects against this complication. It still seems to do so despite the fact that its effect on health in general is waning, or that viral strains isolated from the peripheral blood show resistance to the drug. Alternative antiretroviral drugs, such as zalcitabine or didanosine, which show a much lower CSF/blood concentration ratio, lack this beneficial effect.

One additional disease should be mentioned explicitly. Since the beginning of the AIDS epidemic, a rising incidence of tuberculosis (TB) has been observed, both in Western countries and in the developing countries. The presentation is often an atypical one: extrapulmonary TB is seen as often as the classical pulmonary appearance. Moreover, especially in the USA, outbreaks of TB cases with tubercle bacilli, which are resistant to multiple tuberculostatic drugs, have been reported. Mortality in this group is extremely high.

Clinical staging system

In 1993 the Centers for Disease Control (CDC) (Atlanta, Georgia, USA) and the World Health Organization (WHO) adopted a new clinical staging system for HIV infection. This is a matrix classification (Table 3.1). Three clinical categories are discriminated. Class A harbors the situations without lasting clinical symptoms: the acute HIV infection, the persisting generalized lymphadenopathy, and the fully asymptomatic carrier state. Class B contains all the 'minor' disease states, such as diarrhea or fever for unknown cause, fatigue and weight loss, oral candidiasis, and multidermatomal zoster infection. Patients in Class C have had one or more of the so-called AIDS indicator diseases, consisting of all the 'major' opportunistic infections or the HIV-related malignancies, such as Kaposi's sarcoma, non-Hodgkin lymphoma, or

Table 3.1. WHO clinical classification system for HIV infective disease.

CD4+ lymphocytes (cells/mm³)	Class A	Class B	Class C
≥500	A-I	B-I	C-I
200–499	A-II	B-II	C-II
<200	A-III	B-III	C-III

primary brain lymphoma. Beside the three clinical stages, there are three classes of immunosuppression: I, ≥500/mm³ CD4+ lymphocytes; II, 200–499/mm³ CD4+ lymphocytes; and III, <200/mm³ CD4+ lymphocytes.

Unfortunately, a difference in interpretation has developed between the USA (CDC) and the WHO with regard to the definition of AIDS. Outside the USA the following definition of AIDS is used: a person in Class C-I, C-II, or C-III is considered to have AIDS. These countries stick to a strictly clinical definition of AIDS. The CDC adds another category: a person is also considered to have AIDS if he or she is infected with HIV and has less than 200/mm³ CD4+ lymphocytes. Therefore, in the USA, Class A-III, B-III, C-I, C-II, C-II, and C-III all qualify for the diagnosis. The rationale is an administrative one: in the USA the access to proper health care and social security for large groups of the population is limited, and a diagnosis of AIDS provides extra facilities for an individual.

The list of AIDS indicator diseases, as assessed in 1987 by the CDC, has recently been extended with three diseases: a person is also considered to have AIDS if he or she is infected with HIV and suffers from pulmonary tuberculosis, recurrent bacterial pneumonia, or cervical carcinoma.

Therapy

In HIV infection, therapy consists of two main parts: the actual anti-HIV therapy with compounds which have antiretroviral effects, and therapy against the many complications of the HIV infection. This overview addresses the antiretroviral therapy.

The basis of antiretroviral drug treatment is sought in the interruption of the HIV replication cycle. This cycle can be divided in two parts. The first consists

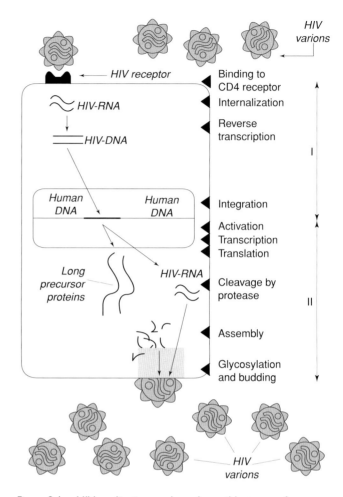

Figure 3.1. HIV replication cycle and possible targets for intervention. The cycle can be divided in the process leading to infection of the cell, i.e. insertion of the viral genome sequence into the human genome (labeled I), and the process leading to the production of new infectious virions (labeled II). Currently, only inhibition of reverse transcription and of the cleavage by protease have been succesfully applied in human trials.

of the events occurring from the binding of an infectious virion to the cell membrane to the insertion of viral nucleic acid material into the genome in the nucleus. The second is from the activation and transcription of the viral genome to the production of new infectious virions by the infected cell (see Figure 3.1). In short, interruption of the first part prevents infection of new cells, and interruption of the second part prevents production of new infectious virions by an infected cell.

Although, theoretically, interruption of the cycle may take place at several points in the cycle, up to now only two methods have demonstrated its clinical utility: inhibition of the virally encoded enzyme reverse transcriptase (RT), which is necessary for the production of viral DNA molecules from the viral RNA genome; and, recently, inhibition of the virally encoded enzyme HIV-protease, which cleaves the first long precursor protein molecules to form smaller parts which are necessary for the construction of whole virions. Without proper cleavage, no infectious viral particles can be assembled.

Currently, two points are being discussed extensively: which is the best antiretroviral therapy, and what is the best moment to start therapy? The RT inhibitors have been studied for 10 years. Of these, the nucleoside analog zidovudine (AZT; 3'-azido-3'-deoxythymidine; Retrovir®) has been in use the longest. AIDS patients treated with this drug showed a longer survival, less new complications, and an improvement in subjective well-being. Their immunity, as measured by the absolute number of CD4$^+$ lymphocytes, also improved. The beneficial results of the first clinical trials were confirmed many times, both in well-controlled settings and in population studies of patients who received routine care. However, the clinical usefulness turned out to be limited in time: after a period of 0.5–1.5 years, the clinical condition again deteriorates. The effect on the CD4$^+$ lymphocytes is even more transient. A moderate rise is seen followed by a return to baseline and further decrease after 4–6 months. This is caused by the development of viral resistance (see later).

A few years after the introduction of zidovudine four other nucleoside analog RT inhibitors were licensed: didanosine (2',3'-dideoxyinosine or DDI), zalcitabine (2',3'-dideoxycytidine or DDC), lamivudine (2'-deoxy,3'-thiacytidine or 3TC), and stavudine (2',3'-dideoxy-2',3'-didehydrothymidine or D4T). They are mainly used in combination with zidovudine, or as alternative antiretroviral treatment in patients who cannot tolerate zidovudine because of its side effects.

In addition to the nucleoside analogs, several other, non-nucleoside RT inhibitors have been developed. These drugs share some characteristics: they are very powerful on a molar basis, both *in vitro* and *in vivo*, they are highly selective HIV-1 inhibitors (e.g. they have no effect on HIV-2), and resistance against them develops quickly, sometimes within 2–4 weeks. Current studies are investigating whether combination with other antiretroviral compounds or a much higher dosing schedule can overcome this resistance problem.

Numerous studies have shown that combination of two or more antiretroviral compounds are more efficacious than monotherapy. The advantages are better efficacy, and postponement or avoidance of resistance. Results up to now show not only a better effect of combination regimens on virological and immunological markers, but also on clinical parameters such as survival or number of new HIV-related complications. However, superiority in clinical effect has still to be demonstrated.

Recently, another class of antiretroviral compounds has begun to be tested in clinical trials: the HIV protease inhibitors. These compounds have very strong antiviral and immunostimulating effects. Some of them are capable of decreasing the plasma viral load (number of HIV-RNA molecules per millilitre of plasma) to 1.5–2 $\log_{10}$ and to increase CD4$^+$ lymphocytes with 100–200 cells/mm^3 when administered as monotherapy. These results are superior to those obtained with nucleoside analog monotherapy. Combining nucleoside analogs with protease inhibitors yields even stronger effects, which are also more durable. In some recent studies with a triple combination (one protease inhibitor and two nucleoside analogs) a 2–2.5 $\log_{10}$ decline in viral load is seen, lasting for more than one year.

Resistance against antiretroviral compounds

Soon after the introduction of zidovudine into clinical practice, it became clear that the clinical benefits, as well as the beneficial changes in laboratory markers, were of limited duration. In 1989 it was shown for the first time that clinical virus isolates from patients who had been treated with zidovudine for prolonged periods, showed diminished sensitivity to the drug. In a transsectional sample, the drug resistance began to develop after 6 months of therapy. Analysis of the RT gene from clinical isolates revealed multiple nucleotide changes conferring specific amino-acid substitutions in the enzyme. Subjects with higher CD4$^+$ lymphocytes counts and those with less advanced HIV infection developed reduced susceptibility at slower rates, reaching lower levels of drug resistance. The dose of zidovudine did not influence the development of resistance. By constructing infectious HIV variants containing the mutations found in the RT gene in the clinical isolates, it was possible to reproduce the diminished zidovudine sensitivity.

In the search for identification of a subgroup which would do better on zidovudine treatment than others, the difference in biological phenotype was found. Some HIV isolates were able to infect multiple sorts of cells, to replicate at higher speed, and to induce the formation of syncytia on cocultivation with donor lymphocytes, when compared to other types. These types have been called syncytium-inducing (SI) strains, whereas the other types are called non-syncytium-inducing (NSI) strains. Generally, subjects with SI types have a more rapid clinical course than subjects harboring only NSI types.

Meanwhile, development of resistance has been found against all antiretroviral compounds currently under investigation. Both the RT and the protease gene mutate easily and, under antiretroviral drug pressure, selection of resistant viruses can be expected within a short period of time. However, in some combination regimens it appears that resistance against one drug counteracts the development of resistance against the other drug. The combination of zidovudine and 3TC seems to represent such a fortunate coupling, which may explain its strong and long-lasting antiretroviral effect (see above).

The occurrence of resistant HIV mutations during antiretroviral therapy may result from two processes: (1) selection of pre-existent resistant strains; or (2) *de novo* mutation during treatment. In order to avoid the former, a multiple drug combination should be applied, in the hope that forcing the virus to become resistant against two, three or even four drugs will result in a loss of virulence. This still has to be demonstrated. Prevention of *de novo* mutation is best achieved by powerful suppression of viral replication, since the chance of development of a given mutation is dependent on the rate of replication.

For a long time the clinical importance of the *in vitro* resistance of clinical isolates has been unclear. However, the expected negative relation between development of resistance against zidovudine during single-agent treatment with the drug and the clinical course has recently been confirmed.

When to start treatment?

Soon after the first proof of the efficacy of zidovudine in symptomatic HIV patient was published, several trials were started to evaluate the compound in the earlier stages of HIV infection, varying from mildly symptomatic to asymptomatic. It was felt that there was no clear reason why treatment should not start as early as possible, as is preferred in all kinds of infectious diseases. The lower the load of micro-organisms that has to be eliminated, the easier the task. Many trials have now been completed but the results are somewhat conflicting. The outcome of several large placebo-controlled trials shows a slight clinical benefit for so-called early treatment (i.e. treatment before symptoms develop, or before the patient shows a steep decline in $CD4^+$ lymphocytes, e.g. less than $200/mm^3$). This benefit consists of a postponement of the diagnosis of AIDS, but not a clear effect on overall survival. Especially interesting is the outcome of the Concorde study, a large French–British placebo-controlled trial in asymptomatic patients. After one year, a slight advantage for the zidovudine group, not reaching significance, was found, which had completely disappeared after 3 years. However, all these studies were performed using zidovudine monotherapy, a form of treatment now considered to be weak and prone to the rapid development of resistance.

Recently, it was found that, whilst patients were asymptomatic carriers, the turnover of HIV virions and $CD4^+$ lymphocytes must be extremely high. Some of the novel powerful antiretroviral agents succeeded in increasing the $CD4^+$ cells to $200–400/mm^3$ within a few days. Many investigators consider this a strong argument to start treatment in this phase instead of waiting until the immunity has almost completely disappeared, as is the case when serious HIV-related disease develops. As a compromise, the CDC has proposed to initiate antiretroviral therapy if the peripheral blood CD4 cell count falls beneath $500/mm^3$ and/or the plasma viral load exceeds 5,000–10,000 copies/ml and/or the patient has HIV-related symptoms.

Antiretroviral treatment in prevention of maternal–infant transmission of HIV

Maternal–infant transmission is the primary means by which young children become infected with HIV. Percentages of infected children born from seropositive mothers vary from 15 to 40. During the last few years, much experience has been obtained of using zidovudine during pregnancy. In April 1991 a multicenter, randomized, double-blind, placebo-controlled trial was started on the efficacy and safety of zidovudine in reducing the risk of maternal–infant HIV transmission. HIV-infected women were eligible if they were in their 14th to 34th week of gestation, had $\geq 200/mm^3$ CD4 cells and had received no prior antiretroviral therapy during the current pregnancy. They were treated from the 14th week of gestation up to the moment of clamping the umbilical cord, whereafter the newborn was treated for an additional 6 weeks. Up to the first interim analysis, 477 pregnant women were enrolled. During that period, 409 of them gave birth to 415 live-born infants. HIV infection status was known for 363 births (180 in the zidovudine group and 183 in the placebo group). Thirteen infants in the zidovudine group and 40 in the placebo group were infected with HIV. Proportions infected at 18 months as estimated by the Kaplan–Meier method were 8.3% (95%CI 3.9–12.8) in the zidovudine group and 25.5% (95%CI 18.4–32.5) in the placebo group. This corresponds to a 67.5% (95%CI 40.7–82.1) reduction in relative risk of HIV transmission ($p = 0.00006$). Toxic effects observed were minimal, only the hemoglobin level at birth in the zidovudine group was slightly lower. The study was stopped after this interim analysis.

Given the fact that most maternal–infant transmissions probably occur very late in pregnancy or during delivery, at present the effect of much shorter courses of therapy (combination therapy instead of zidovudine monotherapy) is being studied. This would have the additional advantage of lowering the costs considerably, bringing this prevention strategy into the reach of the health care systems in developing countries where the incidence of this mode of HIV transmission is high.

Further reading

d'Aquila RT, Johnson VA, Welles SL et al. Zidovudine resistance and HIV-1 disease progression during antiretroviral therapy. *Ann Intern Med* 1995; **122**: 401–408.

Concorde Coordinating Committee. Concorde: MRC/ANRS randomised double-blind controlled trial of immediate and deferred zidovudine in symptom-free HIV infection. *Lancet* 1994; **343**: 871–881.

Connor EM, Sperling RS, Gelber R et al. Reduction of maternal–infant transmission of human immunodeficiency virus type 1 with zidovudine treatment. *N Engl J Med* 1994; **331**: 1173–1180.

Ho DD, Neumann AU, Perelson AS, Chen W, Leonard JM, Markowitz M. Rapid turnover of plasma virions and CD4 lymphocytes in HIV-1 infection. *Nature* 1995; **373**: 123–126.

Larder BA, Darby G, Richman DD. HIV with reduced sensitivity to zidovudine isolated during prolonged therapy. *Science* 1989; **243**: 436–441.

Lange JMA. Combination antiretroviral therapy: back to the future. *Drugs* 1995; **49**(suppl 1): S32–S37.

Mofenson L. Epidemiology and determinants of vertical HIV transmission. *Semin Pediatr Infect Dis* 1994; **5**: 252–265.

Portegies P. AIDS dementia complex: a review. *J AIDS* 1994; **7**: S38–S49.

Volberding PA, Lagakos SW, Grimes JW et al. The duration of zidovudine benefit in persons with asymptomatic HIV infection. Prolonged evaluation of protocol 019 of the AIDS Clinical Trials Group. *JAMA* 1994; **272**: 437–442.

Wein-Hobson S. Virological mayhem. *Nature* 1995; **373**: 102.

Wilde MI, Langtry HD. Zidovudine. An update of its pharmacodynamic and pharmacokinetic properties, and therapeutic efficacy. *Drugs* 1993; **46**: 515–578.

Ho DD. Time to hit HIV, early and hard. *N Engl J Med* 1995; **333**: 450–451.

4 SURVEILLANCE AND EPIDEMIOLOGY OF HIV/AIDS

Patrick J.E. Bindels
Roel A. Coutinho

The start

In June 1981, five unusual cases of *Pneumocystis carinii* pneumonia were reported in previously healthy young men without any clinically apparent underlying immunodeficiency [1]. One month later, another report described the diagnosis of Kaposi's sarcoma, an uncommonly reported malignancy in the USA, among 26 young men [2]. All men were residents of California and New York City. These reports have turned out to be the first cases to be described of a disease complex now known as the acquired immune deficiency syndrome (AIDS).

The young men had in common that they were all homosexual and had a large number of sexual partners. Consequently, AIDS was at first considered to be a disease restricted to the homosexual community. However, in the following years, AIDS was recognized among intravenous drug users and Haitians [3,4]. Later on, recipients of blood or blood products [5], children of mothers at risk for AIDS [6], heterosexual partners of AIDS patients [7] and Africans [8] were also found to suffer from AIDS.

The epidemiological spread and pattern of AIDS made it clear that an agent transmissible via blood and sexual contact should be sought. In 1983, a French group at the Pasteur Institute in Paris reported the isolation of a new retrovirus from the blood of a homosexual man with lymphadenopathy [9]. They named the virus lymphadenopathy associated virus (LAV). In 1984, investigators from the National Institute of Health (NIH) also reported the isolation of a retrovirus, human T-cell leukemia virus type III (HTLV-III) [10]. Later, both viruses appeared to be similar and were called the human immune deficiency virus type 1 (HIV-1). HIV is a retrovirus belonging to the lentivirus subfamily and considered to be the causative agent for AIDS [11–13]. Following the isolation of HIV-1, a related retrovirus was detected from

individuals with AIDS [14]. This human immune deficiency virus type 2 (HIV-2) is predominantly found in West Africa. By now, ten genetically distinct subtypes (A–J) of HIV-1 have been identified and at least five subtypes of HIV-2.

Transmission, infection and disease

HIV is transmitted through sexual contact with an infected person, through exposure to HIV-infected blood or blood products, and from an infected mother to her child (Table 4.1). Transmission does not occur through household or social contact, vaccines, or contact with insects or body fluids, such as sweat or tears. HIV infection through contaminated blood has been eradicated almost completely since HIV antibody screening of blood products has become routine practise in most Western countries since 1985. Nevertheless, persons donating blood while in the 'window-phase' (time between infection and the presence of HIV antibodies) can still infect recipients.

The infectiousness of HIV is considered to be rather low but varies by stage of infection. It is estimated to be highest in the early and late stage of HIV infection [15]. The risk of transmission of HIV among homosexual men in the USA was estimated to be 0.5–3.0% per receptive anal exposures to ejaculate [16]. Among heterosexuals, HIV transmission appears to be more likely from man to woman than from woman to man. Transmission of HIV from man to woman occurs through semen and from woman to man through exposure to vaginocervical secretion and menstrual blood. Anal intercourse carries a higher risk than vaginal intercourse. Overall, the probability of HIV transmission from an infected person to his or her heterosexual partner was estimated to be 0.1% per

Table 4.1. Routes of transmission of HIV.

Sexual:
- Homosexual between men.
- Heterosexual from men to women and from women to men.

Exposure to blood:
- Drug user needle sharing.
- Transfusion of blood, plasma, packed cells, platelet, and factor concentrates.
- Occupational needle-stick injury

Perinatal:
- Prepartum, intrapartum and postpartum (breast feeding).

sexual contact [17]. The presence of sexually transmissible diseases (STD), especially genital ulcers, is known to increase the risk of HIV transmission dramatically. Therefore, prevention and treatment of STD may have a significant influence on the transmission of HIV.

After infection with HIV, acute clinical symptoms may occur. These symptoms have been described as mononucleosis-like syndrome but a variety of other symptoms may also occur, e.g. flu, skin rash, arthralgia, fever, etc.. These symptoms, however, are not specific and are not necessarily present. Many people recently infected with HIV have noticed no symptoms at all. Detection of HIV antibodies with enzyme-linked immunosorbent assay (ELISA) techniques, but also with the nowadays available rapid tests, is usually possible 3–6 months after infection. With more advanced and expensive techniques, such as RNA polymerase chain reaction, it is feasible to detect HIV infection at an earlier stage.

The median incubation period between the time of infection with HIV and the development of clinical AIDS is approximately 8–10 years [18–20] and less than 10% of HIV-infected persons will be still free of AIDS 15 years after infection. During the incubation period, an infected person is symptom-free and no clinical signs of infection are present. Transmission of the virus to uninfected persons is possible, and effective measures to prevent further spread of the virus are essential.

HIV-1 infection causes a loss and functional impairment of CD4+ lymphocytes, which finally results in a defect in the cellular and humoral immune systems.

The individual becomes susceptible to a spectrum of opportunistic infections and certain malignancies [21,22]. After the first occurrence of one of these specific manifestations, an HIV-infected individual is considered to have the clinical disease AIDS. Advanced HIV-2 infection is associated with similar signs and symptoms as advanced HIV-1 infection but HIV-2 infected individuals have a longer incubation period to AIDS [14,23,24]. HIV-2 spreads at a lower rate in the (African) heterosexual population than HIV-1 [25–27] and mother–child transmission rarely occurs after infection with HIV-2 [26,28–30]. In contrast, the transmission rate among HIV-1-infected pregnant women is found to be 15–40% [31]. However, the use of zidovudine started orally during pregnancy, continued intravenously during delivery and administered to the newborn in the first weeks has shown substantially to decrease the transmission rate of HIV-1 in comparison with placebo (8.3% vs 25.5%, a 67.5% reduction) [32,33].

CDC AIDS case definitions

There can be no adequate epidemiological surveillance without a good case definition. Ideally, a case definition has a high specificity and sensitivity, is simple to use, consistent over time, permits comparisons between regions and allows for the monitoring of trends through the years [34]. No case definition will be entirely satisfactory and also the AIDS case definition has its limitations.

In 1982, even before the isolation of HIV, the Centers for Disease Control (CDC) in Atlanta, Georgia, USA, developed a case definition for AIDS. Diseases included in this first definition were *Pneumocystis carinii* pneumonia (PCP), Kaposi's sarcoma, and some other serious opportunistic infections [35]. In 1985, the AIDS case definition was revised for the first time [36] because serological assays to detect antibodies against HIV became available [37–39], and more HIV-related opportunistic diseases and malignancies were identified (e.g. non-Hodgkin lymphoma). The World Health Organization (WHO) adopted the 1985 definition for world-wide use, predominantly in industrialized countries.

In 1987, after a second revision of the CDC AIDS case definition [40], extrapulmonary tuberculosis, HIV encephalopathy, HIV wasting syndrome and also the presumptive diagnosis of some selected diseases

Table 4.2. Classification system of HIV-1 infection of the CDC, 1987.

Group I	Acute infection
Group II	Asymptomatic infection
Group III	Persistent generalized lymphadenopathy
Group IV	Other disease
Subgroup A	Constitutional disease*
Subgroup B	Neurologic disease†
Subgroup C	Secondary infectious diseases
Category C-1	Specified secondary infectious diseases listed in the CDC surveillance definition of AIDS‡
Category C-2	Other specified secondary infectious diseases§
Subgroup D	Secondary cancers¶
Subgroup E	Other conditions

* One or more of the following: fever >1 month, involuntary weight loss >10% of baseline, diarrhea >1 month.
† Dementia, myelopathy, peripheral neuropathy.
‡ *Pneumocytis carinii* pneumonia, chronic cryptosporidiosis, toxoplasmosis, extraintestinal strongyloidiasis, isosporiasis, candidiasis, (esophageal, bronchial, or pulmonary), cryptococcosis, histoplasmosis, mycobacterial infection with M. *Avium* or M. *kansasii*, cytomegalovirus infection, chronic mucocutaneous or disseminated herpes simplex virus infection, and progressive multifocal leukoencephalopathy.
§ Oral hairy leukoplakia, multidermatomal herpes zoster, recurrent *Salmonella* bacteremia, nocardiosis, tuberculosis, or oral candidiasis.
¶ Kaposi's sarcoma, non-Hodgkin lymphoma (small, non-cleaved lymphoma or immunoblastic sarcoma, or primary lymphoma of the brain).

(i.e. PCP and Kaposi's sarcoma) were included. Because the 1987 AIDS case definition was predominantly of use for surveillance purposes and had less relevance for clinicians, a clinical HIV classification system used to stage HIV-infected patients was developed [41] (Table 4.2).

In 1993, CDC decided to change the AIDS case definition for adolescents and adults for the third time [42,43] (Table 3). In this new definition, the classification system for HIV infection and the AIDS case definition were combined. The main reason for the change was to emphasize the clinical importance of the CD4+ lymphocyte count in the categorization of HIV-related clinical conditions [34,43]. Besides patients who were diagnosed with one of the already defined clinical AIDS indicators, HIV-infected individuals with one CD4+ T-lymphocyte count $<200 \times 10^6$/litre were also included in the AIDS case definition (or a CD4+ T-lymphocyte percentage of total lymphocytes of <14 or total lymphocyte count

<1000, as a less expensive alternative). Three indicator diseases were added to the definition as well: pulmonary tuberculosis, recurrent pneumonia, and invasive cervical cancer. The increased number of HIV infections in other risk groups besides homosexual men (especially intravenous drug users and women who acquired HIV heterosexually) and the subsequent identification of infections seen in these groups [44–48] justified the inclusions of these three new indicator diseases.

In children, the clinical course of the HIV/AIDS infection is in some aspects different from the infection in adolescents and adults. For children (<13 years of age), a separate HIV/AIDS case definition(s) has been developed [49,50].

The 1985 and 1987 revised CDC AIDS case definitions were accepted and used by most industrialized countries. However, the introduction of the 1993 CDC expanded surveillance case definition has been subject to much debate. After due consideration, the European countries decided not to follow the USA in the inclusion of CD4+ T-lymphocyte as an indicator of AIDS, although CD4+ cell count is a marker of severe immunodeficiency. The decisive factor was the fact that lymphocyte typing is not sufficiently standardized [51,52] or sufficiently available in the European countries. Additionally, the inclusion of CD4+ T-lymphocytes would cause a selection bias depending on access to medical care and lymphocyte monitoring facilities and it would cause difficulties in analysis of trends [53,54]. Moreover, the inclusion of a CD4+ cell count would mean the labeling of asymptomatic HIV-infected individuals as having (epidemiologically) AIDS. This might cause needless emotional and psychological stress in these individuals [55,56].

The 1993 European AIDS case definition, including only the three new indicator diseases, was accepted in most European countries from mid-1993 onwards (Category C in Table 4.3).

Impact of the revisions of the AIDS case definition

In the USA, after the 1985 revision, the reported incidence of AIDS increased by 3–4% [57,58]. The 1987 revision caused an overall increase of 28% in the number of cases reported in 1988, predominantly

Table 4.3. Revised classification system of HIV disease of the CDC, 1993.

Clinical categories

CD4 count categories	A (Acute, asymptomatic, or PGL)*	B (Symptomatic, not A or C conditions)	C (AIDS indicator conditions)
1 >499/mm^3	A1	B1	C1
2 200–499/mm^3	A2	B2	C2
3 <200/mm^3	A3	B3	C3

Category B
Bacillary angiomatosis
Candidiasis
  Oral
  Recurrent vaginal
Cervical dysplasia
Constitutional symptoms,
  e.g. fever or diarrhea >1 month
Oral hairy leukoplakia
Herpes Zoster
  Recurrent
  Multidermatomal
Idiopathic thrombocytopenia purpura
Listeriosis
Pelvic inflammatory disease
Peripheral neuropathy

Category C
Candidiasis
  Pulmonary
  Esophageal
Cervical cancer
Coccidiodomycosis
Extrapulmonary cryptococcosis
Cytomegalovirus
HIV encephalopathy
Herpes simplex
  >1 month
  Esophageal
Histoplasmosis
Isosporiasis
Kaposi's sarcoma
Lymphoma
Mycobacterium avium
Mycobacterium kansasii
Mycobacterium tuberculosis
Pneumocystis carinii
Recurrent pneumonia
Progressive multifocal leukemia
Salmonellosis

Shaded area (C1–C3, A3, B3): AIDS

* PGL persistent generalized lymphadenopathy.

caused by the inclusion of a presumptive diagnosis (e.g. PCP), HIV wasting syndrome, and HIV dementia [59]. In Europe, the implementation of the revised 1987 CDC case definition resulted in an estimated increase in reported cases ranging from 0% to 28% for the different European countries [60].

The impact of the 1993 revision is, of course, different for the USA and Europe. In the USA, the CDC predicted that the 1993 revision would increase AIDS reports in 1993 to approximately 75% above previously expected numbers [42]. In fact, the number of cases reported in 1993 increased to 111% compared to 1992. The proportionate increase in case reporting was higher among injection drug users (IDU) and persons infected through heterosexual contact [61,62]. One year after the introduction of the 1993 revision in European countries, an analysis of reported AIDS cases revealed that overall 7% was meeting the revised definition only [54]. The impact varied considerably between countries, from 3% in Finland to 21% in Spain. The substantial impact of the revision in the latter country is caused by a high prevalence of tuberculosis. Like in the USA, the impact seems predominantly to affect heterosexual men and women, and IDU [54,63]. However, a substantial part of the reported patients meeting the 1993 revised criteria only would have reported with other 'old' clinical AIDS criteria at a later point in time. So the impact will, in fact, be less in the long term. However, some patients diagnosed as having AIDS because of severe impairment of the immune system will no longer be reported as having a clinical AIDS manifestation.

The impact of the revision has to be taken into account in the analysis of trends of the AIDS epidemic and forecasting of AIDS cases to be expected. Depending upon the magnitude of the impact, there will be an effect on incubation time from HIV sero-conversion to AIDS [64] and on the length of survival from AIDS onwards [62,65]. Both because of an earlier diagnosis owing to the inclusion of CD4+ cell counts <200.

Other AIDS case definitions

In 1986, the WHO developed a clinical case definition for AIDS, also known as the 'Bangui definition' [66]. It became widely used for clinical diagnosis in countries lacking adequate laboratory facilities for reliable HIV testing and/or sophisticated diagnostic facilities, especially Africa. In the absence of a positive HIV test and also other known causes of immunosuppression, such as severe malnutrition and cancer, the definition is based on the presence of generalized Kaposi's sarcoma or cryptococcal meningitis or on 'major' and 'minor signs'. An individual was considered to have AIDS by the existence of two major signs and at least one minor sign. However, the WHO clinical definition did have important drawbacks [34]. Some minor signs were more predictive of HIV infection than AIDS and patients with tuberculosis, but HIV negative, fulfill the criteria (poor specificity, predominantly caused by the inclusion of the non-specific symptom 'persistent cough').

Other definitions proposed were the revised Caracas AIDS case definition, proposed in 1989 in its original form, requiring an HIV-positive test in combination with a points scoring system for various manifestations of HIV infection [67,68] and the 1991 Abidjan AIDS case definition, in a modified version proposed in 1992, combining a positive HIV antibody test with one or more of five clinical syndromes/diagnosis [69].

Although useful for surveillance purposes in countries in Africa, Asia and South America with limited diagnostic facilities, the Caracas, Abidjan AIDS case definition and the WHO clinical definition have their limitations because of poor sensitivity and specificity [68,70].

Epidemiological HIV/AIDS surveillance

Adequate epidemiological surveillance is considered to be the cornerstone of good public health. With the use of the abovementioned (revised) case definitions, surveillance systems have supplied the information for which they were implemented: high-risk groups for HIV infection were identified; prevention and educational programs were developed, both for professionals and the general public, and adapted after the availability of new information; funds were allocated; trends in the HIV/AIDS epidemic were described in monthly and quarterly reports (for the USA by the CDC, for Europe by the European Centre for the epidemiological monitoring of AIDS in Paris, and global overviews are published regularly by the WHO in their Weekly Epidemiological Record). The data were used to predict the number of AIDS cases to be expected and to estimate the prevalence of HIV-infected individuals (using the back calculation method) [71–73], thus helping to plan the future need for health care.

AIDS surveillance

The effectiveness and usefulness of AIDS surveillance depends on its accuracy and overall completeness. Therefore, when evaluating or interpreting AIDS figures provided by surveillance systems, the completeness of case reporting or underreporting and reporting delay (time between AIDS diagnosis and time of reporting to the surveillance department) in particular have to be taken into account. Both elements directly influence the quality of the data because of an underestimation of the number of cases.

Other factors that influence AIDS surveillance data, although less direct or pronounced, are pre-AIDS mortality in HIV-positive individuals causing an underestimation [74], underdiagnosis (i.e. failure to diagnose AIDS) [45,75], and possibly the effect of prophylactic treatment on the delay of the first clinical AIDS manifestation causing a temporal decrease in the number of reported AIDS cases (e.g. antiretroviral therapy, PCP prophylaxis) [76–78].

Underreporting has directly affected the AIDS incidence through the years and has occurred because of different reasons [79,80]: insufficient (passive) reporting systems, case definitions with poor sensitivity (poor specificity may give an overreporting of AIDS cases), moderate cooperation of physicians diagnosing clinical AIDS, concerns of confidentiality of reports, inadequate detection of persons with AIDS because of poor accessibility of health services, and even complete denial of the HIV/AIDS epidemic or deliberate reduction of the number of cases. Especially in some African countries, it is known that AIDS case reporting is not carried out at all or has just started recently.

The underreporting of AIDS cases varies in different areas of the world. In 1990, the CDC has estimated the rate of underreporting of AIDS in the USA to be 15% nationwide [81]. In Europe, the degree of underreporting varies between countries and over time. From 6 of the 12 European Community (EC) countries estimates varying from 0% to 20% are reported [60]. In most western European countries, AIDS surveillance is based on voluntary confidential reporting of cases by physicians to health care authorities. However, in some European countries, such as Sweden, Norway and Denmark [82], Switzerland [83] and also in some states in the USA, reporting of cases is required by law [84]. Some consider compulsory notification of cases by physicians an essential tool of AIDS surveillance [85], while others have stressed that compulsory notification would be counterproductive. Voluntary AIDS case reporting is already more complete than other infectious diseases, which are part of a compulsory notification scheme [86]. The additional benefit of an active surveillance policy, i.e. where the health authorities systematically contact the reporting physician at regular intervals, compared with a passive system, where the reporting depends exclusively on the physician to automatically report cases, is now beyond doubt [87–91].

Reporting delay predominantly influences the most recent AIDS incidence data. The influence of reporting delay on AIDS incidence of earlier years is less since more time has elapsed to allow for 'late-reporting'. The reporting delay differs between countries and transmission groups, and can vary between one month up to several years. In Europe, overall approximately one-third of the cases are reported by the end of the quarter within which they were diagnosed and 12–15% are reported more than one year after diagnosis [50]. There are mainly two methods used to cope with reporting delay. The first method, often applied nowadays, is to adjust the most recent figures for the delay with the use of mathematical models. The European AIDS surveillance data are adjusted for reporting delay for the 12 previous quarters using the method of Heisterkamp et al [92]. A second way to deal with this problem, although less accurate, and used in quarterly surveillance reports (CDC quarterly AIDS reports, USA), is to compare patients by year of reporting and not by year of diagnosis. When assuming no difference in reporting delay over time in this way, more recent trends can be interpreted without adjustment.

HIV surveillance

A disadvantage of AIDS surveillance is that it reflects the HIV situation of several years ago. HIV surveillance may reveal more complete and up-to-date information about the spread of HIV. HIV seroprevalence data can be obtained through sentinel or (serial) cross-sectional surveillance studies. However, a stable or even declining HIV prevalence can mask a high HIV incidence [93]. Therefore, an even better way to monitor the HIV epidemic would be through monitoring HIV incidence and thus focusing directly on the occurrence of new infections. HIV incidence studies require the follow-up of a group of people over time, making these study designs more difficult to perform and more costly. However, prospective cohort studies among homosexual men and injecting drug users, started during the 1980s and still continuing, have revealed important information on the natural history of HIV/AIDS. Discussion of the numerous results from these cohort studies is beyond the scope of this chapter.

In several countries in Europe, the USA and other parts of the world, HIV surveillance programs have been developed and implemented among pregnant women, STD clinic visitors, blood donors, and female sex workers. Substantial differences in HIV prevalence between risk groups in different countries have been presented [94]. Comparison of HIV surveillance data between countries is often only possible to a limited extent because of different sampling strategies or different requirements concerning HIV testing.

The HIV/AIDS epidemic

Classical distribution

During the early years of the epidemic, world-wide, three geographic patterns in the routes of transmission of HIV were distinguished [95]. In each pattern, the main routes in the transmission of HIV explained the distribution among the different risk groups in these countries.

Pattern I was typical of industrialized countries with large numbers of reported cases (North America, Europe, Australia, New Zealand, and parts of Latin America). In these countries, most cases of AIDS were found among homosexual and bisexual men, and intravenous drug users (sharing of needles). Heterosexual transmission of HIV had only occurred in a relatively small group, although their number was growing. Perinatal transmission was relatively uncommon. Transmission of the virus through blood transfusion or blood products was extremely rare since the availability of tests to detect HIV-antibodies (1985), and the subsequent routine screening of donated blood and, on top of this, the request to persons from the known risk groups to withdraw as blood donors.

In pattern II countries, sub-Saharan Africa and some Caribbean countries, the majority of the cases occurred among heterosexual persons. Men and women were equally affected and transmission from a mother to her child was common. Transmission of the virus through homosexual activity or needle-sharing in intravenous drug users is rare. Transmission of the virus through contaminated blood products was a considerable problem, mainly owing to a lack of testing facilities. The high prevalence of (ulcerative) sexually transmitted diseases in most of the pattern II countries played a role in HIV transmission [96,97]. HIV seroprevalence

in the overall population was estimated at more than 1% and had reached 25% in the sexually active adult population in some capitals. Pattern II countries were also called 'AIDS endemic countries'.

In a third group of countries, only a few AIDS cases have been reported. The virus was probably introduced in these countries in the mid-1980s and, therefore, the epidemic was in an early stage, and the course of the epidemic was yet undetermined. Pattern III countries were Eastern European countries, Asia, and the Pacific.

However, these patterns are no longer restricted to the abovementioned countries, limiting their value. Interregional differences and shifts have occurred. The spread and routes of transmission of HIV is a dynamic situation. For example, Brazil, with a rapid increase of heterosexual AIDS cases, represents a mixture of Pattern I and II (homosexual and heterosexual transmission, and intravenous drug users). The former pattern III countries, Thailand and India, seem to have shifted to patterns I and II, respectively.

Global AIDS figures

The world-wide number of AIDS cases reported to WHO was 1 393 649 by the end of June 1996 [98]. Since the end of June 1995, the number of reported cases has increased 19%. In Figure 4.1, the total number of reported AIDS cases in adults and children from the start of the epidemic in the late 1970s/early 1980s until mid-1996 are presented together with the estimated number of cases among adults and children [98]. The estimated figure is corrected for under diagnosis, incomplete reporting and reporting delay, and also based on available HIV incidence and prevalence data around the world, making it a more realistic figure of the number of world-wide AIDS cases. The most

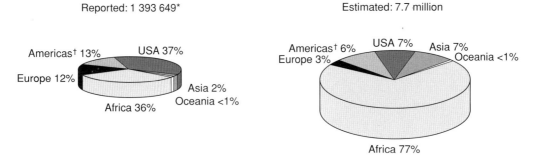

Figure 4.1. Total number of AIDS cases in adults and children from the late 1970s/early 1980s until mid-1996. *AIDS cases reported to WHO as of 30 June 1996. †Excluding USA.

striking difference between the reported and estimated number of cases is seen in Africa, 77% of the world-wide cases instead of 36%. Also the estimated number of cases in Asia, 7% of the world total, where HIV was introduced at a later time point in the pandemic, is already equaling the number of cases in the USA and has more than twice the number in Europe (3% of the cases).

Global HIV figures

Overall, the WHO estimates the cumulative number of HIV-infected persons from the start of the epidemic until mid-1996 to be 27.9 million, including 25.5 million adults and 2.4 million children (Figure 4.2). The world-wide number of persons living with HIV/AIDS was estimated to be 21.8 million by mid-1996 [98].

With 19 million HIV-infected individuals, sub-Saharan Africa is, by far, the most affected region in the world. This is followed by south and south-east Asia with an estimated cumulative number of 5 million HIV-infected individuals, and the Americas and the Caribbean with 3.1 million persons infected with HIV.

Europe

In Western Europe, the entry of HIV into the male homosexual community is thought to have happened in the second half of the 1970s, some years later than in the USA. Retrospective analysis of sera from homosexual men participating in a hepatitis B vaccine trial in Amsterdam revealed that 0.7% were infected with HIV in 1980 [99]. In Britain, among a group of homosexual men tested for hepatitis B infection, 5.5% were HIV infected in 1980, rising to 34% in 1984 [100].

A rapid increase in HIV infection among IDU occurred, in some areas, from the late 1970s/early 1980s onwards. In Amsterdam, the prevalence of HIV infection among IDU increased from 7% in 1982 to approximately 30% in 1985 [101].

Transmission of HIV to heterosexual populations will most likely occur through sexual contacts between IDU and their heterosexual partners, through sexual contacts with heterosexual individuals from high endemic areas, and through sexual contacts between bisexual males and heterosexual females. From the late 1980s/early 1990s onwards, studies among patients

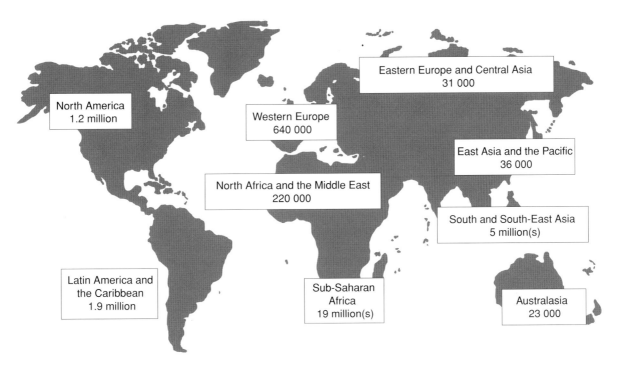

Global total 27.9 million*

Figure 4.2. Estimated cumulative distribution of HIV-infected persons from the late 1970s/early 1980s until mid-1996. *Totals may not add up owing to rounding up. Source: Joint United Nations Program on HIV/AIDS.

attending STD clinics, female sex workers and their clients, and pregnant women show increasing HIV prevalences. In countries such as Italy and Spain, where IDU are the most important risk group, heterosexual transmission has increased rapidly in the past few years [102]. Although regional differences exist, the prevalence in these groups are still much lower than in the IDU and homosexual risk groups.

A reliable way to describe the trends in the HIV epidemic for the whole of Europe is to use AIDS surveillance data. With a cumulative number of 179 445 AIDS patients, adjusted for reporting delay and reported up to 31 March 1996 (including 6532 pediatric cases), the WHO European region accounted for about 12–13% of the world-wide number of cases [102]. In the first years of the AIDS epidemic in the European region, homosexual/bisexual men were the most important risk group but, since 1990, IDU account for the highest number of yearly diagnosed cases (42% of adult/adolescent cases in 1995) (Figure 4.3). Between 1994 and 1995 the number of AIDS cases in Europe, adjusted for reporting delay, in homosexual/bisexual men decreased by 7% and that in IDU by 2%. The number of cases among heterosexually infected persons increased by 9%.

The overall increase of IDU cases and heterosexually acquired cases caused an increase in the proportion of female cases. This proportion was 12% in 1986 and increased to 21% in 1995. Of the women diagnosed with AIDS in 1995, 46% were IDU and 43% had been heterosexually infected (32% of the heterosexually infected women had a IDU sexual partner) [102]. The cumulative adult/adolescent male to female ratio was 5 : 1 by the end of March 1996, but was already 4.3 : 1 for AIDS cases diagnosed in 1994, further decreasing to 4 : 1 in 1995.

The AIDS incidence rates in Europe vary by country. The adjusted AIDS incidence rate in 1995 (number of cases per million population) was highest for Spain with 183, followed by Italy with 103 and France with 89. In Spain and Italy, IDU account for approximately two out of three of the cases [103]. while in most northern European countries, homosexual/bisexual men account for the majority of reported cases. A continuing increase in cases in the IDU risk group in the southern European countries is causing a persistent increase in the AIDS incidence rates and no indication that the AIDS epidemic has leveled off has been noticed [102,104]. However, the implementation of the 1993 European AIDS case definition has predominantly caused an increase in the number of IDU cases and is thus affecting these countries the most. In contrast, the AIDS incidence has stabilized in recent years in countries in the northern part of Western Europe (Austria, Belgium, Denmark, Germany, Netherlands, Switzerland and UK), owing

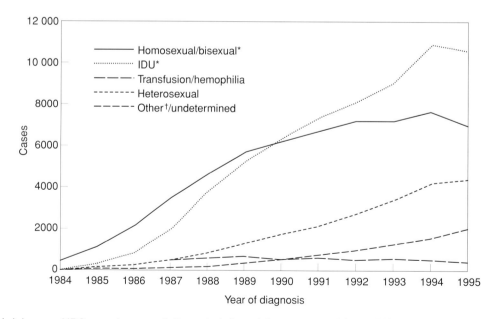

Figure 4.3. Adult/adolescent AIDS cases by year of diagnosis (adjusted for reporting delays, 1993–1995) and transmission group, WHO European Region, 31 December 1995. *Excludes homosexual/bisexual IDU. †Excludes nosocomial infection. Reproduced from *HIV /AIDS Surveillance* 1995; no. 48: 36.

to a stabilization in the incidence of homosexually acquired cases in these countries.

In Eastern European countries, where HIV was probably introduced in the mid-1980s (former pattern III region), the AIDS epidemic is at an early stage, reflected in the much lower AIDS incidence rates compared to Western Europe (e.g. 0.2 and 0.9 for the Russian Federation and the Ukraine in 1995, respectively). However, the number of newly diagnosed AIDS cases has increased from 1994 to 1995 by 23% from 849 to 1048 [102]. The high and increasing number of STDs reported from the Eastern European countries might cause a rapid increase of sexually transmitted HIV infections in the next years.

In Europe, 4% of the total number of cases occurred among children under 13 years of age (2736 cases by the end of March 1996, of whom over 50% were reported from a Romanian nosocomial epidemic detected in 1989). Of these paediatric AIDS cases, 44.3% were infected through mother–child transmission. When evaluating the transmission group of these mothers, the largest proportion of the pediatric cases were born to an IDU mother. The observed increase in the number of AIDS cases among women in the European region may cause, without proper intervention, a continuous increase in the number of paediatric cases.

North America

In the USA, at the time of the first identified cases of AIDS in 1981, substantial spread of HIV had already occurred. A random sample of stored sera of homosexual men in San Francisco who were enrolled in hepatitis B studies between 1978 and 1980, and retrospective analysis revealed that HIV prevalence rose from 4.5% in 1978 to an estimated 44% by the end of 1981 [105–107]. In New York, 43.7% of the participants of a cohort study were infected in 1984 [108] and in Los Angeles almost 50% of the participants were HIV positive in 1983. From this and other studies, it appeared that the introduction of HIV in the large urban centers of the USA took place in the mid-1970s. After 1985, a striking decrease in the incidence rates among homosexual men occurred both in the USA and in Europe. The documented change in the sexual behavior among homosexual men influenced by targeted preventive campaigns is thought to have caused this decrease [109–111].

Among IDU, the virus was introduced in the USA during or shortly after the mid-1970s [112]. The sharing of needles, caused by a lack of sterile 'shooting' equipment and/or a sharing 'tradition' in certain subcultures, facilitated a rapid spread of the virus. In New York City, for example, seroprevalences rates went from 9% in 1978 to 60% in 1984 [112].

By 31 October 1995, a total of 501 310 AIDS cases in the USA were reported to CDC [113], accounting for ~37% of the world-wide number of reported cases but 'only' 7% of the estimated number of cases (Figure 4.1). The epidemic among homosexual/bisexual men continued to account for the largest proportion of reported AIDS cases. However, as in Europe, the AIDS epidemic is increasing more rapidly among IDU and persons infected through heterosexual contact. Therefore, there is also an increase in AIDS cases reported in women [114]. Differences in the proportionate increases in reported cases exist between the Midwest, Northeast and West of the USA. In contrast with Europe, the epidemic in the USA affects Blacks and Hispanics disproportionately [115,116]. Blacks and Hispanics accounted for 51% of the cumulative AIDS cases reported up to October 1995 while they make up only 18% of the American population. Between 1981–1987 and 1993–October 1995, the proportion of cases among Whites decreased from 60% to 43%, while the proportion of cases among Blacks and Hispanics increased from 25% to 38% and 14% to 18%, respectively [113]. Socioeconomic factors and a higher number of IDU among ethnic minorities are the underlying cause of the overrepresentation of Blacks and Hispanics among the AIDS cases. This shift in emphasis towards the minorities in the USA will probably continue in the years to come and will demand extra (governmental) funds and preventive measures for these groups.

By mid-1996, of the estimated cumulative number of 1.2 million HIV-infected persons in North America, approximately 400 000 had died by mid-1996 [98]. Data on mortality attributable to HIV infection in the USA, including provisional mortality data for 1993 and 1994, have demonstrated the enormous impact of HIV/AIDS on mortality statistics and premature mortality in the USA [117]. Nationwide, HIV infection became the leading cause of death for Black men aged 25–44 years in 1991, for all men aged 25–44 years (all races) in 1992 (Figure 4.4), and for White men aged 25–44 years in 1994. Also in 1994, HIV infection was the eighth leading cause of death overall,

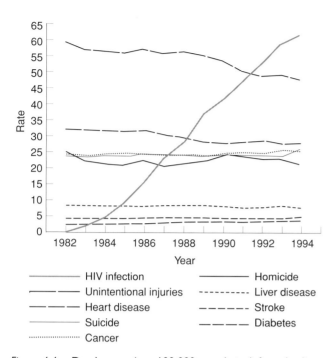

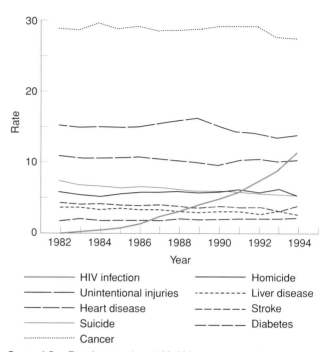

Figure 4.4. Death rates (per 100 000 population) from leading causes of death among men aged 25–44 years, by year, USA, 1982–1994. (National vital statistics based on underlying cause of death, using final data for 1982–1992 and provisional data for 1993–1994.) Reproduced from *MMWR* 1996; **45**: 121–125.

Figure 4.5. Death rates (per 100 000 population) from leading causes of death among women aged 25–44 years, by year, USA, 1982–1994. (National vital statistics based on underlying cause of death, using final data for 1982–1992 and provisional data for 1993–1994.) Reproduced from *MWWR* 1996; **45**: 121–125.

accounting for 2% of all deaths and the fourth leading cause of years of potential life lost before age 65. For women aged 25–44 years, HIV infection became the third leading cause of death in 1994 (Figure 4.5). A comparable impact on premature mortality has been described in European cities, such as Amsterdam. In the period 1984–1992, AIDS became the leading cause of death in this city for men aged 25–54 years from 1990 onwards and the leading cause of working years of potential life lost before 65 years (WYPPL) for men in the 15–64 age group [118].

Latin America and the Caribbean

In Latin America and the Caribbean especially, heterosexual transmission is increasing, although IDU and homosexual men are important risk groups in some countries as well. Sexual contact between female sex workers and their clients, and bisexual men and their female partners is causing the virus to spread in the general heterosexual population. In the Caribbean, heterosexual transmission has been the major route from the start [119]. In Haiti, about 8–10% of the urban population and 5% of the rural population are

infected, again mostly through heterosexual contact [120].

Brazil is another country where predominantly heterosexual transmission is increasing. The percentage of reported heterosexually acquired AIDS cases increased from 7.5% in 1987 to 26% in 1994 [121]. The prevalence of HIV among IDU in some of the countries in this region is equal to the situation in North America and Europe. In Argentina and Brazil, the prevalence among IDU ranges from 30% to 50% and 20% to 60% respectively [122].

Africa

With 499 037 officially reported AIDS patients by mid-1996, accounting for 36% of the global number, and an estimate of 19 million HIV-infected persons, the impact of the epidemic on this continent is evident. The enormous difference between officially reported number of AIDS cases and the estimated number is the result of the lack of HIV-testing facilities in many African countries, a basis for non-diagnosis, logistical problems causing insufficient reporting systems, and, of course, poor access to health care. HIV infection and AIDS predominantly occurs in urban centers and to a lesser extent in the rural parts where most Africans (roughly 80%) are living.

In the sub-Saharan region of Africa, classically known as the 'AIDS endemic region', or pattern II region, and predominantly limited to central and east Africa, heterosexual transmission is the most important route of transmission of HIV, accounting for more than 80% of the cases. This is followed by transfusion of HIV-contaminated blood (10%; although declining since routine screening of blood is now implemented in several countries) and mother–child transmission (one million African children are estimated to have been infected through mother–child transmission and the number of AIDS orphans is already enormous). Intravenous drug use and homosexual transmission do not play an important role in the spread of HIV in this region. The number of male and female HIV/AIDS cases in Africa is approximately equal.

Rwanda is one of the countries in central Africa where HIV has spread at an alarming rate among the general adult population. In early 1993, the HIV prevalence was 33% among pregnant women in the antenatal clinic of the largest hospital in Kigali with an HIV incidence of 3.5 per 100 women years in those HIV-seronegative women followed after delivery [123], indicating that one of three pregnant women was HIV positive. Similar high HIV prevalences are reported from other capitals in central and eastern Africa. Among commercial sex workers in the major cities in this region, HIV seroprevalences above 80% are more a rule than an exception.

In the northern countries of Africa, low incidence data are reported. In the southern and western parts of Africa (Nigeria, South Africa), both prevalence and incidence data among the adult population, especially among commercial sex workers and their clients, and STD clinic visitors, the core groups that play an important role in the heterosexual spread of HIV in an evolving epidemic, have risen in the most recent years [122].

The role of STD in the transmission of HIV and thus the importance of STD prevention has already been stressed in this overview. In 1995, a community-based study performed in Tanzania showed that improved STD case management, a syndromic approach to the treatment of symptomatic STDs, is successful in lowering the incidence of HIV by 40% [124].

In conclusion, the HIV/AIDS epidemic in Africa is placing an increasing pressure on the already over-strained health care systems in many countries. It will also have an impact on the age distribution of the population, the social development and the economic growth of the continent. However, some grounds for cautious optimism for HIV in Africa have been shown in recent data from Uganda. In a cohort study in 15 villages in rural Uganda, a decline in HIV-1 prevalence was noticed among young men and women aged 13–24 years between 1990 and 1994 (3.4% to 1.0% and 9.9% to 7.3%, respectively) [125]. The Ugandan national HIV surveillance among pregnant women suggests that the epidemic seems to have at least levelled off in some parts of Uganda. AIDS control measures (sexual behavior changes, condom promotion, AIDS awareness campaigns) have probably contributed to the observed decline in Uganda. Since these are the first results that describe a decline in HIV prevalence, extreme caution is still necessary. It does not reflect the situation in other parts of this large continent.

Asia

From the earlier figures of HIV and AIDS in Asia, and the knowledge that the virus was introduced in this area at a later point in time than in the rest of the world, it is clear that an explosive growth in the number of infected persons has occurred on this continent, and that this rapid growth is continuing. The number of officially reported AIDS cases is still relatively small (almost 30 000 by mid-1996) but this number is expected to be 4–5 times higher than the number of AIDS cases in the developed countries by the end of this century. Besides Thailand and India, emerging HIV epidemics have been documented from countries, such as Cambodia, Indonesia, China, Vietnam, Taiwan, and the Philippines [126]. In more developed countries, such as Japan, South Korea, and Hong Kong, a steady, less rapid increase in the number of HIV/AIDS cases might be expected.

The first cases in this region were reported among IDU in 1988. Especially in the 'golden triangle', extremely high HIV prevalence data (<45%) were described among IDU in China, Myanmar (Burma), and Thailand [127,128]. Shortly after HIV infections were documented among female sex workers, increasing prevalence among their clients was found with a subsequent spread in the general population. From Thailand, although variable by region, HIV prevalence of >30% among female sex workers was found [126]. Also in Thailand, between 1989 and 1993, an increase at a national level in HIV prevalence among military recruits was seen from 0.5% to 4%, with a prevalence as high as 15% in some regions [122]. At first it was thought that HIV had spread in Thailand from IDU into the general heterosexual population. The discovery of two distinct subtypes of HIV-1 in Thailand, subtype B especially among IDU and subtype E among heterosexuals, invalidated this assumption and indicates distinctly separate introductions into these two groups. It is suggested that subtype E is associated with a higher transmission risk than subtype B, partly explaining the rapid spread among the heterosexual population [129].

Alarming data have been presented from India as well. In Pune, Maharashtra, 22% of 4202 screened STD patients were infected with HIV. Of the non-infected patients, 851 were followed up and the overall seroincidence for HIV-1 was 10.2% per year and the incidence among commercial sex workers 26.1% [130,131]. In Bombay, surveys of sex workers have shown an increase in HIV prevalence from 40% in 1992 to 51% in 1994–1995. Besides heterosexual spread, infection through HIV-infected blood is a serious problem in India. It is estimated that in some regions only 30% of the blood is tested for HIV. Therefore, without immediate intervention through extensive educational and awareness programs, the consequences for India will be catastrophic [132].

In Thailand, the fast spread of HIV has been the main reason for the government to implement a '100% condom campaign', especially focusing on commercial sex workers and their clients [133]. If a brothel does not adhere to this rule, police sanctions follow. In Thailand it is common practice among males to visit commercial sex workers. Recently, a study among 21-year-olds who were conscripted into the army and were from Northern Thailand, the part of Thailand most affected by the HIV epidemic, showed a declining HIV prevalence between the 1991 and 1993 cohort (10.4–12.5%) and the 1995 cohort (6.7%) [134]. There was also a decline over the study period in the number of men who had visited a commercial sex

worker, an increase in condom use, and a marked decrease in the number of men with a history of sexually transmitted diseases (15% in 1995 compared with 42% in 1991) [134]. These results and the results of surveys that revealed an increase in condom use among prostitutes from 14% in 1989 to 94% in 1993 [135], indicate that the public health programs in Thailand are effective. However, more preventive measures must be taken in the battle against HIV because the number of HIV-infected prostitutes in Thailand is still very high and many of the young men infected with HIV will transmit the virus to their wives. Comparable condom promotion campaigns should start in other countries with an emerging epidemic.

Projection of HIV/AIDS cases

To develop public health care policies, and to plan and evaluate preventive measurements, predictions of the course of the AIDS epidemic are necessary. The first projections were based on extrapolation of the observed incidence of AIDS cases and predicted an exponential growth of the number of cases in the early years. This led to an overestimate of the expected number of cases. Now, more sophisticated mathematical models have been developed in which a variety of factors, depending on the region and the purpose for which a prediction is performed, can be incorporated. This brings about another problem that, even in the short-term prediction, the different models may produce significantly different results. However, the predictions still have to be interpreted with caution, taking into account the assumptions and limitations of the mathematical model used. WHO estimates that by the year 2000, the global prevalence of HIV (including AIDS cases) will be approximately 20 million and the cumulative number of HIV infections that have occurred since the beginning of the epidemic is 30–40 million [98]. The number of orphaned children under 10 years will exceed 5 million by the end of the 1990s.

References

1 Centers for Disease Control. Pneumocystis pneumonia – Los Angeles. *MMWR* 1981; **30**: 250–252.

2 Centers for Disease Control. Kaposi's sarcoma and pneumocystis pneumonia among homosexual men – New York City and California. *MMWR* 1981; **30**: 305–308.

3 Centers for Disease Control. Update on Kaposi's sarcoma and opportunistic infections in previously healthy persons – United States. *MMWR* 1982; **31**: 294–301.

4 Centers for Disease Control. Opportunistic infections and Kaposi's sarcoma among Haitians in the United States. *MMWR* 1982; **31**: 353–361.

5 Centers for Disease Control. Possible transfusion-associated acquired immune deficiency syndrome (AIDS) – California. *MMWR* 1982; **31**: 652–654.

6 Centers for Disease Control. Unexplained immunodeficiency and opportunistic infections in infants – New York, New Jersey, California. *MMWR* 1982; **31**: 665–667.

7 Centers for Disease Control. Immunodeficiency among female sexual partners of males with acquired immune deficiency syndrome (AIDS) – New York. *MMWR* 1983; **31**: 697–698.

8 Clumeck N, Mascart-Lemone F, De Maubeuge J, Brenez D, Marcelis L. Acquired immune deficiency syndrome in black Africans. *Lancet* 1983; **i**: 642.

9 Barré-Sinoussi F, Chermann JC, Rey F et al. Isolation of a T-lymphotropic retrovirus from a patient at risk for acquired immune deficiency syndrome (AIDS). *Science* 1983; **220**: 868–871.

10 Gallo RC, Salahuddin SZ, Popovic M et al. Frequent detection and isolation of cytopathic retroviruses (HTLV-III) from patients with AIDS and at risk for AIDS. *Science* 1984; **224**: 500–503.

11 Schechter MT, Craib KJP, Gelmon KA, Montaner JSG, Le TN, O'Shaughnessy MV. HIV-1 and the aetiology of AIDS. *Lancet* 1993; **341**: 658–659.

12 Ascher MS, Sheppard HW, Winkelstein W, Vittinghoff E. Does drug use cause AIDS? *Nature* 1993; **362**: 103–104.

13 Weiss RA. How does HIV causes AIDS? *Science* 1993; **260**: 1273–1279.

14 Barin F, M'Boup S, Denis F et al. Serological evidence for virus related to simian T-lymphotropic retrovirus III in residents of West Africa. *Lancet* 1985; **ii**: 1387–1389.

15 Daar ES, Moudgil T, Meyer RD, Ho DD. Transient high levels of viremia in patients with primary human immunodeficiency virus type 1 infection. *N Engl J Med* 1991; **324**: 961–964.

16 Bindels PJE, Hillemans PHM, Bilkert-Mooyman MAJ, van den Hoek JAR, Coutinho RA, van Wijngaarden JK. De epidemiologie van AIDS in Nederland bij personen geïnfecteerd door heteroseksueel contact. *Ned Tijdschr Geneeskd* 1992; **136**: 1865–1870.

17 Downs AM, de Vincenzi I. European Study Group on Heterosexual Transmission of HIV. Probability of heterosexual transmission of HIV: relationship to the number of unprotected sexual contacts. *J Acquir Immune Defic Syndr Hum Retrovirol* 1996; **11**: 388–395.

18 Hendriks JCM, Medley GF, van Griensven GJP, Coutinho RA, Heisterkamp SH, van Druten HA. The treatment-free incubation period of AIDS in a cohort of homosexual men. *AIDS* 1993; **7**: 231–239.

19 Rutherford GW, Lifson AR, Hessol NA et al. Course of HIV-1 infection in a cohort of homosexual and bisexual men: an 11 year follow up study. *Br Med J* 1990; **301**: 1183–1188.

20 Bacchetti P, Moss AR. Incubation period of AIDS in San Francisco. *Nature* 1989; **338**: 251–253.

21 Fahey JL, Taylor JMG, Detels R et al. The prognostic value of cellular and serologic markers in infection with human immunodeficiency virus type 1. *N Engl J Med* 1990; **322**: 166–172.

22 Crowe SM, Carlin JB, Stewart KI, Lucas R, Hoy JF. Predictive value of CD4-lymphocyte numbers for the development of opportunistic infections and malignancies in HIV-infected persons. *J Acquir Immune Defic Syndr* 1991; **4**: 770–776.

23 de Cock KM, Oudehouri K, Coldebunders RL et al. A comparison of HIV-1 and HIV-2 infections in hospitalized patients in Abidjan, Côte d'Ivoire. *AIDS* 1990; **4**: 443–448.

24 Marlink R, Kanki P, Thior I et al. Reduced rate of disease development after HIV-2 infection as compared to HIV-1. *Science* 1994; **265**: 1587–1590.

25 Kanki PJ, Travers KU, M'Boup S et al. Slower heterosexual spread of HIV-2 than HIV-1. *Lancet* 1994; **343**: 943–946.

26 de Cock KM, Adjorlolo G, Ekpini E et al. Epidemiology and transmission of HIV-2. Why there is no HIV-2 pandemic. *JAMA* 1993; **270**: 2083–2086 [Published erratum appears in *JAMA* 1994; **271**: 196.]

27 Donnelly C, Leisenring W, Kanki P, Awerbuch T, Sandberg S. Comparison of transmission rates of HIV-1 and HIV-2 in a cohort of prostitutes in Senegal. *Bull Math Biol* 1993; **55**: 731–743.

28 Gayle HD, Gnaore E, Adjorlolo G et al. HIV-1 and HIV-2 infection in children in Abidjan, Côte d'Ivoire. *J Acquir Immune Defic Syndr* 1992; **5**: 513–517.

29 Poulsen AG, Kvinesdal BB, Aaby P et al. Lack of evidence of vertical transmission of human immunodeficiency virus type 2 in a sample of the general population in Bissau. *J Acquir Immune Defic Syndr* 1992; **5**: 25–30.

30 Andreasson PA, Dias F, Naucler A, Andersson S, Biberfeld G. A prospective study of vertical transmission of HIV-2 in Bissau, Guinea-Bissau. *AIDS* 1993; **7**: 989–993.

31 Gayle H, Coutinho RA. Epidemiology of HIV infection with a focus on mother-to-mother-child transmission and among drug users. *Curr Opin Infect Dis* 1993; **6**: 200–204.

32 Connor EM, Mofenson LM. Zidovudine for the reduction of perinatal human immunodeficiency virus transmission: pediatric AIDS clinical trials group protocol 076-results and treatment recommendations. *Ped Infect Dis J* 1995; **14**: 536–541.

33 Connor EM, Sperling RS, Gelber R et al. Reduction of maternal–infant transmission of human immunodeficiency virus type 1 with zidovudine treatment. *N Engl J Med* 1994; **331**: 1173–1180.

34 Buehler JW, de Cock KM, Brunet JB. Surveillance definitions for AIDS. *AIDS* 1993; **7** (Suppl 1): S73–S81.

35 Centers for Disease Control. Acquired immune deficiency syndrome (AIDS) – United States. *MMWR* 1982; **31**: 507–514.

36 Centers for Disease Control. Revision of the case definition of acquired immunodeficiency syndrome for national reported – United States. *MMWR* 1985; **34**: 373–375.

37 Sarngadharan MG, Popovic M, Schuepbach J, Gallo RC. Antibodies reactive with human T-lymphotropic retroviruses (HTLV-III) in the serum of patients with AIDS. *Science* 1984; **224**: 506–508.

38 Brun-Vezinet F, Barré-Sinoussi F, Saimot AG et al. Detection of IgG antibodies to lymphadenopathy associated virus in patients with AIDS or lymphadenopathy syndrome. *Lancet* 1984; 1253–1256.

39 Kalyanaraman VS, Cabradilla CD, Getchell JP et al. Antibodies to the core protein of lymphadenopathy-associated virus (LAV) in patients with AIDS. *Science* 1984; **225**: 321–323.

40 Centers for Disease Control. Revision of the CDC surveillance case definition for acquired immunodeficiency syndrome. *MMWR* 1987; **36**: 1S–15S.

41 Centers for Disease Control. Classification system for human T-lymphotropic virus type III/lymphadenopathy-associated virus infections. *MMWR* 1986; **35**: 334–339.

42 Centers for Disease Control and Prevention. 1993 revised classification system for HIV infection and expanded surveillance case definition for AIDS among adolescents and adults. *MMWR* 1992; **41**(no. RR-17): 1–19.

43 Buehler JW, Ward JW, Berkelman RL. The surveillance definition for AIDS in the United States. *AIDS* 1993; **7**: 585–587.

44 Farizo KM, Buehler JW, Chamberland ME et al. Spectrum of disease in persons with human immunodeficiency virus infection in the United States. *JAMA* 1992; **267**: 1798–1805.

45 Stoneburner RL, Des Jarlais DC, Benezra D et al. A larger spectrum of severe HIV-1 related disease in intravenous drug users in New York City. *Science* 1988; **242**: 916–919.

46 Selwyn PA, Alcabes P, Hartel D et al. Clinical manifestations and predictors of disease progression in drug users with human immunodeficiency virus infection. *N Engl J Med* 1992; **327**: 1697–1703 [Published erratum appears in *N Engl J Med* 1993; **328**: 671.]

47 Mientjes GHC, van Ameijden EJC, van den Hoek JAR, Coutinho RA. Increasing morbidity without rise in non-AIDS mortality among HIV-infected intravenous drug users in Amsterdam. *AIDS* 1992; **6**: 207–212 [Published erratum appears in *AIDS* 1992; **6**: following 525.]

48 Schafer A, Friedmann, W, Mielke M, Schwartlander B, Koch MA. The increased frequency of cervical dysplasia–neoplasia in women infected with the human immunodeficiency virus is related to the degree of immunosuppression. *Am J Obstet Gynecol* 1991; **164**: 593–599.

49 Anonymous. 1994 revised classification system for human immunodeficiency virus infection in children less than 13 years of age. *MMWR* 1994; **43**: 1–10.

50 European Centre for the Epidemiological Monitoring of AIDS. *HIV/AIDS surveillance in Europe*. 1995; **48**: 1–53.

51 Mientjes GHC, van Ameijden EJC, Roos MTL et al. Large diurnal variation in CD4 cell count and T-cell function among drug users: implications for clinical practice and epidemiological studies. *AIDS* 1992; **6**: 1269–1272.

52 Veugelers PJ, Schechter MT, Tindall B et al. Differences in time from HIV seroconversion to CD4+ lymphocyte end-points and AIDS in cohorts of homosexual men. *AIDS* 1993; **7**: 1325–1329.

53 Ancelle-Park R. Expanded European AIDS case definition. *Lancet* 1993; **341**: 441.

54 Ancelle-Park RA, Alix J, Downs AM, Brunet JB. Impact of 1993 revision of adult/adolescent AIDS surveillance case-definition for Europe. National coordinators for AIDS surveillance in 38 European countries (letter). *Lancet* 1995; **345**: 789–790.

55 van Griensven GJP, Boucher EC, Roos MTL, Coutinho RA. Expansion of AIDS case definition (letter). *Lancet* 1991; **338**: 1012–1013.

56 Sheppard HW, Ascher MW, Winkelstein W et al. Use of T lymphocyte subset analysis in the case definition of AIDS. *J Acquir Immune Defic Syndr* 1993; **6**: 287–294.

57 Centers for Disease Control. AIDS and human immuno-deficiency virus infection in the United States: 1988 update. *MMWR* 1989; **38**: 1–38.

58 Rutherford GW, Payne SF, Lemp GF. Impact of the revised AIDS case definition on AIDS reporting in San Francisco. *JAMA* 1988; **259**: 2235.

59 Selik RM, Buehler JW, Karon JM, Chamberland ME, Berkelman RL. Impact of the 1987 revision of the case definition of acquired immune deficiency syndrome in the United States. *J Acquir Immune Defic Syndr* 1990; **3**: 73–82.

60 Anonymous. *AIDS Surveillance in Europe* 1989; no. 23 (abstract).

61 Centers for Disease Control. Update: trends in AIDS diagnosis and reporting under the expanded surveillance definition for adolescents and adults – United States, 1993. *MMWR* 1993; **43**: 826–836.

62 Chaisson RE, Stanton DL, Gallant JE, Rucker S, Bartlett JG, Moore RD. Impact of the 1993 revision of the AIDS case definition on the prevalence of AIDS in a clinical setting. *AIDS* 1993; **7**: 857–862.

63 Mientjes GHC, van Ameijden EJC, Keet IPM, van Deutekom H, van den Hoek JAR, Coutinho RA. Disproportional impact of the revised AIDS surveillance definition on the AIDS incidence among drug users compared to homosexual men. *Eur J Public Health* 1995; **5**: 288–290.

64 Brettle RP, Gore SM, Bird AG, McNeil AJ. Clinical and epidemiological implications of the Centers for Disease Control/World Health Organization reclassification of AIDS cases. *AIDS* 1993; **7**: 531–539.

65 Vella S, Chiesi A, Volpi A et al. Differential survival of patients with AIDS according to the 1987 and 1993 CEC case definitions. *JAMA* 1994; **271**: 1197–1199.

66 World Health Organization. Acquired immune deficiency syndrome (AIDS): WHO/CDC case of AIDS definition for AIDS. *Week Epidemiol Rec* 1986; **61**: 69–73.

67 Weniger BG, Quinhoes EP, Sereno Borges A et al. A simplified surveillance case definition of AIDS derived

from empirical clinical data. *J Acquir Immune Defic Syndr* 1992; **5**: 1212–1223.

68 Gallant JE, Somani J, Chaisson RE, Stanton D, Smith M, Quinn TC. Diagnostic accuracy of three clinical case definitions for advanced HIV disease. *AIDS* 1992; **6**: 295–299.

69 de Cock KM, Selik RM, Soro B, Gayle H, Colebunders RL. AIDS surveillance in Africa: a reappraisal of case definitions. *Br Med J* 1991; **303**: 1185.

70 Bélec L, Brogan T, Keou FX, Georges AJ. Surveillance of acquired immunodeficiency syndrome in Africa. An analysis of evaluations of the World Health Organization and other clinical definitions [review]. *Epidemiol Rev* 1994; **16**: 403–417.

71 Heisterkamp SH, de Haan BJ, Jager JC, van Druten JAM, Hendriks JCM. Short and medium term projections of the AIDS/HIV epidemic by a dynamic model with an application to the risk group of homo/bisexual men in Amsterdam. *Stat Med* 1992; **11**: 1425–1441.

72 Hendriks JC, Medley GF, Heisterkamp SH et al. Short-term predictions of HIV prevalence and AIDS incidence. *Epidemiol Infect* 1992; **109**: 149–160.

73 Day NE. The incidence and prevalence of AIDS and prevalence of other severe HIV disease in England and Wales for 1995 to 1999: projection using data to the end of 1994. *Commun Dis Rep* 1996; **6**: R1–R24.

74 van Haastrecht HJA, van den Hoek JAR, Coutinho RA. High mortality among HIV-infected injecting drug users without AIDS-diagnosis: implications for HIV-infection epidemic modellers? *AIDS* 1994; **8**: 363–366.

75 McCormick A. Excess mortality associated with the HIV epidemic in England and Wales. *Br Med J* 1991; **302**: 1375–1376.

76 Graham NMH, Zeger SL, Park LP et al. The effects on survival of early treatment of human immunodeficiency virus infection. *N Engl J Med* 1992; **326**: 1037–1042.

77 Gail MH, Rosenberg PS, Goedert JJ. Therapy may explain recent deficits in AIDS incidence. *J Acquir Immune Defic Syndr* 1990; **3**: 296–306.

78 Longini IM, Scott Clark W, Karon JM. Effect of routine use of therapy in slowing the clinical course of human immunodeficiency virus (HIV) infection in a population-based cohort. *Am J Epidemiol* 1993; **137**: 1229–1240.

79 Buehler JW, Berkelman RL, Stehr-Green JK. The completeness of AIDS surveillance. *J Acquir Immune Defic Syndr* 1992; **5**: 257–264.

80 Jones JL, Meyer P, Garrison C, Kettinger L, Hermann P. Physician and infection control practitioner HIV/AIDS reporting characteristics. *Am J Public Health* 1992; **82**: 889–891.

81 Anonymous. Estimates of HIV prevalence and projected AIDS cases: summary of a workshop, October 31–November 1, 1989. *MMWR* 1990; **39**: 110–119.

82 Smith E, Rix BA, Melbye M. Mandatory anonymous HIV surveillance in Denmark: the first results of a new system. *Am J Public Health* 1994; **84**: 1929–1932.

83 Engel RR. Evaluating modifications in epidemic surveillance systems: a method and an application to AIDS surveillance in Switzerland. *Int J Epidemiol* 1993; **22**: 321–326.

84 Seage GR, Oddleifson S, Carr E et al. Survival with AIDS in Massachusetts, 1979 to 1989. *Am J Public Health* 1993; **83**: 72–78.

85 Gertig DM, Marion SA, Schechter MT. Estimating the extent of underreporting in AIDS surveillance. *AIDS* 1991; **5**: 1157–1164.

86 Evans BG. Estimating underreporting of AIDS: straight forward in theory – difficult in practice. *AIDS* 1991; **5**: 1261–1262.

87 Elcock M, Simon T, Gilbert BP, Copello AG, Kelzer PJ. Active AIDS surveillance: hospital-based case finding in a metropolitan California county. *Am J Public Health* 1993; **83**: 1002–1005.

88 Conway GA, Colley-Niemeyer B, Pursley C et al. Underreporting of AIDS cases in South Carolina, 1986 and 1987. *JAMA* 1989; **262**: 2859–2863.

89 Trino R, McAnaney J, Fife D. Laboratory-based reporting of AIDS. *J Acquir Immune Defic Syndr* 1993; **6**: 1057–1061.

90 Jones JL, Rion P, Hermann P, Kettinger L, Gamble WB. Improvement in AIDS case reporting South Carolina. *JAMA* 1991; **265**: 356.

91 Modesitt SK, Hulman S, Fleming D. Evaluation of active versus passive AIDS surveillance in Oregon. *Am J Public Health* 1990; **80**: 463–464.

92 Heisterkamp SH, Jager JC, Downs AM, van Druten JAM, Ruitenberg EJ. Correcting reported AIDS incidence: a statistical approach. *Stat Med* 1989; **8**: 963–976.

93 van Haastrecht HJA, van den Hoek JAR, Bardoux C, Leentvaar-Kuijpers A, Coutinho RA. The course of the HIV epidemic among intravenous drug users in Amsterdam, The Netherlands. *Am J Public Health* 1991; **81**: 59–62.

94 European Centre for the Epidemiological Monitoring of AIDS. *Surveillance of AIDS/HIV in Europe, 1984–1994* 1994.

95 Centers for Disease Control. Update: acquired immune deficiency syndrome (AIDS) world-wide. *MMWR* 1988; **37**: 286–295.

96 Pepin J, Plummer FA, Brunham RC, Piot P, Cameron DW, Ronzald AR. The interaction of HIV infection and other sexually transmitted diseases: an opportunity for intervention. *AIDS* 1989; **3**: 3–9.

97 Laga M, Nzila N, Goeman J. The interrelationship of sexually transmitted diseases and HIV infection: implications for the control of both epidemics in Africa [review]. *AIDS* 1991; **5**(Suppl 1): S55–S63.

98 Anonymous. Acquired immunodeficiency syndrome (AIDS) – data as at 30 June 1996. *Week Epidemiol Rec* 1996; **27**: 205–208.

99 Coutinho RA, Krone WJA, Smit L et al. Introduction of lymphadenopathy associated virus or human T lymphotropic virus (LAV/HTLV-III) into the male homosexual community in Amsterdam. *Genitourin Med* 1986; **62**: 38–43.

100 Mortimer PP, Jesson WJ, van der Velde EM, Pereira MS. Prevalence of antibody to human T-lymphotropic virus type III by risk group and area, United Kingdom 1978–1984. *Br Med J* 1985; **290**: 1176–1178.

101 van Haastrecht HJA, van den Hoek JAR, Mientjes GHC, Coutinho RA. Did the introduction of HIV among homosexuals precede the introduction of HIV among injecting drug users in The Netherlands? *AIDS* 1992; **6**: 131–32.

102   European Center for the Epidemiological Monitoring of AIDS. *HIV/AIDS Surveillance in Europe* 1996; **49**: 4–33 (abstract).

103   European Center for the Epidemiological Monitoring of AIDS. *HIV/AIDS Surveillance in Europe 1995; 47.*

104   Franceschi S, Dal Maso L, La Vecchia C, Negri E, Serraino D. AIDS incidence rates in Europe and the United States. *AIDS* 1994; **8**: 1173–1177.

105   Jaffe HW, Coutinho RA. AIDS 92/93. Epidemiology: overview [review]. *AIDS* 1993; **7**: (Suppl. 1): S63–S5.

106   Jaffe HW, Darrow WW, Echenberg DF et al. The acquired immunodeficiency syndrome in a cohort of homosexual men: a six year follow up study. *Ann Intern Med* 1985; **97**: 362–366.

107   Centers for Disease Control. Update: acquired immuno-deficiency syndrome in the San Francisco Cohort Study 1978–1985. *MMWR* 1985; **34**: 573–575.

108   Stevens CE, Taylor PE, Zang EA et al. Human T-cell lymphotropic virus type III infection in a cohort of homosexual men in New York City. *JAMA* 1986; **255**: 2167–2172.

109   Hessol NA, Lifson AR, O'Malley PM, Doll LS, Jaffe HW, Rutherford GW. Prevalence, incidence and progression of human immunodeficiency virus infection in homosexual and bisexual men in hepatitis B vaccine trials, 1978–1988. *Am J Epidemiol* 1989; **130**: 1167–1175.

110   van Griensven GJP, de Vroome EMM, Goudsmit J, Coutinho RA. Changes in sexual behavior and the fall in incidence of HIV infection among homosexual men. *Br Med J* 1989; **298**: 218–221.

111   Coutinho RA, van Griensven GJP, Moss A. Effects of preventive efforts among homosexual men. *AIDS* 1989; **3**(Suppl): S53–S56.

112   Des Jarlais DC, Friedman SR, Novick DM et al. HIV-1 infection among intravenous drug users in Manhattan, New York City, from 1977 through 1987. *JAMA* 1989; **261**: 1008–1012.

113   Centers of Disease Control. First 500,000 AIDS case – United States, 1995. *MMWR* 1995; **44**: 849–853.

114   Centers for Disease Control. Update: AIDS among women – United States, 1994. *MMWR* 1995; **44**: 81–85.

115   Thomas PA, Weisfuse IB, Greenberg AE, Bernard GA, Tytun A, Stellman SD. Trends in the first ten years of AIDS in New York City. The New York City Department of Health AIDS surveillance team. *Am J Epidemiol* 1993; **137**: 121–133.

116   Anonymous. AIDS among racial/ethnic minorities – United States, 1993. *MMWR* 1994; **43**: 644–655.

117   Centers for Disease Control. Update: mortality attributable to HIV infection among persons aged 25–44 years – United States, 1994. *MMWR* 1996; **45**: 121–125.

118   Bindels PJE, Reijneveld SA, Mulder-Folkerts DK, Coutinho RA, van den Hoek JAR. Impact of AIDS on premature mortality in Amsterdam, 1982–1992. *AIDS* 1994; **8**: 233–237.

119   Wheeler VW, Radcliffe KW. HIV infection in the Caribbean [editorial]. *Int J STD AIDS* 1994; **5**: 79–89.

120   Pape J, Johnson WD. AIDS in Haiti: 1982–1992 [review]. *Clin Infect Dis* 1993; **17**(Suppl. 2): S341–S345.

121   World Health Organization. Acquired immunodeficiency syndrome (AIDS). *Week Epidemiol Rec* 1995; **70**: 353–360.

122   World Health Organization. The HIV/AIDS pandemic: 1994, overview. *Global Program on AIDS* (Abstract). Geneva: WHO, 1994.

123   Leroy V, van de Perre P, Lepage P et al. Seroincidence of HIV-1 infection in African women of reproductive age: a prospective cohort study in Kigali, Rwanda, 1988–1992. *AIDS* 1994; **8**: 983–986.

124   Grosskurth H, Mosha F, Todd J et al. Impact of improved treatment of sexually transmitted diseases on HIV infection in rural Tanzania: randomised controlled trial [see comments]. *Lancet* 1995; **346**: 530–536.

125   Mulder DW, Nunn AJ, Kamali A, Kengeya-Kayondo JF. Decreasing HIV-1 seroprevalence in young adults in a rural Ugandan cohort. *Br Med J* 1995; **311**: 833–836.

126   Kaldor JM, Sittitrai W, John TJ, Kitamura T. The emerging epidemic of HIV infection and AIDS in Asia and the Pacific. *AIDS* 1994; **8**: S165–S172.

127   Zheng X, Tian C, Choi KH et al. Injected drug use and HIV infection in southwest China. *AIDS* 1994; **8**: 1141–1147.

128   Brown T, Sittitrai W, Vanichseni S, Thisyakorn U. The recent epidemiology of HIV and AIDS in Thailand [review]. *AIDS* 1994; **8** (Suppl. 2): S131–S141.

129   Kunanusont C, Foy HM, Kreiss JK et al. HIV-1 subtypes and male-to-female transmission in Thailand. *Lancet* 1995; **345**: 1078–1083.

130   Rodrigues JJ, Mehendale SM, Shepherd ME et al. Risk factors for HIV infection in people attending clinics for sexually transmitted diseases in India. *Br Med J* 1995; **311**: 283–286.

131   Mehendale SM, Rodrigues JJ, Brookmeyer RS et al. Incidence and predictors of human immunodeficiency virus type 1 seroconversion in patients attending sexually transmitted disease clinics in India. *J Infect Dis* 1995; **172**: 1486–1491.

132   Lalvani A, Shastri JS. HIV epidemic in India: opportunity to learn from the past. *Lancet* 1996; **347**: 1349–1350.

133   Rojanapithayakorn W, Hanenberg R. The 100% condom program in Thailand. *AIDS* 1996; **10**: 1–7.

134   Nelson KE, Celentano DD, Eiumtrakol S et al. Changes in sexual behavior and a decline in HIV infection among young men in Thailand. *N Engl J Med* 1996; **335**: 297–303.

135   Hanenberg RS, Rojanapithayakorn W, Kunasol P, Sokal DC. Impact of Thailand's HIV-control programme as indicated by the decline of sexually transmitted diseases. *Lancet* 1994; **344**: 243–245.

5 PATHOLOGY OF AIDS

Jan G. van den Tweel
Marguerite E.I. Schipper

Introduction

Human immune deficiency virus (HIV) infection is a multisystem disease resulting in a variety of pathologic lesions that are generally either a direct result of HIV infection or secondary to the immunodeficiency status following the viral infection. The majority of the pathologic lesions is of infectious or degenerative origin, but a considerable number of proliferative lesions, both benign and malignant, is also seen. Various tissues and organs can be affected by these processes.

In this chapter, the most important opportunistic infections and tumors that are associated with HIV infections are discussed first. Subsequently, there is an overview of the pathology of the most relevant organ systems.

Opportunistic infections

Opportunistic infections are mainly caused by bacteria, viruses, protozoa and fungi. Table 5.1 gives an overview of the infections that are most frequently encountered in HIV disease. Some of them are also seen in patients without immunodeficiency. They are mainly found in three organ systems: the respiratory tract, the digestive tract, and the central nervous system (CNS). General aspects of these infections are addressed here, whereas the organ-specific aspects will be dealt with under the respective headings.

Bacterial infections

Tuberculosis

Although tuberculosis strictly speaking is not an opportunistic infection, its incidence and the number of AIDS patients dying from tuberculosis seems to be increasing [1]. Moreover, if there is extrapulmonary dissemination of the disease in HIV-positive patients, it is regarded as diagnostic of AIDS [2]. In this situation, the disease is probably the result of reactivation of a previous infection rather than being a primary infection. Disseminated tuberculosis involves the respiratory tract, followed by spleen, lymph nodes, liver and genitourinary tract. Less common sites of involvement are the bone marrow, gastrointestinal tract, the kidneys (Figure 5.1), and the adrenals [3].

Mycobacterium avium intracellulare

Among the atypical mycobacterial infections, *Mycobacterium avium intracellulare* (MAI) is the most frequent one encountered in AIDS. These microorganisms are located in the cytoplasm of macrophages, where large numbers of MAI can be seen both in the H & E staining, and in special stainings such as Ziehl–Neelsen (ZN), PAS, Giemsa, and methenamine silver. The size of the macrophages can be up to 50 μm. Many organs can be affected, with the lymph nodes (Figure 5.2), spleen and liver most frequently involved. Other organs affected by this infection include the bone marrow, gastrointestinal and respiratory tract, and the genitourinary tract. It is rarely seen in the CNS, skin, and heart [1]. Even widespread MAI-infection is infrequently a cause of death.

Viral infections

Cytomegalovirus infection

Cytomegalovirus (CMV) is a DNA virus belonging to the family of the herpes viruses. It is a world-wide ubiquitous pathogenic agent that only gives serious complications in immunodeficient patients, either after primary infection or after reactivation of a latent infection. Although CMV infection can be localized, it usually is a systemic disorder in HIV patients. In a

Table 5.1. Frequency of opportunistic infections and tumors in 400 patients with AIDS during the total course of their disease (modified after Klatt [3]).

	Number of patients	%
Agent		
Pneumocystis carinii	224	56
Cytomegalovirus	201	50
Candida albicans	97	24
M. avium intracellulare	66	17
Herpes simplex/zoster	57	14
Cryptococcus neoformans	46	12
Toxoplasma gondii	42	11
M. tuberculosis	39	10
Cryptosporidium	23	6
Histoplasma capsulatum	9	2
Other infections	16	4
Tumor		
Kaposi's sarcoma	94	24
Malignant lymphoma	52	13

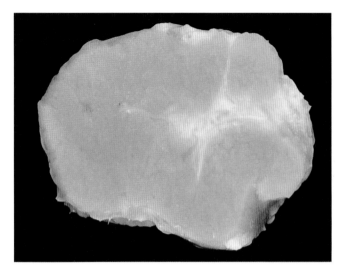

Figure 5.2.   Cut surface of a lymph node affected by *Mycobacterium avium-intracellulare*. The yellow color is typical for this type of infection.

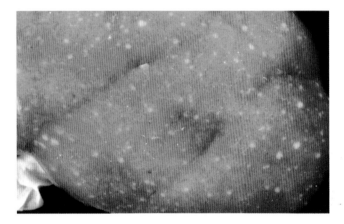

Figure 5.1.   Kidney with multiple, small white lesions on the surface from a patient with miliary tuberculosis.

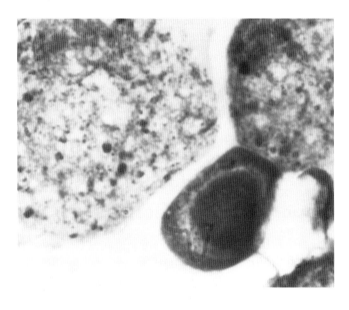

Figure 5.3.   BAL with a CMV-infected alveolar cell, showing a characteristic inclusion body surrounded by a clear thin halo.

large autopsy series, CMV most frequently occurred in the adrenals, respiratory tract, and gastrointestinal tract, followed by the CNS and the retina. Other organs are infrequently the source of infection [1]. Infected cells are enlarged and show large, violaceous to dark-red, intranuclear inclusions, surrounded by a clear thin halo (Figure 5.3). Usually CMV is not an aggressive disease. It is the immediate cause of death in approximately 10% of AIDS cases, the majority dying from pulmonary involvement and CNS infection.

Herpes simplex virus and Herpes zoster virus

Although herpes infections are not only seen in immunocompromised patients, the presence of mucocutaneous herpes virus infections for more than one month duration satisfies the criteria for AIDS in HIV-positive patients. Other than mucocutaneous localizations, dissemination of the disease is very uncommon. Particularly, the perianal region is frequently involved. Oropharyngeal and oesophageal infections are less common. Macroscopically, the lesions are characterized by vesicles or ulcers. Microscopically, the infected cells show small eosinophilic intranuclear inclusions. Secondary infection of the ulcers is common.

Human papilloma virus

This virus is a DNA virus that is found in many proliferative epithelial lesions. In AIDS patients it is associated with dysplasia and with carcinomas of the anorectal epithelium and also with condyloma accuminatum. It is also seen in hairy leukoplakia, a white lesion that is usually present on the lateral border of the tongue.

Protozoal infections

Pneumocystis carinii

Infections by *Pneumocystis carinii* are only seen in severely debilitated or immunocompromised patients. They consist of small cysts that on maturation contain up to eight sporozoites. After rupturing of the cyst, the released sporozoites differentiate into throphozoites. They form cysts and repeat the cycle. Microscopically, they can be recognized in a Grocott staining and by methylene blue, although the experienced eye is usually able to recognize the protozoa in routine H & E sections and Giemsa-stained cytological preparations. The lungs are the organs that are most often involved with these organisms. Extrapulmonary localizations are rare, although they can be found in hilar lymph nodes and very occasionally in one or more other organs [4].

Cryptosporidium

Cryptosporidium results in a gastrointestinal infection that is not accompanied by specific macroscopic lesions. The microorganisms are small, 2–6 μm in diameter, and are found along the mucosal brush border of the stomach and the small and large intestine. Since they are acid-fast, they can be recognized in a Z-N staining. These microorganisms are rarely seen in other organs, although their presence is also reported in the biliary system and the respiratory tract [5].

Toxoplasma gondii

Toxoplasmosis is an infectious disease that is encountered in a wide variety of mammals and birds. It is a very common parasitic infection in the USA and a few thousand children are annually infected at birth.

In adults it usually manifests itself as a lymphadenopathy. Microscopically, the disease is best diagnosed by finding 50 μm-sized cysts filled with bradyzoites. Free protozoa, tachyzoites, are only 1–2 μm and very difficult to find. Only ruptured cysts induce an inflammatory response. In HIV patients, the CNS is often involved in cases of an infection. Extracerebral toxoplasmosis is infrequent, although the respiratory and gastrointestinal tract are sometimes involved, but usually as an autopsy finding [6].

Other protozoa

Among other protozoal infections, those due to *Isospora belli* and *Microsporidium* should be mentioned. They are mainly located in the small intestine and produce their symptoms there. Isosporiasis is an intestinal infection that can occasionally invade the intestinal wall and disseminate to lymph nodes.

Fungi

Candida albicans

Candida albicans is an ubiquitous yeast that can be found in the skin and in the oral cavity of healthy individuals. To fulfill the criteria for candidiasis, the fungus must invade the mucosa of the esophagus or respiratory tract. This is grossly manifested by white plaques or patches. Dissemination beyond these organs is very rare. Microscopically, the invading microorganisms are mainly surrounded by granulocytes. The *Candida* is identified by buds and pseudohyphae without branching or true septations. Death from candidiasis is rare in AIDS, although it can be demonstrated in nearly 25% of the patients (Table 5.1).

Cryptococcus neoformans

Cryptococcus neoformans organisms are small budding yeasts with a diameter of approximately 4–7 μm. The cells have a prominent capsule that can be easily recognized in routine histological stainings. The organisms form pale, mucoid areas in affected tissues. Sometimes the only expression of infection is the presence of multinucleated giant cells with the organisms in their cytoplasm. The CNS is frequently involved, as is the lung. In disseminated disease, other organs such as lymph nodes, spleen, bone marrow and liver can also become affected.

Neoplasms

Malignant lymphomas

Non-Hodgkin lymphomas

Approximately 3% of HIV-positive patients present themselves with a non-Hodgkin lymphoma. The risk of developing lymphoma is increased 100-fold, 6–8 years after infection, and the risk approaches 1% per year once the diagnosis of AIDS has been established [7].

The same authors predict that by 1994, 10% of all non-Hodgkin lymphomas is AIDS-related. Lymphomas of the CNS (Figure 5.4) were considered part of the spectrum of AIDS from the outset, but systemic non-Hodgkin lymphoma is regarded a rather late manifestation of the disease [8,9]. The majority of the lymphomas are (intermediate or) high-grade B-cell lymphomas, including immunoblastic lymphoma, small non-cleaved lymphomas (Burkitt type), and large non-cleaved diffuse lymphomas (centroblastic type). The primary CNS lymphoma carries a particularly poor prognosis. The other patients usually have widespread, often extranodal disease involving many organs.

Hodgkin's disease

Although several reports suggest an association between Hodgkin's disease and HIV infection, Hodgkin's disease is still not considered a criterion for the diagnosis of AIDS. Most patients present with advanced disease (82% with stage III or IV) and with mixed cellularity histology. The response to therapy is poor and more than two-thirds die within one year of diagnosis [10]. Gold and colleagues (1991) did a statistical analysis of a large group of patients and found that HIV-associated Hodgkin's disease had a strong tendency to be out of the normal age range for Hodgkin's disease [11].

Kaposi's sarcoma

The aggressive epidemic disseminated form of Kaposi's sarcoma [12–16]. is a mesenchymal tumor probably of vascular origin, manifesting itself in the skin, the mucous membrane of the bronchial tree, the oropharyngeal, gastrointestinal, and anal mucosa, and in the lymphatic tissue with a preference for MALT (mucosa-associated lymphoid tissue). The tumor is also described in HIV-seronegative individuals and in patients receiving immunosuppressive therapy. The frequent simultaneous occurrence on many different localizations suggests

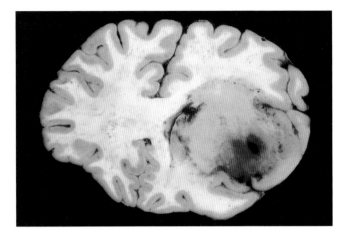

Figure 5.4. Cut surface of the cerebrum showing a centrally necrotic, non-Hodgkin lymphoma.

a multifocal genesis. The early lesions are fine red nodules of 1–2 mm diameter. Later, macular and plague-like lesions occur. The proliferating cell is of vascular or lymphatic endothelial origin. The cytonuclear pleomorphism is slight to moderate and mitoses can be found. The tumor cells show erythrophagocytosis, and contain red blood cells and their cytoplasm. The surrounding tissue contains an aspecific mononuclear inflammatory infiltrate and iron. Slit-like vessels are recognized, containing red blood cells and a marked extravasation of erythrocytes is present. These lesions are not only confined to the upper dermal layer or the mucous membranes, but show an expansive growth along the preexisting (lymphatic) vessels in the deeper layers and surrounding support tissues. This growth pattern is in special present in the lungs, the liver (Figure 5.5), the heart, and the kidneys. In the CNS, Kaposi's sarcoma lesions are not reported.

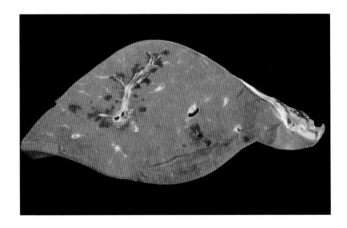

Figure 5.5. Liver with multiple small nodules of Kaposi's sarcoma, around a large portal vein tract.

Organ system pathology

Respiratory tract

The respiratory tract is frequently involved in patients with AIDS. In large autopsy series, 60–80% of the AIDS patients die of pulmonary infections or malignancies. The chest X-rays reveal mostly diffuse bilateral interstitial and alveolar infiltrates. The clinical features of the different diseases can be indistinguishable, although infections generally cause a more diffuse interstitial pattern. Malignancies, like Kaposi's sarcoma, have a more nodular appearance.

Pneumocystis carinii

Among the infections, *Pneumocystis carinii* pneumonia (PCP) is the most frequent opportunistic infection in AIDS patients. A large majority of AIDS patients will have at least one episode of PCP during the course of their disease. The mortality per single episode ranges from 10%–20%. Clinically, the presence of a PCP is suggested by a history of dyspnea on exertion or a non-productive cough and a diffuse bilateral interstitial infiltrate on chest X-ray. The pathologic features of PCP are those of a widespread involvement of the alveolar spaces, with the gross appearance of pneumonic consolidation. In the early phase of the disease, the surface is pale, salmon pink with scattered areas of hemorrhage or congestion. Later in the disease, the lung becomes rubbery and the cut surface is often slimy, similar to the morphological changes in the adult respiratory distress syndrome. In the end stage, the lungs show a fleshy appearance caused by fibrosis and organization of the lung tissue (Figure 5.6). Microscopic investigation shows a foamy alveolar exudate. With the help of special stainings, large numbers of *Pneumocystis carinii* sporozoites can be demonstrated.

To diagnose PCP, a bronchoalveolar lavage (BAL) is a type of investigation with a high sensitivity. If combined with a transbronchial biopsy, the diagnostic sensitivity approaches 100% [17,18].

Cytomegalovirus

Cytomegalovirus can often be found in microscopic specimens of lungs in AIDS patients. The presence of the characteristic inclusion bodies does not always

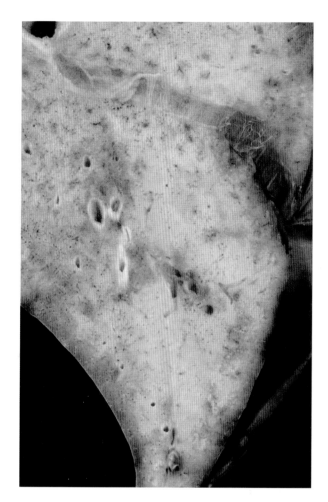

Figure 5.6. Lung tissue with end-stage *Pneumocystis carinii* infection. The tissue is consolidated as a result of fibrosis.

indicate the presence of an active pneumonia. Apart for the presence of viral inclusions other features should be present, such as signs of diffuse alveolar damage, inflammatory infiltrates, and/or areas of hemorrhage. In florid cases, the infiltrates are present in the alveolar spaces and areas of patchy to confluent consolidation can be seen.

Other infections

Cryptococcus neoformans, *Candida*, and *Histoplasma capsulatum* are fungal diseases (Figure 5.7) that are occasionally seen in the lungs of HIV-positive or AIDS patients. Usually, there are interstitial granulomas in the presence of a minimal inflammatory infiltrate. The Grocott stain and the PAS stain are suitable for the demonstration of these microorganisms.

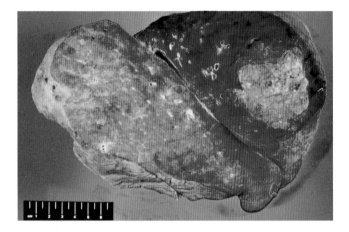

Figure 5.7. Cut surface of the lower lobe of a left lung showing an abscess caused by *Aspergillus* infection.

Cardiovascular system

Gross abnormalities of the heart are rare in AIDS. If a malignant lymphoma is present, approximately 20% of the patients show cardiac involvement.

Kaposi's sarcoma here is even rarer. Only very occasionally is cardiac involvement with Kaposi's sarcoma seen in patients.

A congestive cardiomyopathy is sometimes diagnosed in patients with AIDS [19,20].

Gastrointestinal tract

A wide range of opportunistic infections can involve the gastrointestinal (GI) tract in HIV-seropositive patients, all establishing the diagnosis AIDS, following the Centers for Disease Control and Prevention, Atlanta, Georgia, USA (CDC) criteria. Oral and esophageal invasive candidiasis are present in most patients in the prephase of their full-blown AIDS. In biopsies of the stomach and the upper gastrointestinal tract, cryptosporidiosis and microsporidiosis seem to be related to the diagnoses of diarrhea, weight loss, and malabsorption. These tiny organisms live intracellularly in an extracytoplasmic niche of the surface epithelial cells. The main morphologic abnormality of these infected cells is atrophy of the microvilli. Microsporidium is merely detected by electron microscopical examination.

CMV infections can be present in different stages of the disease, anywhere in the GI tract. The early phases are characterized by a few intraepithelial inclusion bodies in the deep part of the mucous membrane, with or without an associated inflammatory infiltrate.

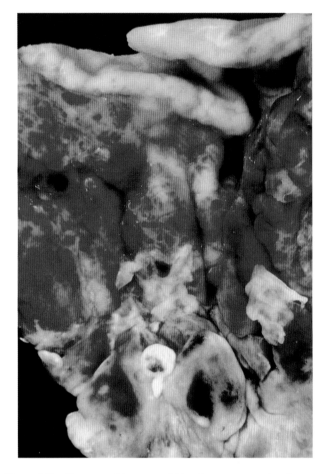

Figure 5.8. Rectum with mucosal bleedings as a result of a CMV infection. The anal mucosa shows submucosal Kaposi's sarcoma lesions.

In the full-blown phase, the mucosa shows multiple, confluent erosions and deep ulcerations with glossy red margins (Figure 5.8). The CMV is mainly present in the endothelial cells and causes local vascular damage resulting in necrosis of the mucous membrane. In the end phase, after treatment with high doses of antiviral therapy, the viral inclusion bodies are easily detected in endothelial and epithelial cells. In this phase, the mucous membrane shows atrophy.

Mycobacterium avium gives the mucous membrane at endoscopy and on gross appearance a glistening yellow colour (Figure 5.9), owing to the presence of histiocytes, loaded with numerous acid-fast microorganisms in the cytoplasm. An inflammatory infiltrate is usually absent. Very often the regional lymph nodes are also infected.

Kaposi's sarcoma occurs frequently in the GI tract and can be present from the oropharyngeal area to the anal mucosa. Early Kaposi's lesions occur in the

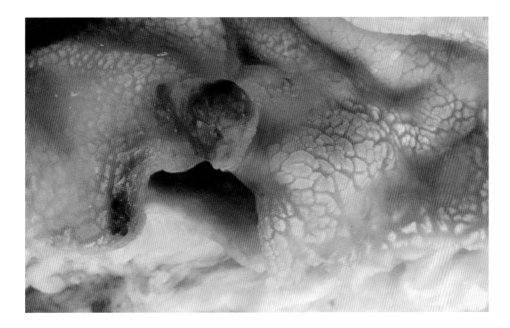

Figure 5.9. *Mycobacterium avium* infection of the large intestine. The small yellow plaques are the result of conglomerates of macrophages filled with MAI.

mucous membrane, covering lymphoid tissue and Peyer's plaques. The lesions present as multiple small red, sometimes pinpoint, noduli in the mucous membrane. Later, large areas of the mucosa can be affected by this disease.

Malignant lymphoma of the GI tract is a less frequent complication of HIV infection than Kaposi's sarcoma. However, it is one of the most common sites of involvement by malignant lymphoma in patients with AIDS. The lymphomas usually occur in the small intestine and the anorectal region. On gross appearance, they are usually symptomatic lesions with obstruction, perforation, or bleeding.

Hepatobiliary system

Although opportunistic infections and neoplasms involve the liver in approximately 30% of AIDS cases, they are often of minor clinical importance, since they almost never result in liver failure [21]. Among the infections that can be found in the liver are *Mycobacterium avium*, and fungal infections like *Cryptococcus* and *Histoplasma*. Kaposi's sarcoma is rare and, when present, located in the connective tissue around the large portal vein branches and the large biliary tracts. Malignant lymphomas of the liver are rarely seen as primary tumors. They usually occur in association with lymphomas elsewhere [22].

CMV infection and cryptosporidial cholecystitis has been reported by Himant et al. [23].

Hematopoietic organs

Several causes can result in (generalized) lymphadenopathy. An AIDS-specific reaction to HIV infection is characterized by extreme follicular hyperplasia with many 'starry-sky' macrophages. Later in the disease, the follicles are destroyed and, finally, the lymph node is characterized by a complete depletion of follicle centers [24].

The mesenterial lymph nodes are often involved in *Mycobacterium avium* infections. Malignant lymphoma is also an important cause of lymphadenopathy, although extranodal lymphoma localizations are much more frequent than nodal ones.

The most important feature of HIV infection in the bone marrow are dysplastic features of hematopoiesis. In addition, opportunistic infections can have localizations in the bone marrow, although they are infrequent [25].

Kaposi's sarcoma is very rare but lymphoma localization is quite frequent.

Central nervous system

The CNS can be affected by HIV infection with the clinical manifestation of an HIV encephalopathy/AIDS

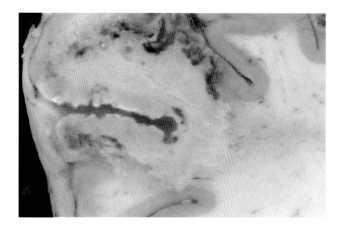

Figure 5.10. Part of the cerebral cortex with extensive necrosis resulting from HIV encephalopathy.

dementia complex [26] or by secondary opportunistic lesions, including the localization of an intracerebral non-Hodgkin lymphoma.

The morphological spectrum of the HIV encephalopathy is either characterized by multiple perivascular accumulations of multinucleated giant cells with inflammatory cells and focal necrosis, or by diffuse white matter damage of cerebral and cerebellar hemispheres (Figure 5.10). Since the presence of HIV antigens has also been demonstrated within vacuolar lesions of the spinal cord, the vacuolar myelopathy has to be considered as an HIV-induced disease.

Among the opportunistic non-viral infections, toxoplasmosis is the most frequent lesion localized in the cerebral hemispheres, the basal ganglia, and the brainstem. The main appearances are multiple areas of ill-defined necrosis, a slight inflammatory infiltrate with multiple macrophages, and, on microscopical examination, a large number of *Toxoplasma gondii* tachyzoites in the periphery of the necrosis. A second pattern is widespread nodular microgliosis with encysted bradyzoites without evidence of necrosis or inflammation. Fungal infections are mainly caused by *Cryptococcus neoformans*, *Candida* species, and *Aspergillus*.

Different types of opportunistic viral infections are localized in the brain causing white matter damage, demyelination, as well as fulminant encephalitis. Infection with polyomavirus (JC-virus or SV 40)

leads to the so-called 'progressive multifocal leukoencephalopathy' (PML), characterized by multiple confluent areas of demyelination in both hemispheres, the cerebellum and the brainstem. Viral inclusion bodies are detected both in cells of oligodendroglial and astrocytic origin.

CMV causes both a diffuse encephalitis and microglial noduli. The CMV inclusion bodies are predominantly located in the ependyma and subependymal regions and in a small number of the microglial nodules. In a few patients, a concomitant infection with *Herpes simplex* virus type I is reported. Both viral infections appear to be systemic and are found in multiple extracerebral localizations at autopsy. Destruction of retinal cells owing to CMV causes 'cotton wool' spots in the retina.

Non-Hodgkin lymphomas (Figure 5.4) are frequently located primarily within the CNS in HIV-seropositive individuals, whereas it is a rare condition in the normal population. These intermediate and high-grade B-cell lymphomas show a predominantly perivascular arrangement in small nodules. Metastatic lymphomas are characterized by diffuse leptomeningeal infiltration.

In liquor samples, some of the intracerebral abnormalities associated with the HIV-infection can be established. The primary HIV-infection in the cerebral cortex results in an increased number of lymphocytes and plasma cells.

The secondary intracerebral non-Hodgkin lymphomas with preferential spread in leptomeningeal space are detected early in liquor samples. On the contrary, primary non-Hodgkin lymphomas are detected only in the terminal phase of the disease.

Opportunistic infections with bacteria, fungi, and protozoa are almost always associated with an increased amount of inflammatory cells in the cerebrospinal fluid, mainly neutrophils and monocytes.

The opportunistic microorganisms, such as *Cryptococcus neoformans*, *Mycobacterium*, *Candida*, or *Toxoplasma*, can be demonstrated with special staining procedures. Apart from increased cellularity of the liquor, viral opportunistic infections sometimes show characteristic intranuclear inclusion bodies.

References

1   Barnes PF, Bloch AB, Davidson PT, Sinder DE Jr. Tuberculosis in patients with human immunodeficiency virus infection. *N Engl J Med* 1991; **324**: 1644–1650.

2   Centers for Disease Control. Classification system for human T-lymphocytotropic virus type III/lymphadenopathy-associated virus infections. *MWWR* 1986; **35**: 334–339.

3   Klatt EC. *Practical AIDS Pathology*. Chicago: ASCP Press, 1992.

4   Radin DR, Baker EL, Klatt EC et al. Visceral and nodal calcification in patients with AIDS-related *Pneumocystis carinii* infection. *AJR* 1990; **154**: 27–31.

5   Klatt EC. Diagnostic findings in patients with acquired immune deficiency syndrome. *J Acquir Immune Defic Syndr* 1989; **5**: 459–465.

6   Tschirhart DL, Klatt EC. Disseminated toxoplasmosis in the acquired immunodeficiency syndrome. *Arch Pathol Lab Med* 1988; **112**: 1237–1241.

7   Biggar RJ, Rabkin CS. The epidemiology of acquired immunodeficiency syndrome-related lymphomas. *Curr Opin Oncol* 1992; **4**: 883–893.

8   Levine AM. Epidemiology, clinical characteristics, and management of AIDS-related lymphoma. *Hematol Oncol Clin North Am* 1991; **5**: 331–342.

9   Levine AM. AIDS-associated malignant lymphoma. *Med Clin North Am* 1992; **76**: 253–268.

10 Ames ED, Conjalka MS, Goldberg AF et al. Hodgkin's disease and AIDS. *Hematol Oncol Clin North Am* 1991; **5**: 343–356.

11 Gold JE, Altarac D, Ree HJ, Kahn A, Sordillo PP, Zalusky R. HIV-associated Hodgkin disease: a clinical study of 18 cases and review. *Am J Hematol* 1991; **39**: 93–99.

12 Palca J. Kaposi's sarcoma gives on key fronts. *Science* 1992; **225**: 1352–1355.

13 Tappero JW, Conant MA, Wolfe SF, Berger TG. Kaposi's sarcoma. Epidemiology, pathogenesis, histology, clinical spectrum, staging criteria and therapy. *J Am Acad Dermatol* 1993; **72**: 245–261.

14 Haverkos HW, Freidman-Kien AE, Drotman DP, Morgan WM. The changing incidence of Kaposi's sarcoma among patients with AIDS. *J Am Acad Dermatol* 1990; **22**: 1250–1253.

15 Roth WK, Brandstetter H, Sturzl M. Cellular and molecular features of HIV-associated Kaposi's sarcoma. *AIDS* 1992; **6**: 895–913.

16 Ensoli B, Barillari G, Gallo RC. Pathogenesis of AIDS-associated Kaposi's sarcoma. *Hematol Oncol Clin North Am* 1991; **5**: 281–295.

17 McKenna RJ, Campbell A, McMurtrey MJ et al. Diagnosis of interstitial lung disease in patients with acquired immunodeficiency syndrome (AIDS): A prospective comparison of bronchial washing, alveolar lavage, transbronchial lung biopsy and open-lung biopsy. *Ann Thorac Surg* 1986; **41**: 318–321.

18 Gal AA, Klatt EC, Koss MN et al. The effectiveness of bronchoscopy in the diagnosis of *Pneumocystis carinii* and *Cytomegalovirus* pulmonary infections in acquired immunodeficiency syndrome. *Arch Pathol Lab Med* 1987; **111**: 238–241.

19 Cohen IS, Anderson DW, Virmani R et al. Congestive cardiomyopathy in association with the acquired immunodeficiency syndrome. *N Engl J Med* 1986; **315**: 628–630.

20 Grody WW, Cheng L, Lewis W. Infection of the heart by the human immunodeficiency virus. *Am J Cardiol* 1990; **66**: 203–206.

21 Cappell MS. Hepatobiliary manifestations of the acquired immune deficiency syndrome. *Am J Gastroenterol* 1991; **86**: 1–15.

22 Caccamo D, Pervez NK, Marchevsky A. Primary lymphoma of the liver in the acquired immunodeficiency syndrome. *Arch Pathol Lab Med* 1986; **110**: 553–555.

23 Öst A, Baroni CD, Biberfeld P et al. Lymphadenopathy in HIV-infection: histological classification and staging. *Acta Pathol Microbiol Immunol Scand Suppl* 1989; **8**: 7–15.

24 Hinnant K, Schwartz A, Rotterdam H et al. Cytomegalovirus and cryptosporidial cholecystitis in two patients with AIDS. *Am Surg Pathol* 1989; **107**: 133–137.

25 Sun NCJ, Shapshak P, Lachant NA et al. Bone marrow examination in patients with AIDS and AIDS-related complex. *Am J Clin Pathol* 1989; **92**: 589–594.

26 Budka H. Human immunodeficiency virus (HIV)-induced disease of the central nervous system: pathology and implications for pathogenesis. *Acta Neuropathol* 1989; **77**: 225–236.

Further reading

Reik RA, Rodriguez MM, Hensley GT. Infections in children with human immunodeficiency virus/acquired immunodeficiency syndrome: an autopsy of 30 cases in south Florida. *Pediats Pathol Lab Med* 1995; **15 (2)**: 269–81.

Schwartz RA. Kaposi's sarcoma: advances and perspectives. *J. Am. Acad. Dermatol.* 1996; **34 (5 Pt 1)**: 804–14.

Chang AD, Drachenberg CI, James SP. Bacillary angiomatosis associated with extensive esophageal polyposis: a new muco-cutaneous manifestation of acquired immunodeficiency disease (AIDS).

Yachnis AT, Berg J, Martinez-Salazar A et al. Disseminated microsporidiosis especially infecting the brain, heart, and kidneys. Report of a newly recognized pansporoblastic species in two symptomatic AIDS patients. *Am J Clin Pathol* 1996; **106 (4)**: 535–43.

Lanjewar DN, Anand BS, Genta R et al. Major differences in the spectrum of gastrointestinal infections associated with AIDS in India versus the west: an autopsy study. *Clin Infect Dis* 1996 **23 (3)**: 482–5.

Nosari A, Cantoni S, Oreste P et al. Anaplastic large cell (CD30/Ki-1+) lymphoma in HIV+ patients: clinical and pathological findings in a group of ten patients. *Br J Haematol* 1996; **95 (3)**: 508–12.

Camilleri-Broet S, Davi F, Feuillard J et al. AIDS-related primary brain lymphomas: histopathologic and immunohistochemical study of 51 cases. The French Study Group for HIV-Associated Tumors. *Hum Pathol* 1997 **28 (3)**: 367–74.

CYTOPATHOLOGY IN AIDS

Norman H. Chan

Introduction

The application of routine cytology and fine-needle aspiration (FNA) cytology has enjoyed a tremendous gain in popularity in the diagnosis and management of AIDS-related diseases [1,2]. Good results in FNA cytology require cooperation between the interventional radiologists and the cytologists. Both routine and FNA cytology are rapid and safe diagnostic procedures. In concert with radiology, FNA biopsy of virtually any deep-seated organs can be achieved, allowing diagnoses which would otherwise require operating room time and hospitalization (Table 6.1). A rapid, accurate diagnosis of opportunistic infection or malignancy can be made as outpatient procedures at the doctor's office or at the radiology suite, often within the same day of the biopsy procedure.

In the clinical setting of AIDS, where catastrophic events can occur quickly, the ability to perform an unscheduled FNA biopsy quickly without requiring operating room time is a clear advantage over a conventional biopsy procedure. Cytology also allows for safe, repeated sampling of a particular organ. In fact, repeat open biopsy has become impractical in certain recurrent infections, such as *Pneumocystis carinii* pneumonia (PCP), where cytological diagnosis has virtually replaced open biopsy [3,4]. The disease seen in AIDS is almost always accompanied by florid pathologic changes, facilitating cytological diagnoses. This chapter will discuss the AIDS-related diseases commonly requiring cytological diagnosis.

Localization and aspiration

Localization and fine-needle aspiration biopsy (FNAB) of a mass lesion can be achieved by palpation when the lesion is superficial. This is a commonly used technique for the aspiration of enlarged subcutaneous lymph nodes. This procedure can be easily performed in the office when a patient presents with an enlarging mass. FNAB of deep-seated organs requires imaging guidance. Depending on the site of the target lesions, fluoroscopy, computed tomography (CT) or ultrasound (US) are radiological techniques commonly used to locate and confirm the placement of the biopsy needle tip in a target lesion.

Interdisciplinary team

A well-trained interdisciplinary team is necessary to ensure the proper handling of specimens. A cytotechnologist should always be present at the time of aspiration. This ensures the optimal preparation of fresh specimens, avoidance of artefacts caused by preparation delay and for the proper division of the specimens to ensure accurate diagnosis. After aspiration, the biopsy needle and syringe are passed directly from the radiologist to the cytotechnologist for the preparation of smears, which are stained and examined immediately. At this point, the proper handling of the aspirate is pivotal, as the amount of aspirate is small and in the clinical setting of AIDS, the diagnostic possibilities are multiple. Guided by the quick stains, the subsequent aspirates are triaged into the proper diagnostic channels; for example, bacterial or tuberculosis (TB) culture when the quick stain appears inflammatory, for flow cytometry in cases where the smear is composed of suspected lymphoma cells, or to obtain adequate material for cell block. Failure to channel the aspirate properly may seriously affect the sensitivity and the outcome of the FNAB. Precautions must be taken by the cytotechnologist in handling the specimens of HIV-infected patients. Universal precautions [5,6]. should be adopted when handling bloody specimens or body fluids. The essentials should include gloving or when indicated double gloving, masks, and

Table 6.1.   Common target organs in the HIV-infected requiring imaging guidance.

Location	Mode of imaging for biopsy	Pathology	Comments
Thorax	Fluoroscopy or CT	Mass lesions, such as lymphoma or fungal infections	*P. carinii* infections are usually diagnosed by lung lavage (BAL) from bronchoscopy
Liver	Ultrasound	Lymphoma, fungal infections or abscess drainage, MAC infection	A common site for lymphoma
Retroperitoneal lymph node	Ultrasound, CT	Malignant lymphoma, MAC infection	Differential diagnosis of lymphoma vs MAC infection
Brain	CT (stereotactic biopsy)	Lymphoma, abscess, toxoplasmosis	Differential diagnosis of lymphoma v. toxoplasmosis

protective eye wear, and water-resistant gowns or aprons when attending a FNA procedure. Extreme care should be taken when handling needles and sharp instruments in order to avoid contact between skin and mucous membrane with contaminated specimens. Preparation of the specimens should be performed under the protection of a laminar flow hood, especially when centrifugation of a particular sample is required. Equipment must be cleaned and sterilized before reuse.

Cytology equipment and methods of preparation

No expensive equipment is necessary to perform FNA. The basic components include syringe holders, disposable plastic syringes, fine-gauge needles (varying lengths), glass slides, stains, and a microscope for interpretation. For the biopsy of cutaneous masses, we prefer the use of a Cameco syringe holder (Cameco, Burbank, CA, USA). This device allows for aspiration by a single hand, thus freeing the second hand of the aspirator for palpation and guidance. The calibre of the fine needle used varies from 18 to 25 gauge and the length varies from 1 to 20 cm. Longer fine needles are flexible and require a needle guide or stylet to increase the stiffness. The stylet also allows for the expulsion of clotted specimens within the fine needle for the preparation of a cell block. The selec-

tion of the length of the fine needle will depend on the depth of the target. A variety of biological stains are successfully employed. In general, Europeans favor the use of air-dried smears stained by the Romanowsky stains, such as the May–Grünwald Giemsa or the Diff Quik stain (Baxter Scientific Products, Mcgaw Park, IL, USA), used commonly by hematopathologists for the interpretation of bone marrow aspirates. This is the preferred stain for the interpretation of lymphoproliferative disorders. North Americans prefer the use of either hematoxylin and eosin (H&E) or the Papanicolaou (PAP) stain on fixed smears. We recommend the use of modified Clarke's solution (87.5% absolute alcohol, 12.5% glacial acetic acid) over 95% alcohol as a fixative because glacial acetic acid serves as an agent for the lysis of red blood cells, giving a clearer background in bloody aspirates. If possible, both fixed and air-dried smears should be made. Air-dried smears can be reserved for a Gram stain for bacteria, Giemsa stain for a malignant lymphoma, or a Kinyuon stain (Difco Lab., Detroit, MI, USA) for acid-fast organisms. Bronchial washing and lavage specimens can be prepared by cytospin (Cytospin II, Shandon Instruments, Sewickley, PA, USA) or by the Millipore filter (Millipore Corp., Bedford, MA, USA) and stained by the PAP stain. Although, any of the commonly used biological stains are adequate for interpretation, the final results depend ultimately on the familiarity and experience with the specific stains used by the interpreters [7].

Immunochemistry and molecular diagnostics

Immunochemistry refers to the localization and identification of an *in situ* cellular component determined by its antigenic properties by using fluorescent monoclonal antibodies. The target component could be a tumor marker, a cell-surface protein, or antigens relating to a specific infectious agent. These targets are identified by using a target-specific tagged antiserum, with the eventual formation of an antigen–antibody complex. Finally, the localization of this specific complex is achieved by precipitating a color reaction involving the tagged antisera so it can be visualized. Currently, this is achieved by using antibodies tagged with horseradish peroxidase, followed by the addition of hydrogen peroxide and a chromogen, resulting in color precipitation at the site of a specific antigen–antibody reaction that can be seen with an ordinary light microscope. The two most commonly used techniques of localization today are the peroxidase–antiperoxidase and the avidin–biotin methods. Readers are referred to specialized texts for further technical details [8,9]. The advantage of immunochemistry is the increase in specificity, as an antigen–antibody reaction is more specific than a chemical reaction, the guiding principle behind histochemistry.

In situ hybridization refers to the *in situ* detection and identification of a specific nucleic acid sequence, through the use of a tagged complimentary DNA/RNA sequence (DNA/RNA probe) and its subsequent hybridization with the host nucleic acid (target). In the denaturing step, after addition of a specific probe, denaturation of the host DNA is allowed to occur by raising the temperature of the environment of the substrate, causing the host's double-stranded DNA to dissociate. By lowering the temperature in the hybridization step, the tagged probe and the complimentary DNA sequence in the host genome are allowed to anneal. Factors affecting the hybridization step include the temperature of the reaction, the pH, and the degree of base-pair mismatch between the probe and the target. After hybridization is complete between the target genome and the probe tagged with horseradish peroxidase, the addition of hydrogen peroxide and a chromogen results in a color reaction that can be seen under a light microscope. This technique is highly specific and allows for the recognition and localization of a specific segment of DNA in the host genome [10]. Both immunochemistry and *in situ* hybridization can easily be applied to appropriately fixed paraffin-embedded tissue, smears, cytocentrifuge slides (cytospins) and cell blocks processed for routine diagnostic purposes.

Lastly, commercial kits of numerous antisera and DNA probes are readily available, opening the door for these two techniques to be adapted for everyday use in histology and cytology. For the purpose of this chapter, applications pertaining to the diagnosis of infectious organisms will be discussed. Commercially available monoclonal antibodies are available for localization of HIV antigens by immunohistochemistry, such as the HIV viral protein p17 or p24 (Chemicon International Inc., Temecula, CA, USA). Radiolabeled DNA probes (Du Pont Diagnostic Imaging Division, North Billerica, MA) are also available for the detection of the HIV viral genome for research purposes. Commercially available monoclonal antibodies are successfully used in the detection of cytomegalovirus (CMV), the herpes virus (HSV), the Epstein Barr virus (EBV), the human papilloma virus (HPV), *Pneumocystis carinii* and the protozoan *Toxoplasma gondii*. The employment of DNA probes (Gen-probe Inc., San Diego, CA, USA) to identify and distinguish between the mycobacterial species is a major advance in the field of microbiology, by providing rapid colony identification which was formerly not possible. *In situ* hybridization is theoretically the most sensitive method to detect viral infections; practically, in many viral infections, such as CMV, HSV, and HPV infections, both hybridization and immunochemistry are equally effective.

Clinical applications

A list of AIDS-associated diseases commonly encountered in a cytology laboratory will be discussed. This is by no means an exhaustive list, but rather represents an overview of these conditions and the role played by cytology in their diagnosis.

Pneumocystis carinii

No discussion of opportunistic infection in AIDS is complete without the mention of *Pneumocystis carinii* pneumonia, as this disease constitutes the most important opportunistic infection in AIDS. The first reports occurred during World War II in central Europe in epidemic forms, involving debilitated and malnourished children. A second wave of PCP reemerged in tandem with the AIDS epidemic [11–13]. It is the most common opportunistic infection in AIDS, caused by a unicellular organism that defies classification. PCP is also a well-recognized form of opportunistic infection in immunosuppressed hosts, such as leukemic patients following chemotherapy or transplant recipients. This organism has not been grown successfully in culture, thus morphological identification remains the only means of diagnosis. Cytological diagnosis has virtually replaced open lung or transbronchial biopsy in the diagnosis of PCP [3,4]. Diagnosis is usually achieved by interpreting bronchial brushing, washing and bronchoalveolar lavage (BAL) specimens obtained via fiberoptic bronchoscopy. A combination of brushings, washings, and BAL has been used successfully in our institution for the diagnosis of PCP for the last 10 years. Although known mainly as a pulmonary infection, the incidence of extrapulmonary pneumocystis infection is apparently on the rise with the prophylactic use of aerosolized pentamindine [14].

Morphology

In the lungs, *P. carinii* (PC) proliferates in three stages: cysts, sporozoites, and trophozoites. The cysts are oval or round, cup- or crescent-shaped structures measuring 5–10 mm. Owing to its size and the ease of identification of the cyst capsule by special stains (Grocott's methenamine silver, toluidine blue), this is the easiest structure of PC to identify. PC cysts can contain up to eight internal sporozoites (intracystic bodies) measuring 1–2 mm, seen best with the Giemsa stain. They are formed by internal division within the larger cyst. The sporozoites mature within the mother cyst and following its rupture, mature sporozoites are released into airspaces as trophozoites (thin-walled cysts) where they mature into mother cysts, completing the reproductive cycle. In the BAL specimens, PC alveolar casts have a typical appearance using PAP or H&E stains, [4,15] and appear as acellular, granular, or foamy casts (Figure 6.1). In scanty specimens, such as induced sputum or BAL of patients who have had previous aerosolized pentamidine prophylaxis, the use of monoclonal antibodies [16] may be necessary in order to increase the diagnostic yield.

Specimens

1. Bronchoalveolar lavage (BAL).
2. Induction and collection of sputum.

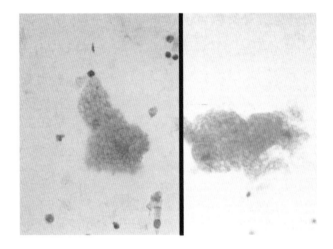

Figure 6.1. Foamy, alveolar casts of *P. carinii* (PAP stain)

3. FNA biopsy of mass lesion for extrapulmonary disease.

Cytological methods and comments

1. Smears, Millipore filters (Millipore Corp., Bedford, MA, USA) or cytospin preparations (Shandon Instruments, Sewickley, PA, USA) made from bronchial wash, brush or BAL specimens.
2. Standard and special stains including:
   - Papanicolaou stain (PAP)
   - Grocott's methenamine silver (GMS), Giemsa or toluidine blue stain [17,18].
   - Autofluorescence [19,20].
3. Immunoperoxidase stains (Dako Corp., Carpinteria, Cal, USA) used in induced sputum specimens.
4. *P. carinii* has not been successfully cultured and no serological tests are yet available for diagnosis.

Bronchoscopy and BAL

Through a bronchoscope wedged into a lobar or segmental bronchus, normal saline (20–100 ml) is instilled into the corresponding airways, and later reaspirated and sent for culture and cytology. Specimens can also be obtained by using a disposable brush. Bronchial washing and BAL specimens have all shown excellent results, with sensitivity ranging from a low of 59% for bronchial washing [21] to 90% for both washing and BAL specimens [22].

Sputum induction

Some authors have reported success in the detection of PCP by the induction of sputum rather than by bronchoscopy [23]. Following induction by nebulizing a 3–5% saline mist through an ultrasonic nebulizer, the collected sputum is processed by staining with either a Giemsa or GMS stain. Sensitivity is reported in the range of 50–60% [23,24]. However, this technique has a limited role in the management of patients on aerosolized prophylactic agents for PCP where only a small number of organisms can be identified.

Mycobacteria group

Mycobacterium tuberculosis and *Mycobacterium avium complex* (MAC) are the significant mycobacterial infections which cause morbidity and mortality in AIDS. Although *M. tuberculosis* and MAC appear morphologically similar, their distinction is clinically important as different drug regimens are used for their treatment. Infections caused by *M. tuberculosis* usually show a good response to drug therapy whereas MAC infections do not [25]. The incidence of *M. tuberculosis* is high in particular subgroups of the HIV-infected population, frequently involving Haitians, [26]. Africans as well as inner-city Black Americans [27] and intravenous drug abusers (IVDA) [28]. The disease profile of *M. tuberculosis* is different in the HIV-positive population. The lack of significant pulmonary pathology with atypical presentation is common, such as disseminated or extrapulmonary disease involving lymph nodes and bone marrow [26,28].

MAC are ubiquitous saprophytes existing in soil and water. They can frequently be isolated from multiple body sites in asymptomatic subjects and do not cause disease in the immunocompetent population. Prior to the AIDS epidemic, disease caused by MAC was almost unheard of. In AIDS, MAC infection is invariably disseminated at the time of diagnosis, usually with positive blood culture, bone marrow, and lymph node involvement, and no evidence of pulmonary disease. Gastrointestinal involvement can lead to a chronic malabsorption syndrome, with a morphological pattern of small bowel involvement mimicking Whipple's disease.

To the practising cytologist, FNA aspirates of enlarged regional lymph nodes infected by either organism are common. Although differences in disease pattern exist between *M. tuberculosis* and MAC, such as a large numbers of organisms and the lack of a granulomatous response in MAC infection, [29] the definitive diagnosis is made by the isolation and culture of the organisms. Since both *M. tuberculosis* and MAC are both slow-growing organisms, identification of the species takes from 3–8 weeks, causing delay in treatment. Recent advances in molecular biology, with the introduction of commercially available DNA probes (Gen-Probe Inc.) capable of distinguishing between these two species, have been successfully introduced and have drastically decreased the time requirement for the identification of these species.

Morphology

There are differences in the pattern of tissue response between MAC and *M. tuberculosis*. A granulomatous pattern is seen in *M. tuberculosis* and the number of organisms identified are far less, usually requiring a careful search under the oil immersion lens before any acid-fast organisms are identified. Macrophages congested with intracytoplasmic mycobacteria, the so-called 'pseudogaucher' cells [30] are seen in aspirates of MAC. The organisms can be visualized by a multitude of stains listed below, as well as seen as negative images in the Diff Quik stain [31–33]. Occasionally, a spindle cell proliferative pattern simulating a sarcoma, is encountered in MAC-infected tissue [34]. These organisms are best described as acid-fast, short to filamentous, beaded bacillary forms, found lying freely in the background, within a granuloma or inside the cytoplasm of a macrophage/histiocyte.

Specimens

1. FNA specimen of lymph nodes and other mass lesions.
2. Bone marrow biopsy and aspiration.
3. Bronchoscopy specimens.
4. Endoscopic biopsies.

Cytological methods and comments

1. Smears, cytospins and cell blocks made from specimens listed above
2. Special stains:
   (a) Ziehl–Neelsen (ZN).
   (b) Kinyuon stain (Difco Lab., Detroit, MI, USA).
   (c) Rhodamine-Auramine stain (fluorescent microscopy).
   (d) Commercially available DNA probes (Gene-probe Inc.).
   (e) Non-specific staining with periodic acid–Schiff (PAS) and GMS stains in instances of MAC infections.
3. The atypical mycobacteria group (MAC) can be visualized with the Diff Quik and other stains as negative images, but not *M. tuberculosis*.

4. Culture of the aspirate is essential. DNA probes of culture can shorten the time requirement to differentiate between species.

Fungal infections

General comments

Patients with AIDS are at risk of developing fungal infections, which require intact T-cell function for containment. At presentation, fungal infections tend to be disseminated. Deep mycoses presenting as mass lesions can be successfully diagnosed by FNA [35,36]. Histologically, a large number of organisms are usually seen within the cytoplasm of macrophages and accompanied by a poor granulomatous response. The cytology of these fungal infections corresponds with the histological picture, usually a large number of free organisms are identifiable in an inflammatory background, or within the cytoplasm of macrophages and histiocytes. The organisms vary from 2 mm to up to 100 mm and can easily be identified by special stains. After the morphological identification of any fungal infection, culture confirmation of the diagnosis is essential. The important fungal infections will be discussed individually.

Cryptococcosis

Cryptococcus neoformans is a ubiquitous fungus found in the dropping of pigeons and other birds, and in the soil contaminated by their droppings. In the USA, this fungus accounts for up to 10% of opportunistic infections in patients with AIDS and 50% of these patients have disseminated disease. The lung is the portal of entry when organisms are inhaled via contaminated airborne particles into the respiratory tract. Meningeal involvement is common in disseminated disease [37]. Other common sites of involvement include the peritoneal cavity and the skin [38,39]. Cryptococcosis is frequently diagnosed by cytology in cerebral spinal fluid (CSF), [40]. FNA specimens of the lung and lymph nodes, and in skin biopsies.

Morphology

Cryptococcus neoformans is a budding fungus measuring from 3 to 50 mm, with variable morphology. This organism is characterized by a thick, gelatinous capsule. The capsule stains positively with the PAS, mucicarmine and the GMS stains. The distinct carminophilia of the thick capsule is a diagnostic feature of

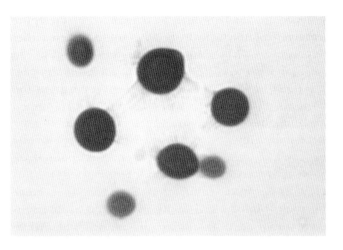

Figure 6.2.   Teardrop-shaped yeasts of varying sizes, typical for *C. neoformans* (Mucicarmine stain)

Cryptococcus (Figure 6.2). Smaller capsular-deficient forms have been described in the AIDS population [41]. In the cytology specimens, *Cryptococcus* is often seen to exhibit budding with a narrow base, where the daughter yeasts are attached by a thin, tapered isthmus. Both the budding and the capsule-deficient forms can be well-visualized by the PAP stain.

Specimens

1. Lumbar puncture.
2. FNA of a mass lesion, often a regional lymph node or a lung mass.
3. Punch biopsy of skin.

Cytological methods

1. Smears, cytospin preparations or Millipore filters, usually from either a bronchoscopy specimen CSF, or from FNA of lymph node or a lung mass
2. Standard and special stains including:
    *   PAP stain
    *   PAS, GMS, or mucicarmine stain
    *   India ink preparation (CSF)
3. A portion of the cytology specimen should be reserved for culture.
4. DNA probes or tissue immunohistochemistry not available for diagnosis (special stains are considered the gold standard).

Candidiasis

Candida species are commonly encountered in cytology specimens. Of these, *Candida albicans* is most frequently associated with human infections. Candidiasis is seldom disseminated or fatal, and tends to be localized to the mouth (oral thrush), and the upper aerodigestive tract, such as the oropharynx and the esophagus. *Candida* esophagitis commonly occurs in AIDS and is included as one of the indicator disease of AIDS [12,42]. Cytology plays a major role in the diagnosis of candidiasis. A combination of biopsy, brushing and washing cytology, as well as culture are successfully employed in endoscopy specimens for the diagnosis of candidiasis. Its presence in pulmonary cytology material is difficult to interpret, and in most instances is clinically insignificant, representing contamination from the oral cavity. Disseminated disease is uncommon but does occur in AIDS, and, when present, is usually associated with the use of intravenous catheters, broad-spectrum antibiotics, and neutropenia [43].

Morphology

In tissue sections, *Candida* exists in two forms, yeast and pseudohyphae, and causes an inflammatory reaction in the background. The yeasts (blastospores) are of uniform size, encapsulated, and measure from 2 to 4 mm in diameter and appear rounded or oval. They elongate into pseudohyphae and appear as slender, filamentous structures without septation and with budding at points of constriction. *Candida* is well-visualized by H&E stains, but the organisms may vary in staining intensity from case to case and may be missed entirely. The capsules are highlighted by the usual fungal stains such as the GMS, PAS, and even the tissue Gram stain.

Specimens

1. Endoscopy specimens consisting of scrapings and smears obtained from the upper aerodigestive tract.
2. *Candida* is frequently a contaminant of bronchoscopy specimen.

Cytological methods

1. Staining and interpretation of smears and scrapings by PAP, PAS, and GMS stains.
2. Tissue immunohistochemistry or DNA probes not necessary for diagnosis.
3. A portion of the aspirate should be reserved for culture.

Histoplasmosis

Histoplasma capsulatum is a pathogenic dimorphic yeast found in temperate regions throughout the world. This disease is rare in Europe and occurs in endemic areas

in North America, some Caribbean islands, and in Africa. In North America, histoplasmosis is prevalent along the Ohio–Mississippi and the St Lawrence River region. In endemic regions of the USA, a positive skin test to *Histoplasma* is found in up to 80% of the population, whereas it is as low as 1% in Europe [44]. Like Cryptococcosis, this fungus is concentrated in pigeon and bat droppings, and soils enriched by their droppings. Infection takes place via the pulmonary route with inhalation of contaminated particles into the lung. Mini-epidemics have been reported surrounding construction sites and following soil excavation [45,46]. In immunocompetent hosts, the primary pulmonary infection is usually asymptomatic. In HIV-infected patients, disseminated disease is common. Both disease reactivation and progression of newly acquired disease are thought to occur. This disease is diagnosed using cytology by recognizing either free organisms in the extracellular space, or by identifying infected macrophages or histiocytes packed with many organisms they cannot kill or eliminate [47]. Histoplasmosis can also be diagnosed by the morphology of infected monocytes on peripheral blood smears [48]. Confirmation by culture of BAL, bone marrow, blood, or lung tissue is necessary.

Morphology

H. capsulatum is a dimorphic fungus with a mycelial and yeast phase. In tissue, *H. capsulatum* exists as yeast forms, appearing round to oval in shape, measuring from 2 to 5 mm in diameter and reproduces by budding. In soil, its natural habitat, it occurs in the mycelial form. In tissue sections, stained by H&E, they appear as tightly packed, rounded structures surrounded by a clear zone, distending the cytoplasm of macrophages or phagocytes. The clear zone superficially resembles the thick capsule of *Cryptococcus*, but is actually an artefact of fixation owing to retraction of cytoplasm from the cell wall. The differential diagnosis of histoplasmosis includes the cysts of toxoplasma and the yeasts of *Cryptococcus*. Any standard fungal stains will stain the cell wall of histoplasma, distinguishing it from *Toxoplasma*. Lastly, the characteristic thick carminophilic capsule of *Cryptococcus* is a contrasting feature from the thin, rigid cell wall of *Histoplasma*.

Specimens

1. FNA specimens of mass lesions.
2. Any cytology specimens containing macrophage/

monocytes, such as sputum or peripheral blood smears.

Cytology methods

1. Staining and interpretation of smears or cytospin preparation by PAP, PAS, Giemsa, or GMS stains.
2. Tissue immunohistochemistry or DNA probe not necessary.
3. Culture and isolation recommended.

Other fungal infections

As a cause of opportunistic infection in AIDS, coccidiomycosis [49] is seen in endemic regions, such as the south-west of the USA. The role of *Aspergillus* in AIDS has not been clearly defined in AIDS [50] and disseminated aspergillosis remains a very rare event in AIDS when compared to other mycoses.

Parasitic infections

Toxoplasma gondii

Toxoplasmosis is caused by an obligate intracellular parasite *Toxoplasma gondii*. This infection has a world-wide distribution, with a high prevalence in warm and humid temperate regions of the world. The life cycle of this parasite is well understood, [51] involving intermediate hosts where asexual reproduction (cysts) occurs and definitive hosts where sexual reproduction (oocytes) takes place. Many species of mammals and birds as well as humans serve as the intermediate host. Domestic cats and a range of wild cats are the definitive hosts of this parasite; thus, the prevalence of this disease is high in regions where domestic or wild cat numbers are numerous, and where moist climate and soil conditions favor the survival of oocytes. In humans, infection occurs with the ingestion of raw or undercooked infected meat, or through the oral–fecal route via soil contaminated by cat feces containing toxoplasma cysts or oocysts. Ingestion of oocysts is followed by the digestion of the cyst capsule in the host's gastrointestinal (GI) tract, liberating organisms which then invade the epithelial cells of the GI tract, followed by blood-borne dissemination. Blood-borne transplacental congenital infections are observed in humans. Lymphadenopathy is a common finding in symptomatic disease of the immunocompetent host.

In the HIV-infected population, central nervous system involvement is common and clinically the most important. Pulmonary infection, although relatively common and reported in up to 36% of cases in one series, [52] is rarely diagnosed before death. Reasons for this low diagnostic rate include the lack of dramatic pulmonary symptoms, the overshadowing symptoms of the central nervous system (CNS) disease and the paucity of organisms in the infected lung tissue. The premortem diagnosis of this disease is usually achieved by identifying toxoplasma cysts in brain tissue [52,53] either by open biopsy or by stereotactically directed FNA specimens. Lymph node biopsy is usually the diagnostic procedure performed in the healthy, where a characteristic pattern of lymph-node-reactive hyperplasia is described.

Morphology

The morphological appearance of *T. gondii* is different in smears from that in tissue sections. Three morphological forms exist: tachyzoites, bradyzoites, and oocysts. The tachyzoites are encountered in acute infections where rapid multiplication of the organisms occur. On smears they measure from 3 to 7 mm in length, 2 to 4 mm in width, and are tear-drop- or crescent-shaped. On tissue sections, they form groups or aggregates within membrane-bound cytoplasmic vacuoles, and appear rounded or oval. They are best seen with the Giemsa–Wright stain. The bradyzoites are encountered in chronic infections. They are slow growing, rounded and are packed tightly into cysts. The cysts are bound by a PAS-positive membrane measuring from 30 to 100 mm and contain numerous bradyzoites. They are readily identified in H&E tissue sections or in smears. Oocysts contain up to eight sporozoites and are found only in the feces of the definitive hosts. Commercially available monoclonal antibodies have been used successfully to identify *T. gondii* in brain tissue and with less success in lung tissue [52].

Specimens

1. Open biopsy of enlarged regional lymph node (symptomatic infection in the immunocompetent hosts).
2. FNA or tissue biopsy of an intracranial mass.
3. Rarely, cysts can be recognized in other cytology specimens, such as BAL.

Histological and cytological method

1. Smears and tissue biopsy from the CNS.
2. Standard and special stains including: Giemsa, H&E, PAP, PAS, and GMS stains.

3. Localization of organisms by monoclonal antibodies with immunoperoxidase stain (Dako Corp., Carpenteria, CA, USA).
4. *T. gondii* cannot be cultured, morphological identification is crucial.

Other parasitic infections

Other protozoans, [54] including cryptosporidium, [55–57] microsporidium, [58] *Isospora belli*, [57] and amoeba cause disease in the AIDS population. An amoebic abscess in the liver is readily diagnosable by cytology but is a relatively rare disease. The helminth *Ascaris lumbricoides* causes disease in the AIDS population as well as the immunosuppressed; the hyperacute infection caused by *A. lumbricoides* can be easily diagnosed in sputum specimens [59]. Cytology plays no significant role in the diagnosis of the remaining protozoan infections.

Viruses

Virtually any form of viral infection can occur in patients with AIDS. Excluding the HIV, the majority fall into two groups of DNA viruses: herpes group (including *Herpes simplex*, *Varicella–zoster*, CMV, and EBV) and the papovaviruses. Of these, CMV is the most commonly encountered. CMV may be present without causing symptoms in up to 90% of AIDS patients [60]. Asymptomatic infections may involve the respiratory, gastrointestinal, and urinary system; most of these infections do not require active treatment. Thus, the clinical significance of a positive result of CMV is often difficult to assess in the HIV-infected patient. A positive result, by either immunohistochemistry or by *in situ* hybridization, does not readily distinguish between chronic smoldering infection and aggressive CMV disease. The interpretation of any positive results must be taken in conjunction with the clinical picture [61]. HSV causes localized or disseminated mucocutaneous disease and is a rare but well-recognized infection of the lower respiratory tract. The EBV is implicated in the pathogenesis of lymphocytic interstitial pneumonia, malignant lymphoma and oral leukoplakia. The HPV (JC virus) is the causative agent of progressive multifocal leukoencephalopathy, a degenerating white matter disease, and is implicated in anal intraepithelial neoplasia and squamous cell carcinoma of the anal regions in AIDS. CMV and herpes infections are readily diagnosable in cytology specimens by the morphological identification of viral inclusions. Diagnostic yield may be increased with the aid of either immunochemistry or *in situ* hybridization.

Morphology

Viral infections are diagnosed in cytological specimens by the identification of viral inclusions; these changes are well described in the DNA viruses. Viral inclusions due to the CMV and the herpes viruses are described. Cells with CMV inclusions are large, up to 3–4 times the size of uninfected cells. They contain eosinophilic intranuclear inclusions of up to half the diameter of the nucleus, surrounded by prominent, clear halos, with margination of nuclear material along the inner surface of the nuclear membrane (Figure 6.3). Multinucleation is less common than in herpetic infection. Multiple small basophilic cytoplasmic granules representing cytoplasmic inclusions may be seen in CMV. These are not seen in herpes infections. Herpetic inclusions are characterized by multinucleation of the nuclei with molding, opaque (ground-glass) nuclei and no cytoplasmic inclusions. Late lesions have smaller, eosinophilic intranuclear inclusions surrounded by a distinct halo. In general, herpes inclusions are seen in squamous cells, and CMV inclusions are seen in glandular epithelium and endothelial cells. Diagnosis of HPV inclusion is also possible by cytology.

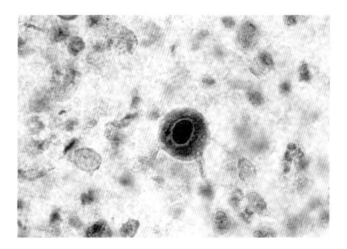

Figure 6.3. Typical intranuclear inclusion of CMV, with "owl's eye" appearance

Specimens

1. Sputum (herpes).
2. Bronchial brush and wash specimens and BAL (herpes and CMV).
3. Smears from skin, oral mucosa, and esophagus (herpes), remaining GI tract (CMV).
4. Tissue biopsies from skin, oral mucosa, esophagus and upper airways (herpes), remaining GI tract (CMV).

Cytologic methods for both herpes and CMV inclusions

1. Smears, Millipore filters, or cytospins preparations stains by PAP, H&E, or Giemsa stains.
3. Commercially available monoclonal antibodies for immunochemistry (both).
4. Commercially available kits for *in situ* hybridization (both).

Progressive generalized lymphadenopathy and lymphoma

Lymphadenopathy is a common finding in HIV-positive patients. The syndrome of persistent generalized lymphadenopathy (PGL), defined as lymphadenopathy involving two or more non-contiguous extrainguinal sites of greater than 3 months duration, [62] is considered by many as an early manifestation of HIV infection. This syndrome is often accompanied by constitutional symptoms, such as fever, malaise, headache, and weight loss. PGL involves a dynamic process, starting with follicular hyperplasia of the germinal centers, and evolving to a final stage characterized by involution of the germinal centers or follicular lysis. Immunohistochemical studies of lymph nodes show changes of T-lymphocytes parallel to that seen in the peripheral blood, with a simultaneous reversal of the T-helper/suppressor ratio, and a polyclonal stimulation of B-lymphocytes. It is in this background that evolution from PGL to frank malignant lymphoma may occur, the great majority of which are high-grade B-cell lymphomas [63]. The definition of AIDS has been expanded to include the occurrence of an intermediate or a high-grade lymphoma of B-cell lineage [64]. At the same time, these patients suffer a progressive impairment of cell-mediated immunity and are also at risk of developing infections requiring intact cell-mediated immunity. Faced with an HIV-positive patient with lymphadenopathy, the differential diagnoses are myriad and can only be clarified by tissue evaluation. Multiple authors have reported success in assessing superficial [2] as well as abdominal lymph nodes [65] by FNA in this clinical setting. Finally, the proper handling of the FNA specimen is crucial and can influence the diagnostic yield, as multiple etiologies must be taken into account when interpreting the aspirate of an enlarged regional lymph node (see cytology preparation below).

Morphology

The diagnosis of PGL is made on negative findings, principally the absence of a malignant lymphoma or an infectious agent. The typical FNA smear pattern consists of a pleomorphic population of lymphocytes, plasma cells, and tingible-body macrophages in a clean background, without the presence of granulomata or necrosis. A necrotic background in an FNA smear should always raise the possibility of either a necrotic malignant lymphoma or an infectious agent such as tuberculosis. The majority of the lymphomas are high-grade lymphomas of either small noncleave cell (Burkitt's-like lymphomas), immunoblastic lymphomas (Figure 6.4), or other unclassified high-grade lymphomas.

Specimen

FNA of any regional lymph nodes, depending on the location of these lymph nodes. These specimens are obtained with or without the help of ultrasound guidance.

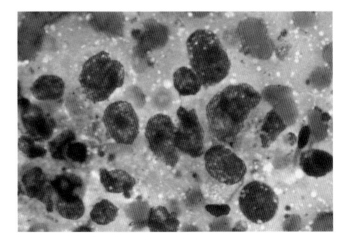

Figure 6.4. Monomorphic, large lymphoma cells with prominent nucleoli, characteristic of immunoblastic lymphoma (Giemsa-Wright stain)

Cytology preparation

1. Initial rapid cytologic assessment of FNA specimen is important.
2. Smears stained by H&E, Diff Quik, ZN (Zeehl-Nielsen) or Giemsa should be interpreted quickly,
3. FNA specimen processing should be guided by the smear appearance. If inflammatory, Gram and ZN stain followed by submitting portion of the specimen for the appropriate culture (bacterial or mycobacterial, fungal). If lymphocytes appear atypical, consider submitting a sample for flow cytometry for cell surface marker analysis.

Kaposi's sarcoma

Described by Moriz Kaposi in 1872, Kaposi's sarcoma (KS) existed in two distinct forms before the AIDS epidemic [66]. The European form afflicts elderly men of Mediterranean extraction, particularly the Italians and the Ashkenazy Jews. This form is an uncommon, indolent cutaneous neoplasm with a predilection of the skin of the lower extremities. The African form involves mostly African male children, and is an aggressive sarcoma where visceral and nodal disease is common and mortality is high.

In the beginning of the AIDS epidemic in 1981, reports of an aggressive form of KS began to surface in young, previously healthy, gay Caucasian males in the USA [11,67]. Since then, KS has been included as one of the indicator diseases of AIDS [42]. This epidemic form of KS occurs in HIV-positive patients in both Africa and the Western world, with a higher incidence in the homosexual population where CMV infection is high. The incidence of AIDS-associated KS has been in the decline since the beginning of the epidemic [68].

Clinically, five different patterns are recognized: early, nodular, aggressive cutaneous, lymphadenopathic, and systemic generalized KS. These clinical patterns include the classical, indolent cutaneous disease seen in the elderly male of Mediterranean extraction to the aggressive, disseminated disease seen in young homosexual men. The clinical picture of African KS spans the entire spectrum. The histological patterns include early, angiomatous, spindle cell, inflammatory, mixed, and pleomorphic variants. Since KS is a highly vascular tumor, cutting biopsies can lead to life-threatening hemorrhage [69]. FNA cytology usually plays no role in the diagnosis of KS, as these aspirates are usually scanty and bloody, owing to the vascular and spindle nature of KS. Occasionally, the diagnosis of KS may be suggested when a percutaneous biopsy of an intraabdominal nodule reveals a spindle cell neoplasm with slit-like vascular spaces.

Conclusion

By providing rapid and accurate diagnoses, cytology plays a significant role in AIDS-related diseases. Cooperation and communication between the radiology and cytology departments, together with the expertise of the radiology and cytology staff will ensure excellent results.

References

1 Bottles K, McPhaul LW, Volberding P. Fine-needle aspiration biopsy of patients with acquired immunodeficiency syndrome (AIDS): experience in an outpatient clinic. *Ann Intern Med* 1988; **108**: 42–45.

2 Suvarna SK, Glazer G, Coleman DV. Use of fine needle aspiration cytology for investigating lymphadenopathy in HIV positive patients. *J Clin Path* 1993; **46**: 564–556.

3 Rorat E, Garcia RL, Skolom J. Diagnosis of *Pneumocystis carinii* pneumonia by cytologic examination of bronchial washings. *JAMA* 1985; **254**: 1950–1951.

4 Stanley MW, Henry MJ, Iber C. Foamy alveolar casts: diagnostic specificity for *Pneumocystis carinii* pneumonia in bronchoalveolar lavage fluid cytology. *Diagnost Cytopathol* 1988; **4**: 113–115, 112.

5 Centre for Disease Control. Recommendations for prevention of HIV transmission in health care settings. *MMWR* 1987; **36** (Suppl. 2): 1S–18S.

6 Gerberding JL, Sande MA. Exposures to HIV in patients and laboratory specimens. In: Cohen PT, Sande MA, Voberding PA (eds) *AIDS Knowledge-base*. Waltham, MA: Medical Publishing Group, 1990: 1–2.

7 Suen KC. *Atlas and Text of Aspiration Biopsy Cytology*. Baltimore, MA: Williams & Wilkins, 1990.

8 Bourne JA. *Handbook of Immunoperoxidase Staining Methods*. Santa Barbara: Dako Corp, 1983.

9 Sternberger LA. *Immunochemistry*, 2nd edn. New York: John Wiley and Sons, 1979.

10 Davis L, Kuehl M, Battey J. *Basic Methods in Moecular Biology*,

2nd edn. Norwalk, CT: Appleton and Lange, 1994.

11 Friedman-Kien AE, Laubstein LJ, Marmor M et al. KS and *PCP* among homosexual men – New York city and California. *MMWR* 1981; **30**: 305–307.

12 Gottlieb MS, Schroff R, Schanker HM et al. *Pneumocystis carinii* pneumonia and mucosal candidiasis in previously healthy homosexual men: evidence of a new acquired cellular immunodeficiency. *N Engl J Med* 1981; **305**: 1425–1431.

13 Masur H, Michelis MA, Greene JB et al. An outbreak of community-acquired *Pneumocystis carinii* pneumonia: initial manifestation of cellular immune dysfunction. *N Engl J Med* 1981 **305**: 1431–1438.

14 Raviglione MC. Extrapulmonary pneumocystosis: the first 50 cases. *Rev Infect Dis* 1990; **12**: 1127–1138.

15 Greaves TS, Strigle SM. The recognition of *Pneumocystis carinii* in routine Papanicolaou-stained smears. *Acta Cytol* 1985; **29**: 714–720.

16 Kovacs JA, Ng VL, Masur H et al. Diagnosis of *Pneumocystis carinii* pneumonia: improved detection in sputum with use of monoclonal antibodies. *N Engl J Med* 1988; **318**: 589–593.

17 Chandra P, Delaney MD, Tuazon CU. Role of special stains in the diagnosis of *Pneumocystis carinii* infection from bronchial washing specimens in patients with the acquired immune deficiency syndrome. *Acta Cytol* 1988; **32**: 105–118.

18 Paradis IL, Ross C, Dekker A, Dauber J. A comparison of modified methenamine silver and toluidine blue stains for the detection of *Pneumocystis carinii* in bronchoalveolar lavage specimens from immunosuppressed patients. *Acta Cytol* 1990; **34**: 511–556.

19 Markowitz S, Leiman G. Cytologic detection of *Pneumocystis carinii* by ultraviolet light examination of Papanicolaou-stained sputum specimens [letter]. *Acta Cytol* 1986; **30**: 79–80.

20 Pfitzer P, Wehle K, Blanke M, Burrig KF. Fluorescence microscopy of Papanicolaou-stained bronchoalveolar lavage specimens in the diagnosis of *Pneumocystis carinii*. *Acta Cytol* 1989; **33**: 557–559.

21 Mones JM, Saldana MJ, Oldham SA. Diagnosis of *Pneumocystis carinii* pneumonia. Roentgenographic pathologic correlates based on fiberoptic bronchoscopy specimens from patients with AIDS. *Chest* 1986; **89**: 522–526.

22 Ognibene FP, Shelhamer J, Gill V et al. The diagnosis of *Pneumocystis carinii* pneumonia in patients with AIDS using subsegmental bronchoalveolar lavage. *Am Rev Respir Dis* 1984; **129**: 929–932.

23 Bigby TD, Margolskee D, Curtis JL et al. The usefulness of induced sputum in the diagnosis of *Pneumocystis carinii* pneumonia in patients with AIDS. *Am Rev Respir Dis* 1986; **133**: 515–518.

24 Pitchenik AE, Ganjei P, Torres A, Evans DA, Rubin E, Baier H. Sputum examination for the diagnosis of *Pneumocystis carinii* pneumonia in the acquired immunodeficiency syndrome. *Am Rev Respir Dis* 1986; **133**: 226–229.

25 Hawkins CC, Gold JW, Whimbey E et al. *Mycobacterium avium* complex infections in patients with the acquired immuno-deficiency syndrome. *Ann Intern Med* 1986; **105**: 184–188.

26 Pitchenik AE, Cole C, Russell BW, Fischl MA, Spira TJ, Snider DE Jr. Tuberculosis, atypical mycobacteriosis, and the acquired immunodeficiency syndrome among Haitian and non-Haitian patients in south Florida. *Ann Intern Med* 1984; **101**: 641–665.

27 Rieder HL, Cauthen GM, Bloch AB et al. Tuberculosis and acquired immunodeficiency syndrome – Florida. *Arch Intern Med* 1989; **149**: 1268–1273.

28 Sunderam G, McDonald RJ, Maniatis T, Oleske J, Kapila R, Reichman LB. Tuberculosis as a manifestation of the acquired immunodeficiency syndrome (AIDS). *JAMA* 1986; **256**: 362–366.

29 Klatt EC, Jensen DF, Meyer PR. Pathology of *Mycobacterium avium-intracellulare* infection in acquired immunodeficiency syndrome. *Hum Pathol* 1987; **18**: 709–714.

30 Solis OG, Belmonte AH, Ramaswamy G, Tchertkoff V. Pseudogaucher cells in *Mycobacterium avium intracellulare* infections in acquired immune deficiency syndrome (AIDS). *Am J Clin Pathol* 1986; **85**: 233–235.

31 Maygarden SJ, Flanders EL. Mycobacteria can be seen as 'negative images' in cytology smears from patients with acquired immunodeficiency syndrome. *Modern Pathol* 1989; **2**: 239–243.

32 Stanley MW, Horwitz CA, Burton LG, Weisser JA. Negative images of bacilli and mycobacterial infection: a study of fine-needle aspiration smears from lymph nodes in patients with AIDS. *Diagnost Cytopathol* 1990; **6**: 118–121.

33 Ang GA, Janda WM, Novak RM, Gerardo L. Negative images of mycobacteria in aspiration biopsy smears from the lymph node of a patient with acquired immunodeficiency syndrome (AIDS): report of a case and a review of the literature. *Diagnost Cytopathol* 1993; **9**: 325–328.

34 Chen KT. Mycobacterial spindle cell pseudotumor of lymph nodes. *Am J Surg Pathol* 1992; **16**: 276–281.

35 Kaw YT, Brunnemer C. Initial diagnosis of disseminated cryptococcosis and acquired immunodeficiency syndrome by fine needle aspiration of the thyroid. A case report. *Acta Cytol* 1994; **38**: 427–430.

36 Molina JM, Oksenhendler E, Daniel MT, Clauvel JP. Fine-needle aspiration and *Cryptococcosis* in the acquired immunodeficiency syndrome (AIDS). *Ann Intern Med* 1988; **108**: 772.

37 Kovacs JA, Kovacs AA, Polis M et al. *Cryptococcosis* in the acquired immunodeficiency syndrome. *Ann Intern Med* 1985; **103**: 533–558.

38 Borton LK, Wintroub BU. Disseminated *Cryptococcosis* pre-senting as herpetiform lesions in a homosexual man with acquired immunodeficiency syndrome. *J Am Acad Dermatol* 1984; **10**: 387–390.

39 Rico MJ, Penneys NS. Cutaneous *Cryptococcosis* resembling *molluscum contagiosum* in a patient with AIDS. *Arch Dermatol* 1985; **121**: 901–902.

40 Katz RL, Alappattu C, Glass JP, Bruner JM. Cerebrospinal fluid manifestations of the neurologic complications of human immunodeficiency virus infection. *Acta Cytol* 1989; **33**: 233–244.

41 Bottone EJ, Toma M, Johansson BE, Wormser GP. Capsule-deficient *Cryptococcus neoformans* in AIDS patients. *Lancet* 1985; **1**: 400.

42 Centres for Disease Control. Revision of the CDC surveil-lance case definition for the acquired immunodeficiency syndrome. *MMWR* 1987; **36**: 1S–15S.

43 Janoff EN, Smith PD. Perspectives on gastrointestinal infections in AIDS. *Gastroenterol Clinics North Am* 1988; **17**: 451–463.

44 Sotgiu G, Mantanovi A, Massoni A. Histoplasmosis in Europe. *Mycopathologia* 1970; **40**: 53–74.

45 Huang CT, McGarry T, Cooper S, Saunders R, Andavolu R. Disseminated histoplasmosis in the acquired immunodeficiency syndrome. Report of five cases from a nonendemic area. *Arch Intern Med* 1987; **147**: 1181–1184.

46 Wheat LJ, Connolly-Stringfield PA, Baker RL et al. Disseminated histoplasmosis in the acquired immune deficiency syndrome: clinical findings, diagnosis and treatment, and review of the literature. *Medicine* 1990; **69**: 361–74.

47 Blumenfeld W, Gan GL. Diagnosis of histoplasmosis in bronchoalveolar lavage fluid by intracytoplasmic localization of silver-positive yeast. *Acta Cytol* 1991; **35**: 710–712.

48 Henochowicz S, Sahovic E, Pistole M, Rodrigues M, Macher A. Histoplasmosis diagnosed on peripheral blood smear from a patient with AIDS. *JAMA* 1985; **253**: 3148.

49 Fish DG, Ampel NM, Galgiani JN et al. Coccidioidomycosis during human immunodeficiency virus infection. A review of 77 patients. *Medicine* 1990; **69**: 384–391.

50 Klapholz A, Salomon N, Perlman DC, Talavera W. Aspergillosis in the acquired immunodeficiency syndrome. *Chest* 1991; **100**: 1614–1618.

51 Binford CH, Connor DH. *Pathology of Tropical and Extraordinary Disease*, Vol. 1. Washington, D.C.: Armed Forces Institute of Pathology, 1976: 284–300.

52 Tschirhart D, Klatt EC. Disseminated toxoplasmosis in the acquired immunodeficiency syndrome. *Arch Pathol Lab Med* 1988; **112**: 1237–1241.

53 Wanke C, Tuazon CU, Kovacs A et al. Toxoplasma encephalitis in patients with acquired immune deficiency syndrome: diagnosis and response to therapy. *Am J Trop Med Hygiene* 1987; **36**: 509–516.

54 Canning EU. Protozoan infections [review]. *Trans Roy Soc Trop Med Hygiene* 1990; **84**: 19–24.

55 Casemore DP, Sands RL, Curry A. Cryptosporidium species a 'new' human pathogen. *J Clin Path* 1985; **38**: 1321–1326.

56 Crawford FG, Vermund SH. Human cryptosporidiosis. *Crit Rev Microbiol* 1988; **16**: 113–159.

57 Soave R. Cryptosporidiosis and isosporiasis in patients with AIDS. *Infect Dis Clinics North Am* 1988; **2**: 485–493.

58 Desportes I, Le Charpentier Y, Galian A et al. Occurrence of a new microsporidan: *Enterocytozoon bieneusi*, in the enterocytes of a human patient with AIDS. *J Protozool* 1985; **32**: 250–254.

59 Vieyra-Herrera G, Becerril-Carmona G, Padua-Gabriel A, Jessurun J, Alonso-de Ruiz P. *Strongyloides stercoralis* hyperinfection in a patient with the acquired immune deficiency syndrome. *Acta Cytol* 1988; **32**: 277–28.

60 Mintz L, Drew WL, Mines RC et al. Cytomegalovirus infections in homosexual men: an epidemiologic study. *Ann Intern Med* 1983; **99**: 326–329.

61 Murray JF, Mills J. Pulmonary infectious complications of human immunodeficiency virus infection. *Am Rev Resp Dis* 1990; **141**: 1356172.

62 Meyer PR, Yanagihara ET, Parker JW, Lukes RJ. A distinctive follicular hyperplasia in the acquired immune deficiency syndrome (AIDS) and the AIDS related complex. A pre-lymphomatous state for B cell lymphomas? *Hematol Oncol* 1984; **2**: 319–347.

63 Raphael MM, Audouin J, Lamine M et al. Immunophenotypic and genotypic analysis of acquired immunodeficiency syndrome-related non-Hodgkin's lymphomas. Correlation with histologic features in 36 cases. French study group of pathology for HIV-associated tumors. *Am J Clin Pathol* 1994; **101**: 773–782.

64 Centres for Disease Control. Revision of the CDC surveillance case definition for the acquired immunodeficiency syndrome. *MMWR* 1987; **36**: 1S–15S.

65 Townsend RR, Laing FC, Jeffrey RB Jr, Bottles K. Abdominal lymphoma in AIDS: evaluation with US. *Radiology* 1989; **171**: 719–724.

66 Friedman-Kien AE, Saltzman BR. Clinical manifestations of classical, endemic African, and epidemic AIDS-associated Kaposi's sarcoma. *J Am Acad Dermatol* 1990; **22**: 1237–150.

67 Friedman-Kien AE, Laubenstein LJ, Rubinstein P et al. Disseminated Kaposi's sarcoma in homosexual men. *Ann Intern Med* 1982; **96**: 693–700.

68 Haverkos HW, Friedman-Kien AE, Drotman DP, Morgan WM. The changing incidence of Kaposi's sarcoma among patients with AIDS. *J Am Acad Dermatol* 1990; B22: 1250–1253.

69 Gottesman D, Dyrszka H, Albarran J, Hilfer J. AIDS-related hepatic Kaposi's sarcoma: massive bleeding following liver biopsy. *Am J Gastroenterol* 1993; **88**: 762–774.

7 RISK OF HIV TRANSMISSION: IMPLICATIONS FOR HEALTH CARE WORKERS

John R. Mathieson
Eric van Sonnenberg

Introduction

The emergence of the acquired immune deficiency syndrome (AIDS) has been a most unusual event in medical history. As we have begun to learn about this mysterious disease, we have found that many basic principles in medicine have been challenged. The impact of AIDS has included a fundamental reappraisal of methods of disease transmission, and the type of risks posed not only to health care professionals, but also to the public seeking medical care.

In the early days of the epidemic, we did not know what the causative agent was, how it was transmitted, or how to test for the presence of AIDS. Understandably, this stage of ignorance often led to confusion amongst the health care professions [1–3]. AIDS patients were regarded with a wide variety of attitudes and prejudices, ranging from a cavalier approach, to a state of excessive fear and even hysteria. The latter state of mind prevailed in many institutions early in the epidemic, including a university-affiliated hospital in the same city as one of the authors (JM). In this case, the hospital administrators publicly refused to allow AIDS patients into their building, fearing transmission of AIDS to their employees. However, since the early 1980s, a great deal has been learned about AIDS, its detection, transmission, and prevention. In this chapter, we will discuss these topics as well as practical safety measures that can be taken so that AIDS patients can be offered the same high standards of compassionate medical care as anyone else, without undue risk to health care workers (HCWs). We will also briefly discuss the issues surrounding the human immune deficiency virus (HIV)-positive HCW, and subsequent risks to the general public.

Risk of infection

When a HCW comes in contact with body fluid from an HIV-positive patient, the risk of acquiring the infection depends upon two factors: the type of body fluid, and the nature of the contact [4]. Table 7.1 lists the body fluids considered infectious and non-infectious, according to the Centre for Disease Control in Atlanta. In general, the risk of infection parallels the amount of virus present in the fluid. It is now known that body fluids from HIV-positive patients are much less infectious than was feared during the early years of the epidemic. Blood is the most infectious fluid, and even when a needle contaminated with HIV-infected blood accidentally punctures the skin of an HIV-negative person, the risk of being infected with HIV is surprisingly low – approximately 0.1 to 0.4% [5–11]. This is probably due to the relatively low number of virus particles in HIV-positive patients' blood, compared to other diseases, such as hepatitis B [12,13]. Despite this surprisingly low risk, the tragic fact is that there were at least 32 well-documented cases of HCWs acquiring HIV infection through occupational exposure in the first decade of the epidemic [14,15]. Further, it is highly likely that this figure underestimates the actual number of such cases [16]. Since infection of HIV is generally considered a universally fatal infection, every possible precaution must be taken to avoid such accidents [9,6,17].

It is also possible, both theoretically and based on case experience, to acquire HIV infection without an actual skin puncture. At least four HCWs have become HIV-positive after mucocutaneous exposure to HIV-positive infected blood [14]. HIV can be transmitted from other body fluids from a mucous membrane or

Table 7.1. Body fluids and risk of HIV transmission.

Infectious
Blood
Semen
Vaginal and cervical secretions
Wound and tissue fluid
Cerebrospinal fluid
Amniotic fluid
Pleural fluid
Pericardial fluid
Peritoneal fluid
Nasal secretions
Synovial fluid

Non-infectious (unless visibly blood-stained)
Urine
Feces
Saliva
Sputum
Vomit
Sweat
Tears

open wounds. Although the risk of such transmission is very low, the additional prognosis of HIV infection makes even a very remote risk unacceptably high [18–20]. It is prudent to recommend strict adherence to the principles of Universal Precautions. Even though certain fluids (Table 7.1) [21] are not felt to pose a significant risk unless visibly blood stained, we find it easiest to treat *all* body fluids (with the exception of sweat and tears) as potentially dangerous.

Universal precautions

Early efforts at protecting HCWs from AIDS centered in part on identifying carriers of the disease, so that appropriate protective measures could then be taken by anyone coming in contact with these known AIDS patients. However, this approach has proven futile, for several reasons. The natural history of HIV infection is such that there are significant periods of time in which an infected individual will be negative to serum testing. Further, many HIV-positive individuals have not been tested, and many are unaware of being at risk for HIV [22]. Even when HIV-positive patients are aggressively investigated, there is no clear risk factor identified in a substantial proportion of patients, perhaps as many as 10%. Also, it is impossible to iden-

tify potential AIDS patients by their outward physical appearance or behavior [22]. Finally, many AIDS patients require treatment on an urgent basis, which may not even allow for an adequate history to be taken, let alone allowing time for obtaining results of serologic testing [8].

Therefore, most public health recommendations adopt some system of Universal Precautions, in which blood and other body fluids from all patients are regarded as potentially hazardous. The fact that hepatitis B is also very common in AIDS patients, and is also much more likely to be accidentally transmitted, has served as a useful further motivation to adopt Universal Precautions [23]. It should be added that while we and others advocate treating all body fluids of every patient as potentially hazardous, there is no doubt that we are even more cautious when we do know we are dealing with an AIDS patient.

Radiology and AIDS

The nature of protective measures required depends upon the nature of the interaction between the patient and the HCW. For example, for casual contact such as routine radiography, ultrasound scanning, or non-contrast computed tomography (CT) and magnetic resonance imaging (MRI), no special precautions are required. For contacts involving intravenous puncture, gloves should be worn, and exquisite care must be taken to the handling of the sharp objects. Needles should never be recapped by hand. All sharp objects should be disposed of immediately after use, using safe point-of-use containers. For radiologists who do not perform interventional procedures, the risk of exposure to HIV is mainly confined to venepuncture for contrast injection. However, radiologists are increasingly asked to perform other more invasive procedures on AIDS patients, and constant vigilance is required to avoid accidental exposure [24,25].

Interventional radiology and AIDS

Percutaneous fine-needle aspiration biopsy

Imaging-guided biopsies are the commonest potential source of accidental infection in most hospital radiology practices, apart from venepuncture. All facets of fine-needle aspiration biopsy (FNAB) procedures must be designed to minimize this possibility. Gloves must be worn routinely. Obviously, gloves help prevent cutaneous contact with body fluids. Also, it has been shown that gloves decrease the volume of blood transferred during accidental needle punctures. 'Double gloving' and changing gloves at intervals during a procedure has been recommended for lengthy procedures in bloody fields. Masks and eye protection should also be worn when there is risk of fluids contacting the face. Masks with attached transparent face shields are available, and we have found these quite convenient to use, as they do not impair vision. The use of impermeable gowns, hats and boots should be considered when appropriate.

Bedside 'sharp' disposal containers should be available in every room where biopsies are performed, and must be kept easily accessible to the radiologist. In practice, we find this is the commonest source of procedural errors, as 'sharps' containers are often stored in inconvenient locations, and may have objects piled on top of then, such as papers and charts. Also, standard size sharps disposal containers may be too small for the longer needles and stylets used in radiology departments. Containers must be taller than the longest sharp object used, and must be emptied regularly. Syringes and needles used for local anesthesia should be disposed of immediately after use. Needles must never be recapped by hand, as this is the commonest cause of accidental puncture injuries. If it is necessary to replace a cap on a needle, it must be done without holding the cap by hand. When sharp objects must be reused, such as in angiographic or other interventional procedures, a system of safe storage must be adopted. One example of such a system is that previously described by one of the authors (EVS). A film cannister is modified with perforations on its top, sized to fit a variety of needles and other sharp objects. Once any sharp object is removed from the patient's body it is immediately inserted into the container, sharp end downwards, and left there until it is needed again. In this way, there are no exposed sharp objects on the equipment tray. Whatever system is used, it must be clearly understood by all personnel and followed without exception.

Although room lighting is kept deliberately low, especially for ultrasound-guided biopsies, there must be sufficient light to see the needle tip and skin puncture marks from local anesthesia. Gauze should always be available to stop any bleeding from the puncture site. Also, gloves and other protective equipment should be available to be worn by any of the attending personnel in the room who may be asked to assist in the procedure. Gloves should be disposed of, and not washed for a second use. It has been shown that 'wicking' may occur with wet gloves, with fluids being drawn through very small holes by capillary action. Also, the act of washing gloves is likely to create holes in them.

When biopsies are done for quick stain cytology, the radiologist will pass the needle and syringe containing the biopsy specimen to the cytopathology technologist for immediate plating on slides. It is while the needle is being passed from one person to another that another substantial risk of accidental puncture occurs. Communication between the radiologist and the cytopathology technologist must be clear and explicit, and the needle should be passed with the sharp tip pointing away from the person receiving it. Another solution is to avoid passing the needle from one person to another altogether, by the person performing the biopsy placing the needle and syringe on a table top, and the technologist then picking up the needle from the table. In one of the authors (JM) hospitals, over 10 000 imaging-guided biopsies have been performed since the beginning of the AIDS epidemic, and to our knowledge, only one accidental puncture with a contaminated needle has occurred. In this instance, the radiologist was punctured with the biopsy needle while attempting to pass the needle to the technologist. Although, fortunately, the individual involved remains well and HIV-negative, this accident emphasizes the importance of rigid adherence to Universal Precautions and safe methods of handling contaminated sharp objects.

Another possible source of accidental contamination occurs when the cytopathology technologist expresses the biopsy specimen from the needle and syringe on to the microscope slides. Sometimes, a plug of material will temporarily occlude the lumen of the needle, and as the plug is dislodged with increasing pressure on the syringe, some material may be sprayed into the air. All personnel in the room should be aware of this potential source of contact. Once the cytopathology technologist has finished plating the material on to the microscope slides, the technologist should directly dispose of the needle and syringes, without passing them to another person.

Consideration must be given to artificial resuscitation procedures, particularly when patients are given narcotic or sedative drugs. Mouth-to-mouth resuscitation is completely abandoned, and a variety of respiration devices with one-way valves should be made easily available throughout the department.

Angiography

Angiography is performed for a wide variety of indications in AIDS patients, and is particularly useful in the diagnosis and treatment of bleeding from the gastrointestinal (GI) tract. Angiography presents the greatest risk for having HIV-infected blood splashed or sprayed on HCWs, thereby coming in contact with mucous membranes or open wounds. There is an obvious risk of exposure during the act of arterial or venous puncture. Presently, many needle manufacturers are attempting to produce self-contained puncture systems to eliminate or minimize this risk. Additionally, every catheter and wire exchange maneuver presents an opportunity for inadvertent spraying of blood. The use of a sheath with a hemostatic valve helps reduce spraying and splashing of blood. When a needle is being removed over a guide wire, many angiographers are in the habit of wiping the guide wire with gauze that is held in the same hand that is being used to remove the needle. This practice increases the risk of accidental needle puncture, and should be avoided. The puncture needle should be held by its hub while it is being removed from the guide wire, and then the guide wire should be wiped with gauze in a separate motion. Care must be taken when removing a guide wire from a catheter so that the guide wire does not spring loose from the operator's hand and inadvertently uncoil, and brush against an exposed area on the HCW's body. Particular care must be taken with nitinol wires with hydrophilic coating, as these wires are not only extremely slippery, but can be very springy when coiled excessively. Glass syringes should not be used, owing to the risk of breakage and subsequent injury and contamination.

Other interventional procedures

The number of non-angiographic interventional procedures performed in AIDS patients continues to grow rapidly. We have performed all manners of interventional procedures on AIDS patients, including abscess draining, nephrostomy, biliary drainage, biliary stone removal, cholecystostomy, gastrostomy, gastrojejunostomy, and chest tube insertion. In many cases,

the indications are no different from those in non-AIDS patients. However, there are some special circumstances that apply to AIDS patients. AIDS patients frequently have an abnormal-appearing gallbladder on ultrasound or CT. When a gallbladder wall is thickened, or when pericholecystic fluid is found, the radiologist should personally perform a careful ultrasound examination to see whether these findings are associated with a sonographic Murphy's sign, indicating cholecystitis, either calculus or acalculous. Gallbladder wall thickening is usually *not* due to acute cholecystitis. However, if the gallbladder is tender as well as thick-walled, indicating acute cholecystitis, prompt performance of a percutaneous cholecystostomy can give a dramatic clinical response, and in the case of acalculous cholecystitis, is usually curative.

Pneumothorax is a complication of repetitive pulmonary infections in AIDS patients. We have found that imaging-guided chest tube insertion is very useful under these circumstances and often small (6–8 French) tubes are satisfactory. However, a collapsed lung often may not reexpand quickly in AIDS patients, owing to underlying chronic lung damage. Pleurodesis may be needed. We have also treated AIDS-related pneumothoraces on an outpatient basis, using a one-way Heimlich valve, rather than underwater suction. Patients being considered for outpatient treatment of pneumothoraces must be carefully selected, and must be thoroughly instructed as to how the valve works, as an improperly connected valve could prove disastrous.

We have not found abscesses to be particularly common in AIDS patients, but abscesses can occur in a wide variety of locations. Both typical and atypical tuberculous infections can cause abscesses, often in musculoskeletal sites including psoas, paraspinal, thigh muscles, and feet.

When a liver abscess is found, the primary site of origin in the GI tract must be sought. In particular, we have found infections arising from the colon, appendix, stomach, and distal ileum to cause liver abscesses.

Nutritional support methods bear special mention. AIDS patients are frequently malnourished and, although the reasons are not always straightforward, we have found that AIDS patients can benefit greatly from supplemental nutrition. The radiologist may become involved with transnasal or oral placement of feeding tubes into the stomach or duodenum. It may be very difficult for a clinician to place a transnasal tube into the duodenum or jejunum at the bedside. However, for a radiologist skilled at enteroclysis, this can be a very simple procedure, particularly with the aid of fluoroscopy. When longer term access for supplemental feeding is required, a fluoroscopically guided percutaneous gastrostomy or gastrojejunostomy is often the fastest, safest, and lest expensive method of achieving external GI tract access.

We have found that a gastrostomy alone is sufficient for feeding most AIDS patients, and we reserve gastrojejunostomies for those patients shown to have gastroesophageal reflux after a gastrostomy, or for patients with significant neurologic impairment. In most cases, we have found that gastrostomies can be removed after a few weeks or months, since after patients have gained weight and improved their nutritional status, and indeed their general condition, they can often eat well enough to do without supplemental feeding.

Accidental exposure to HIV

If a HCW suffers an accidental needle puncture or other exposure to possibly contaminated blood, certain first-aid precautions should be followed immediately:

1. Promote active bleeding from the site of puncture or contamination.
2. Wash the site with antiseptic solution, such as 10% povidone iodine.
3. Irrigate the site with normal saline for up to 15 minutes.

It should also be understood that there are no convincing experimental data to support the above recommendations. However, it is unlikely that this will ever be studied on a randomized, prospective basis, and most authors feel it is sensible to follow these rather elementary measures [26,27].

It has also been proposed that the HCW should then begin on a course of zidovudine (AZT). Although conclusive data are not yet available, some recent reports suggest that AZT is beneficial, and some institutions are beginning to recommend treatment with AZT immediately after exposure [28].

After first-aid measures have been taken, one must then assess the risk of HIV transmission through serologic testing. The source patient from whom the blood or other body fluid was originally obtained must be assessed for HIV infection. If the patient is found

or is known to have HIV infection, or if the patient declines serologic testing for HIV, the HCW should be assumed to have been exposed to HIV. Serologic testing of the HCW for HIV should be performed immediately after the exposure, and if seronegative, testing should be repeated at 6 weeks, and 3, 6, and 12 months after exposure. If the source patient is seronegative on repeated testing, testing of the HCW can cease. In most centers, testing for hepatitis B and C is done at the same time.

Tuberculosis and the health care worker

Until recently, most of the infectious diseases suffered by AIDS patients did not pose a substantial risk to HCWs with a normally functioning immune system. However, since 1990, multidrug-resistant *Mycobacterium* tuberculosis (MTb) has been found with increasing frequency in AIDS patients, and several cases of transmission to HCWs has been described [29–34]. Indeed, in an HIV dental clinic, transmission between two HCWs seems to have occurred, one of whom may have acquired the infection from a patient.

The risk of acquiring MTb from an infected person depends upon the number of organisms they expel into the air, which in turn depends upon the site of the disease within the patient, and the presence of cough, and of cavitary pulmonary disease. Castro et al. point out that AIDS patients with MTb are no more likely than non-AIDS patients with MTb to transmit the mycobacteria to either casual contacts or to HCWs [35]. However, since MTb is more common in AIDS patients, and because of the serious problem posed by the emergence of multidrug-resistant strains, HCWs caring for AIDS patients face a definite risk of acquiring mycobacterial infection. HCWs should be cognizant of these risks, and aware of the importance of identifying patients with tuberculosis as early as possible, so that appropriate protective measure can be instituted [36–38].

The HIV-positive health care worker

With the passage of time, the problem of the HIV-positive HCW has received increasing attention.

Difficult practical and ethical issues have been raised of balancing the rights of the HCW to privacy and security of employment, with the rights of the general public to safe medical care [39]. One highly publicized case of an HIV-positive dentist transmitting HIV to his patients has caused a great deal of alarm and confusion [40–42]. As worrisome and tragic as this case was, it appears to have exaggerated these risks, as the unfortunate patients were probably deliberately infected in this case. However, there have been other cases causing concern and it is difficult to know at the time how this problem should be handled [43].

Certainly, an HIV-positive HCW poses no risk to the patients in the majority of medical circumstances, unless there is a risk of his or her body fluids reaching the patient. Recently, this issue has gone beyond theory and conjecture. In one hospital in the USA, the hospital's administrators have forced a physician to withdraw from their surgical residency program after he was found to be HIV-positive, as a result of occupational exposure to the blood of an AIDS patient. He refused the hospital's offer of a position in another medical residency and appealed the court's decision, but the hospital's position was upheld by the appellate court [44]. The legal and ethical ramifications of this issue are only beginning to emerge.

In practical terms, these concerns do not apply to most of the procedures taking place in the radiology department. The possible exceptions would include procedures in which the operator's hands are most likely to be accidentally injured and subsequently come in contact with a patient, such as in procedures with the operator's hand in the patient's mouth such as sialography. However, further clarification of the limits that should be placed upon HIV-positive HCWs is needed.

References

1   Heilman RS. Doctors and AIDS: double standard and double jeopardy. *RadioGraphics* 1991; **11**: 382.

2   Shelley GA, Howard RJ. A national survey of surgeons' attitudes about patients with human immunodeficiency virus infections and acquired immunodeficiency syndrome. *Arch Surg* 1992; **127**: 206–212.

3   Bird AG, Gore SM, Leigh-Brown AJ et al. Escape from collective denial: HIV transmission during surgery. *Br Med J* 1991; **303**: 351–352.

4   Fauci AS. The human immunodeficiency virus: infectivity and mechanisms of pathogenesis. *Science* 1988; **239**: 617–622.

5   Lowenfels AB, Wormser GP, Jain R. Frequency of puncture injuries in surgeons and estimated risk of HIV infection. *Arch Surg* 1989; **124**: 1284–1286.

6   Marcus R, CDC Cooperative Needlestick Surveillance Group. Surveillance of health care workers exposed to blood from patients infected with the human immunodeficiency virus. *N Engl J Med* 1988; **319**: 1118–1123.

7   Wormser GP, Joline C, Sivak SL, Arlin ZA. Human immunodeficiency virus infections: considerations for health care workers. *Bull N York Acad Med* 1988; **64**: 203–215.

8   Hochreiter MC, Barton LL. Epidemiology of needlestick injury in emergency medical service personnel. *J Emerg Med* 1988; **318**: 86–90.

9   Henderson DK Fahey BJ, Willy M et al. Risk for occupational transmission of human immunodeficiency virus type 1 (HIV-1) associated with clinical exposures. A prospective evaluation. *Ann Intern Med* 1990; **113**: 740–746.

10 Quebbeman EJ, Telford GL, Hubbard S et al. Risk of blood contamination and injury to operating room personnel. *Ann Surg* 1991; **214**: 614–620.

11 Ippolito G, Petrosillo N, Puro V et al. The risk of occupational HIV infection in health care workers: the Italian multicenter study. *Ann Intern Med* 1993; **153**: 1451–1458.

12 Centers for Disease Control. Update: human immunodeficiency virus in health-care workers exposed to blood of infected patients. *MMWR* 1987; **36**: 285–289.

13 Gerberding JL, Bryant-LeBlanc CE, Nelson K et al. Risk of transmitting the human immunodeficiency virus, cytomegalovirus, and hepatitis B virus to health care workers exposed to patients with AIDS and AIDS-related conditions. *J Infect Dis* 1987; **1**: 1–7.

14 Anonymous. Surveillance for occupationally acquired HIV infection – United States, 1981–1992. *MMWR* 1992; **41**: 823–825.

15 Chamberland ME, Conley LJ, Bush TJ et al. Health care workers with AIDS. National surveillance update. *JAMA* 1991; **266**: 3459–3462.

16 Hamory BH. Underreporting of needlestick injuries in a university hospital. *Am J Infect Control* 1983; **11**: 174–177.

17 Gerberding JL. Current epidemiologic evidence and case reports of occupationally acquired HIV and other bloodborne diseases. *Infect Control Hosp Epidemiol* 1990; **11**: 558–560.

18 Gerberding JL, Littell, C, Tarkington A et al. Risk of exposure of surgical personnel to patients' blood during surgery at San Francisco general hospital. *N Engl J Med* 1990; **322**: 1788–1793.

19 Kelen GD, DiGiovanna T, Bisson L et al. Human immunodeficiency virus infection in emergency department patients. Epidemiology, clinical presentations, and risk to health care workers: the Johns Hopkins experience. *JAMA* 1989; **262**: 516–528.

20 Decker MD. The OSHA bloodborne hazard standard. *Infect Control Hosp Epidemiol* 1992; **13**: 407–417.

21 Centers for Disease Control. Update: universal precautions for prevention of transmission of human immunodeficiency virus, hepatitis B virus, and other bloodborne pathogens in health-care settings. *MMWR*, 1988; **37**: 377–382, 387–388.

22 Kelen GD, Fritz S, Qaqish B et al. Unrecognized human immunodeficiency virus infection in emergency department patients. *N Engl J Med* 1988; **318**: 1645–1650.

23 Hersey JC, Martin LS. Use of infection control guidelines by workers in healthcare facilities to prevent occupational transmission of HBV and HIV: results from a national survey. *Infect Control Hosp Epidemiol* 1994; **15**: 243–252.

24 Wall SD, Olcott EW, Gerberding JL. AIDS risk and risk reduction in the radiology department. *AJR* 1991; **157**: 911–916.

25 Williams DM, Marx V, Korobkin M. AIDS risk and risk reduction in the radiology department. *AJR* 1991; **157**: 919–921.

26 Fahey BJ, Beekmann SE, Schmitt J et al. Managing occupational exposures to HIV-1 in the healthcare workplace. *Infect Control Hosp Epidemiol* 1993; **14**: 405–412.

27 Henderson DK. Zeroing in on the appropriate management of occupational exposures to HIV-1. *Infect Control Hosp Epidemiol* 1990; **11**: 175–177.

28 Cardo DM, Srivastava PU, Ciesielski C et al. Case-control of HIV seroconversion in health care workers after percutaneous exposures to HIV-infected blood. *Infect Control Hosp Epidemiol* 1995; **16**: 536.

29 Dooley SW Jr, Castro KG, Hutton MD. Centers for Disease Control and Prevention. Guidelines for preventing the transmission of tuberculosis in health-care settings, with special focus on HIV-related issues. *MMWR* 1990; **391**: 1–29.

30 Centers for Disease Control and Prevention. Nosocomial transmission of multidrug-resistant tuberculosis among HIV-infected persons – Florida and New York, 1988–1991. *MMWR* 1991; **40**: 585–591.

31 Dooley SW, Villarino ME, Lawrence M et al. Nosocomial transmission of tuberculosis in a hospital unit for HIV-infected patients. *JAMA* 1991; **267**: 2632–2634.

32. Daley CL, Small PM, Schecter GE et al. An outbreak of tuberculosis with accelerated progression among persons infected with the human immunodeficiency virus. *N Engl J Med* 1992; **326**: 231–235.

33 Edlin BH, Tokars JI, Grisco MH et al. Nosocomial transmission of multidrug-resistant tuberculosis among hospitalized patients with the acquired immunodeficiency syndrome. *N Engl J Med* 1992; **362**: 1514–1521.

34 Fischl MA, Uttanchandani RB, Daikos GL et al. An outbreak of tuberculosis caused by multiple-drug-resistant tubercule bacilli among patients with HIV infection. *Ann Intern Med* 1992; **117**: 177–183.

35 Castro KG, Dooley SW. Mycobacterium tuberculosis transmission in healthcare settings: is it influenced by coinfection with human immunodeficiency virus? *Infect Control Hosp Epidemiol* 1993; **14**: 65–66.

36 Di Perri G, Cadeo GP, Castelli F et al. Transmission of HIV-associated tuberculosis to healthcare workers. *Infect Control Hosp Epidemiol* 1993; **14**: 67–72.

37 Cleveland JL, Kent J, Gooch BF et al. Multidrug-resistant mycobacterium tuberculosis in an HIV dental clinic. *Infect Control Hosp Epidemiol* 1995; **16**: 7–11.

38 Stroud LA, Tokars, JI, Grieco MH et al. Evaluation of infection control measures in preventing the nosocomial transmission of multidrug-resistant mycobacterium tuberculosis in a New York City hospital. *Infect Control Hosp Epidemiol* 1995; **16**: 141–147.

39 Henderson, DK. Position paper: the HIV-infected healthcare worker. The Association for Practitioners in Infection Control: the Society of Hospital Epidemiologists of America. *Infect Control Hosp Epidemiol* 1990; **11**: 647–656.

40 Anonymous. Update: investigations of persons treated by HIV-infected health-care workers – United States. *MMWR* 1993; **42**: 329–331, 337.

41 Ciesielski CA, Marianos D, Ou CY et al. Transmission of human immunodeficiency virus in a dental practice. *Ann Intern Med* 1992; **116**: 798–805.

42 Mishu B, Schaffner W. HIV transmission from surgeons and dentists to patients: can models predict the risk? *Infect Control Hosp Epidemiol* 1994; **15**: 114–146.

43 Schulman KA, McDonald RC, Lynn LA et al. Screening surgeons for HIV infection: assessment of a potential public health program. *Infect Control Hosp Epidemiol* 1994; **15**: 147–155.

44 Appeals court upholds hospital firing of HIV-positive physician. *Bull Infect Control Hosp Epidemiol* 1995; **16**: 492.

8 NUCLEAR MEDICINE IN AIDS

Eric A. van Royen

Introduction

The major advantage of nuclear medicine is its unique ability to detect functional and physiologic changes in disease that may precede the structural changes detectable by other imaging modalities. Nuclear medicine is an extreme versatile and flexible modality particularly because of the increasing number of radiolabeled chemical probes that are currently being developed.

This chapter focuses on the value of nuclear medicine as a diagnostic method to detect infections, secondary malignancies, and neurologic disease in acquired immune deficiency syndrome (AIDS). The important role of [67]Gallium scintigraphy in pulmonary disease and malignant lymphoma is stressed.

[67]Gallium citrate

[67]Gallium was originally introduced as a bone-seeking radiopharmaceutical. Chemically, it is a metal closely related to aluminum and iron, which is avidly bound by plasma transferrin after intravenous injection. The radionuclide [67]Gallium has a half-life of 78 hours and disintegrates while emitting three gamma quanta of 93, 185, and 300 keV each. Although physically less ideal than [99m]Technetium, it has relatively good properties for external imaging by a gamma camera fitted with a medium energy collimator.

Chemically, the radionuclide is administered as citrate or chloride, which is not critical for its target-seeking properties, since the gallium ion is bound to transferrin. The metallo–protein complex is retained in inflammatory tissue and many malignant tumors. The mechanism by which uptake and fixation of the tracer occur are not precisely understood. Usually it takes 24–48 hours before images can be made. Although the method has a high sensitivity, specificity is low because so many different pathologic conditions are [67]Gallium-positive.

[67]Gallium scintigraphy is the most important nuclear medicine procedure in the diagnosis of AIDS, since many manifestations of the disease are characterized by [67]Gallium uptake. The most common indication is the investigation of patients presenting with fever or other symptoms suggestive of infection. Since whole-body images are always obtained, it is especially helpful as a screening method. Imaging methods which rely on anatomical localization such as ultrasound, X-ray, computed tomography (CT), or magnetic resonance imaging (MRI) are better used when directed to a particular area of the body.

In a recent review of Wassie et al., the results of [67]Gallium scintigraphy in 37 human immune deficiency virus (HIV) antibody-positive patients were analyzed for the clinical usefulness of the test [1]. New and additional information was provided in 53% of the studies, while in 32%, the result had a positive effect on the management of the patient. [67]Gallium was most useful in the differential diagnosis of *Pneumocystis carinii* pneumonia (PCP) from Kaposi's sarcoma of the lung and in the diagnosis of unsuspected lymphoma. Efficacy was found to be diminished by the widespread use of empirically prescribed antibiotics, while early referral of patients improved it.

Pneumocystis carinii pneumonia

During the early and mid-1980s, PCP was the initial manifestation of AIDS in almost two-thirds of patients and it affected about 80% of patients at some stage of the disease. Over the past few years, this number has been declining to about 40%. Bacterial pneumonia, caused by *Streptococcus pneumoniae*, *Haemophilus influenzae*, and Mycobacteria has become more important as the principal complication of HIV infection. Apart from the latter condition, which is characterized by intense ^{67}Gallium uptake, the diagnosis of the former relies on chest X-ray and sputum culture. Nevertheless, PCP is still an important opportunistic infection in AIDS. The diagnosis depends on the demonstration of pneumocysts in sputum or bronchoalveolar lavage fluid. The sensitivity of the latter procedure is 90–95% with a very high specificity.

PCP infection is characterized by a markedly increased, bilateral, diffuse uptake of ^{67}Gallium in the lungs, while normally little or no deposition is found. The generalized pulmonary activity is markedly disproportionate to the clinical and radiologic findings. Numerous reports have been published on the high sensitivity and the lower specificity of ^{67}Gallium scintigraphy to detect interstitial lung disease caused by *P. carinii* [2–5].

In a series of 34 patients, Barron et al. reported an overall sensitivity of 94% and specificity of 74% of the scintigram to detect PCP as confirmed by transbronchial biopsy [4]. The disease prevalence was about 50% in their group. If the chest X-ray was normal or equivocal, the sensitivity was 86% and the specificity 85%. Based on these data, the authors concluded that a negative scan is more reliable to exclude PCP than a positive scan to diagnose the disease. Kramer et al. evaluated 227 scans performed in a group of 180 HIV-seropositive patients with a prevalence of PCP of 37%, and compared the nuclear medicine results with those of chest X-ray and clinicopathologic diagnosis based on biopsy, culture, or response to specific therapy [6]. The intensity of the ^{67}Gallium uptake was graded on a scale of 0–4, with grade 3 being an uptake intensity equal to, and grade 4 greater than liver activity. Moreover, they characterized the uptake pattern as diffuse, focal extrapulmonary, focal intrapulmonary, or ill-defined perihilar activity. They concluded that a heterogeneous intense uptake had an 87% positive predictive value for PCP. The positive predictive value of increased pulmonary activity for pathology of the lung was 93%, while a negative scan had a negative predictive value of 96%. If the intensity of lung uptake is less than liver uptake, the specificity falls to 50%, owing to other diffuse lung diseases, such as cytomegalovirus (CMV) infection.

In view of the many pulmonary disorders during HIV infection, the number of repeated invasive procedures may be quite a burden to the patient. Selection of symptomatic patients for bronchoscopy may be

achieved by ^{67}Gallium scintigraphy in view of the high sensitivity. Another approach to the detection of interstitial lung disease in HIV is the ^{99m}Tc DTPA aerosol scintigraphy. After inhalation, the clearance of this compound by the lung, as measured by the gamma camera, is proportional to the permeability of the lung parenchyma. An increased permeability has been reported in smokers, [7] but also in PCP infection [8]. Rosso et al. reported in a larger series of 88 patients that this test also may be used to detect lung disease in AIDS if chest X-ray and P_aO_2 are normal [8].

The inhalation of aerosolized pentamidine as prophylactic therapy of PCP may influence the distribution pattern of the disease and, therefore, ^{67}Gallium uptake[9]. As a result of poor drug delivery to suboptimal ventilated areas, localized uptake of the radionuclide may be found [10]. Under these circumstances, the scintigram may be useful to guide bronchoscopy to the diseased region of the lung.

Immunoscintigraphy employing a specific radiolabeled monoclonal antibody against *Pneumocystis carinii* has recently been described for imaging PCP infection in AIDS. In a small series of 16 patients, Goldenberg et al. claimed a high sensitivity and specificity. [11]. Moreover, it was reported that the antigen often persisted in the lungs after apparently successful therapy.

Other pulmonary disorders

Increased pulmonary ^{67}Gallium uptake is found in various other pathologic conditions frequently observed in AIDS. CMV infection of the lung is characterized by a pattern of low-grade uptake with perihilar prominence [6]. Adrenal uptake owing to CMV adrenalitis, which may be associated with CMV pulmonary infection, may give a clue to this diagnosis on the ^{67}Gallium scan [12]. No larger series has been published on the sensitivity and specificity of this procedure.

Mycobacterium infection either by *M. tuberculosis* or *M. avium* accumulates ^{67}Gallium avidly. Thadepalli et al. described increased focal accumulation in lung and lymph nodes affected by active tuberculosis [13]. Following the publication of a case report of a diagnosis of disseminated *Mycobacterium* infection by ^{67}Gallium in a patient suffering from AIDS [14], Kramer et al. studied the efficacy in their large series [6]. Nodal uptake strongly suggested *Mycobacterium*

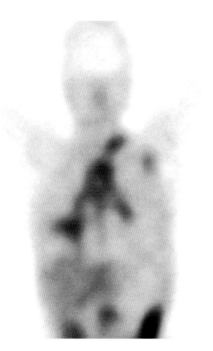

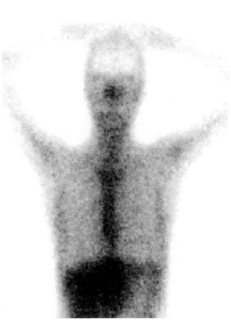

Figure 8.1. Intensive ⁶⁷Gallium uptake in *M. avium* infection in a patient suffering from AIDS. Notice also the uptake in the periaortic lymph nodes just below the liver.

Figure 8.2. A normal ⁶⁷Gallium scintigram of the thorax. There is little or no activity of the radionuclide found in the lung area. Notice the physiologic activity in liver and sternum.

infection or tuberculosis, especially if patchy lung activity is also found. *Mycobacterium avium* infection presents more frequently with extrahilar nodes, especially in periaortic nodes, while tuberculosis tends to be more commonly limited to hilar uptake [12]. Figure 8.1 demonstrates the intense and extensive ⁶⁷Gallium uptake in a patient suffering from AIDS and *Mycobacterium avium* infection in comparison to a normal image of the thorax (Figure 8.2). Figure 8.3 demonstrates the uptake of ⁶⁷Gallium in pulmonary tuberculosis.

Bacterial infections of the lung often show a pattern of localized lobar uptake of ⁶⁷Gallium without nodal uptake. Sometimes this uptake may be useful to guide bronchoscopy to obtain a specific diagnosis (Figure 8.4).

Lymphocytic interstitial pneumonitis (LIP) is a disorder of unknown etiology, which is rare in adults with AIDS and relatively common in children. Zuckier et al. described a 3-year-old child who demonstrated intense diffuse ⁶⁷Gallium uptake as a result of LIP [15]. Therefore, this condition cannot be discerned from PCP on the grounds of scintigraphic findings. In adults with LIP, a lower pulmonary uptake has been reported, although supportive data are lacking [12].

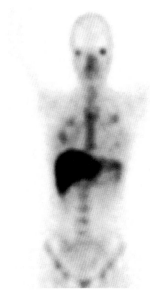
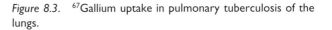

Figure 8.3. ⁶⁷Gallium uptake in pulmonary tuberculosis of the lungs.

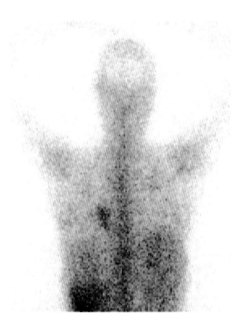

Figure 8.4. Focal pulmonary [67]Gallium uptake in an AIDS patient with fever of unknown origin due to bacterial infection.

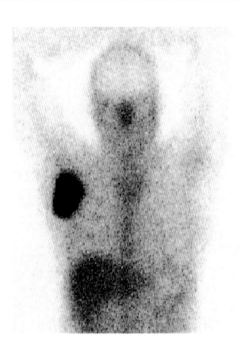

Figure 8.5. [67]Gallium accumulation in a case of AIDS-related malignant lymphoma located in the right axilla.

Malignancies

Several reports confirm that Kaposi's sarcoma (KS) does not accumulate [67]Gallium either in cutaneous [2], pulmonary [5,6], or mediastinal sites. Therefore, it may be used in the differential diagnosis of pulmonary Kaposi's sarcoma from PCP. The radionuclide [201]Thallium has been shown to accumulate in cutaneous, mucosal, and extracutaneous Kaposi's sarcoma, [16] as it does in many other neoplastic lesions. Although it is a non-specific uptake, in some conditions it may be of value to determine the extent of the disease. However, since it also accumulates in PCP, it is not as useful as [67]Gallium. It has also been suggested that, since KS is a highly vascular tumor, ^{99m}Tc labeled red blood cells might be useful in visualizing KS lesions.

Non-Hodgkin lymphoma (NHL) has been recognized as an important complication of AIDS either of central nervous system or peripheral lymphatic origin. The histology of peripheral NHL is usually high-grade, small, Burkitt's type, diffuse large cell or immunoblastic types, which generally are [67]Gallium-positive [17]. [67]Gallium scintigraphy, again, is an effective method of detecting site involvement in malignant lymphoma especially if a higher dose and single photon emission computed tomography (SPECT) [18,19] is applied.

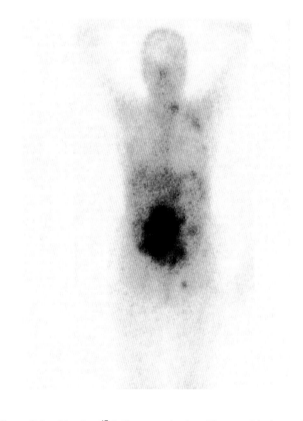

Figure 8.6. Massive [67]Gallium uptake in widespread lesions of NHL in AIDS.

[67]Gallium scintigraphy is especially useful during follow-up after therapy and often superior to CT in detecting or excluding residual tumor or relapse (Figures 8.5 and 8.6).

Central nervous system

The diagnosis of brain lymphoma is particularly difficult in AIDS patients, since lymphoma and toxoplasma encephalitis may have a similar appearance on CT and MRI [20]. Contrast-enhancing mass lesions are often empirically treated for *Toxoplasma gondii*, since it is the most common cause of focal encephalitis. If the patient does not respond, stereotactic biopsy is required to exclude lymphoma. Ruiz et al. in a prospective series of 37 AIDS patients studied the use of [201]Thallium in this differential diagnosis [21]. Intense focal uptake of [201]Thallium in the brain lesions of malignant lymphoma was found, while no activity occurred in toxoplasma. The application of this technique may orient the neurosurgeon to specific sites for biopsy (Figure 8.7). Some role for [111]Indium-labeled leukocyte scintigraphy in the diagnosis has been suggested [12], but few supportive data are available. The role of nuclear medicine procedures is also limited.

A large percentage of patients may develop dementia owing to invasion of the brain tissue by the virus. It

has been stated that nearly two-thirds of patients will eventually develop moderate to severe dementia [22]. The brain tissue itself, apart from the immunologic system, is a target for the retrovirus, which causes structural damage to the white matter and the deep gray nuclei, particularly the basal ganglia [23]. The cells chiefly infected by the HIV-1 virus are the brain macrophages, microglia, and multinucleated giant cells, while the astrocytes are spared. The injury to the neurons themselves is induced by toxins arising from the infected macrophages, which trigger calcium influx to the neuron after activation of the glutamate receptor [24].

Characteristic alterations in regional cerebral glucose metabolism can be detected with nuclear imaging studies, as reported by Rottenberg et al. employing positron emission tomography (PET) and [18]Fluorine-labeled deoxyglucose [25]. In early AIDS-related dementia, hypermetabolism in thalamus and basal ganglia occurred, while later hypometabolism of cortical and subcortical gray matter dominated. The abnormalities of glucose metabolism have been shown to be reversible after azido-dideoxythymidine (AZT) therapy [26]. Regional cerebral blood flow (rCBF) in AIDS dementia has also been studied by SPECT. Patchy focal abnormalities were found [27], which differed from the bilateral temporo-occipital hypoperfusion in dementia of the Alzheimer type. If structural brain damage is present, which will often be the case in these patients, e.g. by toxoplasmosis or

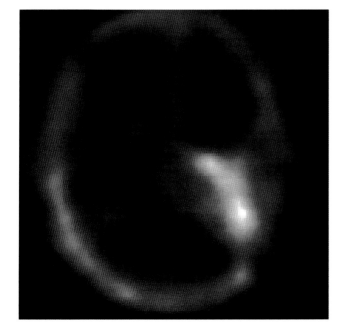

Figure 8.7.   [201]Thallium uptake in SPECT images of the brain in malignant lymphoma.

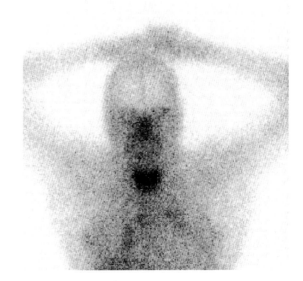

Figure 8.8.   Increased [67]Gallium uptake in thyroiditis.

CMV, the rCBF images will be subject to non-specific changes in affected areas, which is a drawback to a successful use of rCBF SPECT in this category of patients. No data on specificity and sensitivity in larger series are available.

Miscellaneous

Candida esophagitis may show up in the [67]Gallium thoracic images, while CMV esophagitis does not. Bone scintigraphy and [67]Gallium scintigraphy are useful nuclear medicine procedures to demonstrate septic arthritis and osteomyelitis, which often occur in AIDS,

days before radiographic abnormalities are found. AIDS-related myositis, a syndrome characterized by tenderness and weakness of the involved muscle groups, may be visualized on a [99m]Technetium bone scintigraphy by extraosseous deposition of the diphosphonate in the affected muscles [28]. The heart muscle may also be involved in HIV infection, resulting in cardiac dysfunction. Measurement of the myocardial ejection fraction by [99m]Technetium-labeled red cells is indicated in these patients, since dilated cardiomyopathy is associated with a poor diagnosis [29].

Finally, intense thyroidal [67]Gallium uptake has been described in painless thyroiditis in AIDS [30] (Figure 8.8).

References

1   Wassie E, Buscombe JR, Miller RF, Ell PJ. Ga-67 scintigraphy in HIV antibody positive patients – a review of its clinical usefulness. *Br J Radiol* 1994; **67**: 349–352.

2   Woolfenden JM, Carrasquillo JA, Larson SM. Acquired immunodeficiency syndrome: Ga-67 imaging. *Radiology* 1987; **152**: 383–387.

3   Bitran J, Bekerman C, Weinstein R. Patterns of Gallium-67 scintigraphy in patients with acquired immunodeficiency syndrome and the AIDS related complex. *J Nucl Med* 1987; **28**: 1103–1106.

4   Barron TF, Birnbaum NS, Shane LB. *Pneumocystis carinii* pneumonia studied by Gallium-67 scanning. *Radiology* 1985; **154**: 791–793.

5   Rosso J, Guillon JM, Parrot A et al. Technetium-99m-DTPA aerosol and Gallium-67 scanning in pulmonary complications of human immunodeficiency virus infection. *J Nucl Med* 1992; **33**: 81–87.

6   Kramer EL, Sanger JH, Garay SM, Grossman RJ, Tiu S, Banner H. Diagnostic implications of Ga-67 chest scan patterns in human immunodeficiency virus seropositive patients. *Radiology* 1989; **170**: 671–676.

7   Mason GR, Ulzer JM, Effros RM, Reid E. Rapid reversible alteration of pulmonary epithelium permeability induced by smoking. *Chest* 1983; **83**: 6–11.

8   Mason GR, Duane GB, Mena I, Effros RM. Accelerated solute clearance in *Pneumocystis carinii* pneumonia. *Am Rev Respir Dis* 1987; **135**: 864–868.

9   Jules-Elysee K, Stover D, Zaman M. Aerolized pentamidine: effect on diagnosis and presentation of *pneumocystis carinii* pneumonia. *Ann Intern Med* 1990; **112**: 75–757.

10 Katial R, Honeycutt W, Oswald SG. *Pneumocystis carinii* pneumonia presenting as focal bibasilar uptake on Gallium scan during aerosolized pentamidine prophylaxis. *J Nucl Med* 1994; **35**: 1038–1040.

11 Goldenberg DM, Sharkey RM, Udem S et al. Immunoscintigraphy of *pneumocystis carinii* pneumonia in AIDS patients. *J Nucl Med* 1994; **35**: 1028–1034.

12 Ganz WI, Serafini AN. The diagnostic role of nuclear medicine in the acquired immunodeficiency syndrome. *J Nucl Med* 1989; **30**: 1935–1945.

13 Thadepalli H, Rambhatat K, Mishkin FS, and Unknown P. Correlation of microbiologic findings and Gallium-67 scans in patients with pulmonary infections. *Chest* 1977; **72**: 442–448.

14 Malhotra C, Erickson AD, Feinsilver SH, Unknown P. Ga-67 studies in a patient with acquired immunodeficiency syndrome and disseminated mycobacterial infection. *Clin Nucl Med* 1985; **10**: 96–98.

15 Zuckier LS, Ongseng F, Goldfarb CR. Lymphocytic interstitial pneumonitis: a cause of pulmonary Gallium-67 uptake in a child with acquired immunodeficiency syndrome. *J Nucl Med* 1988; **29**: 707–711.

16 Lee VW, Rosen MP, Baum A, Cohen SE, Cooley TP, Liebman HA. AIDS related Kaposi sarcoma: findings on Thallium-201 scintigraphy. *Am J Radiol* 1988; **151**: 1233–1235.

17 Ziegler JL, Beckstead JA, Volberding PA. Non-Hodgkin lymphoma in 90 homosexual men. *N Engl J Med* 1984; **311**: 565–570.

18 Tumeh SS, Rosenthal DS, Kaplan WD, English RJ, Holman BL. Lymphoma: evaluation with Ga-67 SPECT. *Radiology* 1987; **164**: 111–114.

19 Kostakoglu L, Yeh SDJ, Portlock C et al. Validation of Gallium-67 citrate SPECT in biopsy confirmed residual Hodgkin's disease in the mediastinum. *J Nucl Med* 1992; **33**: 345–350.

20 Dina TS. Primary central nervous system lymphoma versus toxoplasmosis in AIDS. *Radiology* 1991; **179**: 823–828.

21 Ruiz A, Ganz WI, Post MJD et al. Use of thallium-201 brain SPECT to differentiate cerebral lymphoma from toxoplasma encephalitis in AIDS patients. *Am J Neuroradiol* 1994; **15**: 1885–1894.

22 Navia BA, Jordan BD, Price RW. The AIDS dementia complex: I Clinical features. *Ann Intern Med* 1986; **19**: 517-524.

23 Navia BA, Cho ES, Petito CK, Price RW. The AIDS dementia complex: II neuropathology. *Ann Intern Med* 1986; **19**: 525–535.

24 Lipton SA, Gendelman HE. Dementia associated with the acquired immunodeficiency syndrome. *N Engl J Med* 1995; **332**: 934–940.

25 Rottenberg DA, Moeller JR, Strother SC et al. The metabolic pathology of the AIDS dementia complex. *Ann Neurol* 1987; **22**: 700–706.

26 Brunetti A, Berg G, DiChiro G. Reversal of brain metabolic abnormalities following treatment of AIDS dementia complex with AZT: a PET FDG study. *J Nucl Med* 1989; **30**: 581–590.

27 Pohl P, Vogl G, Fill H. Single photon emission computed tomography in AIDS dementia complex. *J Nucl Med* 1988; **29**: 1382–1386.

28 Scott JA, Palmer EL, Fischman AJ. HIV associated myositis detected by radionuclide bone scanning. *J Nucl Med* 1989; **30**: 556–558.

29 Currie PF, Jacob AJ, Foreman AR, Elton RA, Brettle RP, Boon NA. Heart muscle disease related to HIV infection: prognostic implications. *Br Med J* 1994: **309**: 1605–1607.

30 Achong DM, Snow KJ. Gallium-avid painless thyroiditis in a patient with AIDS. *Clin Nucl Med* 1994; **19**: 413–415.

9 SURGERY IN AIDS

Esther C.J. Consten
Jan J.B. van Lanschot

General surgical issues concerning HIV-infected and AIDS patients

Surgery in patients with human immune deficiency virus (HIV) infection or acquired immune deficiency syndrome (AIDS) should be aimed at giving optimal care in balance with the ultimately bad prognosis, while limiting the risks for healthcare workers. Involvement of the surgeon may be threefold: (1) diagnostic; (2) provision of supportive care; and (3) surgical management of HIV-related manifestations [1].

1. The diagnosis of AIDS is basically a clinical diagnosis. Surgical procedures may be performed to support the diagnosis of an AIDS-related surgical/clinical manifestation [2]. However, surgical procedures are also carried out in patients not known to be suffering from HIV infection.

2. Patients with AIDS may need supportive care to facilitate medical treatment. Chronic venous access is often needed for long-term antimicrobial therapy, and occasionally for chemotherapy or parenteral nutrition.

3. Patients can also develop complications requiring surgical management, ranging from simple cutaneous abscesses to esophageal obstruction owing to malignant tumors or life-threatening gastrointestinal perforations. Although treatment of AIDS patients must not differ from that of any other patient, it should be kept in mind that the morbidity and the mortality in

Table 9.1. Common surgical complications in the GI tract.

Organ Involvement	Perforation	Obstruction	Hemorrhage
Oropharynx	–	Kaposi's sarcoma	Kaposi's sarcoma
Esophagus	Candida, CMV, Kaposi's sarcoma	Kaposi's sarcoma	Kaposi's sarcoma
Stomach/small bowel	CMV, MAI, *Cryptosporidium*, Kaposi's sarcoma, lymphoma	CMV, Kaposi's sarcoma, lymphoma	CMV, Kaposi's sarcoma, lymphoma
Hepatobiliary tract/	Kaposi's sarcoma, lymphoma	Kaposi's sarcoma, lymphoma	Kaposi's sarcoma
Gallbladder	CMV, *Cryptosporidium*		
Appendix	CMV, Kaposi's sarcoma		
Colon	CMV, MAI, *Cryptosporidium*, Kaposi's sarcoma	CMV, MAI, Kaposi's sarcoma	CMV, MAI, Kaposi's sarcoma
Anorectum	–	Condylomata acuminata Kaposi's sarcoma, lymphoma, squamous cell carcinoma cloacogenic carcinoma	Kaposi's sarcoma, ulcers lymphoma, squamous cell cloacogenic carcinoma

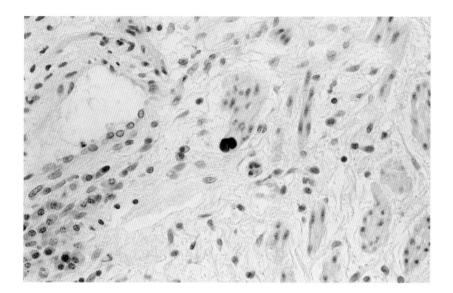

Figure 9.1. Typical picture of immunoperoxidase-positive CMV inclusion bodies in the foveolar cells of the cardiac mucosa.

AIDS patients can be quite different [3,4]. With that in mind, the expected postoperative prognosis should be related to the quality of life [5,6].

Since the clinical syndrome of most infections and tumors is atypical in such patients, surgeons should be acquainted with the manifestations of HIV infection and AIDS in order to make a proper judgment of diagnostic procedures, therapeutic treatment, and/or supportive surgery.

Gastrointestinal manifestations

The gastrointestinal (GI) tract is a major target organ system for life-threatening opportunistic infections and unusual malignancies in patients with AIDS. The patients are susceptible to a spectrum of diseases that may cause a variety of symptoms and complaints [1,7–10].

It should be emphasized that patients with AIDS may well have regular surgical problems, such as peptic ulcer disease, cholecystitis, and appendicitis, although the diagnosis may be obscured because of an unusual presentation or coexistence of other symptoms. The usual as well as the unusual must be considered.

Several major infectious pathogens and neoplastic processes can affect the GI tract in AIDS patients. The most important manifestations will be discussed both in general and in specified terms according to different organs. Ultimately, the infectious or neo-

plastic processes can lead to perforation, obstruction or hemorrhage, for which surgical therapy is indicated (Table 9.1).

Major infectious and neoplastic processes

Cytomegalovirus

Cytomegalovirus (CMV), one of the five members of the herpes virus family causing human disease (CMV, *Herpes simplex* virus, *Varicella zoster* virus, Epstein–Barr virus, and human herpes virus type 6), is one of the most frequent opportunistic pathogens in the GI tract in AIDS patients [11]. Many cell types may be infected, including epithelial cells in mucous membranes and endothelial cells of capillaries in the gut mucosa. This may lead to a diffuse, ulcerative gastroenteritis [12]. The infection may be responsible for stomatitis, esophagitis, gastritis, enterocolitis, cholecystitis, and hepatitis. Severe infections may lead to bleeding, diarrhea and GI perforation [13–15]. The diagnosis of CMV disease is difficult. A definite diagnosis is only obtained if CMV inclusion bodies are found and can be confirmed by immunoperoxidase-staining (Figure 9.1) [16,17]. The disease may be suspected when clinical symptoms coincide with increased CMV antibodies of the IgM and/or IgG type. Thus, the diagnosis always includes the need of a substantial biopsy. In case diagnostic procedures fail, test treatment with intravenous gancyclovir or foscarnet may be instituted.

One of the most acute complications may be intestinal perforation as a result of necrosis, possibly caused by vasculitis of the mucosal and submucosal capillary beds in the gut [18]. After resection of the affected intestine, fecal diversion by ileostomy or colostomy is advised to avoid possible anastomotic breakdown [3].

Mycobacterium avium intracellulare

This is an ubiquitous microorganism rarely associated with disease before the AIDS era. Known sites of extra-pulmonary involvement include the lymph nodes, the ileocecal region, the liver, and the peritoneum. Infection with Mycobacterium avium intracellulare (MAI) is frequently associated with severe abdominal pain, fever, weight loss, and/or hepatosplenomegaly [19]. Enteritis, showing a thickening of the jejunal wall, enlarged lymph nodes, and inflammatory intra-abdominal masses is often found when MAI is present. AIDS patients in whom a terminal ileitis, owing to Crohn's disease, is suspected often turn out to have an MAI infection [20]. The diagnosis of mycobacterial infection is histologically confirmed by the presence of acid-fast microorganisms in feces and/or biopsy specimens. Differentiation from Mycobacterium tuberculosis can be difficult. The recently developed polymerase chain reaction (PCR) techniques for the identification of acid-fast bacilli are promising [21]. Therapy for MAI comprises a combination of 3–5 antimycobacterial drugs, such as clarithromycine and ethambutol, because of the multi-drug resistance of MAI [22–24].

As in CMV infection, MAI enterocolitis can lead to perforation necessitating laparotomy with extensive resection and fecal diversion [3,25].

Cryptosporidium, Microsporidium, and Isospora belli

Infections of the GI tract with protozoa (Cryptosporidium, Microsporidium, Isospora belli) can cause severe diarrhea, weight loss, nausea and cramping abdominal pain. The tiny protozoans that inhabit the microvilli are responsible for a profuse and often bloody mucoid diarrhea [26]. The diagnosis is based on the characteristic oocytes that may be demonstrated by histopathologic examination of rectal biopsy specimens. Some of these infections (isosporiasis) may be treated medically while others (cryptosporidiosis, microsporidiosis) cannot, as yet, be treated effectively. Surgical intervention is rarely indicated unless a life-threatening complication is evident. The protozoa can diffusely infect most of the GI tract and the gallbladder,

including the bile ducts [24,27–29]. Thus, the management of these patients is mainly supportive and should be restricted to nutrition, and maintenance of fluid and electrolyte balance.

Kaposi's sarcoma

The pattern of Kaposi's sarcoma in AIDS patients is different from that in non-HIV-infected patients. Three types can be distinguished [30–32]:

1. The classic form, in elderly men, is generally benign and involves a single lesion that rarely occurs extracutaneously.
2. The form seen in Africans, and sometimes in transplant recipients and other persons receiving immunosuppressive therapy, is also usually a single lesion, but is generally aggressive.
3. The AIDS-associated form is disseminated. Basically any organ system can be affected, but skin, lymph nodes, lungs, and/or GI tract are most often involved [33,34].

Patients may present with dysphagia, protein-losing enteropathy, abdominal pain, diarrhea, tenesmus, severe bleeding, obstruction, or perforation. However, involvement of the GI tract is asymptomatic in 17–47% of patients [35,36].

The diagnosis is established by endoscopy and deep biopsies of the GI tract. Sometimes, Kaposi's sarcoma can present as a solitary lesion, e.g. in the hepatobiliary tract. However, one must realize that in AIDS patients this form of malignancy is always disseminated. Therefore, resection of a Kaposi's sarcoma should only be performed in patients with severe complaints or a life-threatening condition [3,14,15].

Lymphoma

Lymphoma generally involves the central nervous system (CNS), the GI tract, and the bone marrow. The diagnosis requires histologic confirmation. GI lymphomas in AIDS patients are aggressive. Multimodular chemotherapy has resulted in a remission in more than 50%, but is associated with a high recurrence rate and a short disease-free interval [37]. This type of treatment poses a management dilemma because iatrogenic immunosuppression may enhance opportunistic infections. Intestinally located lymphomas sometimes require surgical resection, especially when confined to the stomach. A disadvantage of surgical intervention may be the necessity of having to construct an ileostomy or colostomy after resection of the affected segments of the intestine. Before chemotherapy, surgery may be indicated to prevent intestinal perforation [38].

Organ involvement

Oropharynx

Oral candidiasis and hairy leukoplakia are common opportunistic infections of the mouth [38–40]. Oral candidiasis usually responds to local agents such as nystatin or amphotericin B (chewing tablets) or systemic therapy with ketoconazole and fluconazole [41]. Sometimes oral acyclovir is of benefit for patients with hairy leukoplakia. Cytomegalovirus and *Herpes simplex* virus may also cause oral lesions [42,43]. Therapy consists of either gancyclovir for CMV infection, or acyclovir for *Herpes simplex* virus infections.

Kaposi's sarcoma is commonly found in the mouth and usually becomes manifest on the palate, tongue, gingiva, or tonsillar fossa. Oropharyngeal lesions have been reported to cause pharyngeal obstruction, ulceration, life-threatening bleeding, dysphagia, and gagging, for which either local therapy (laser treatment, surgical resection, intralesional injection of alkylating agents) or systemic polychemotherapy may be indicated [35,44].

HIV-associated parotid gland disease is characterized by parotid gland enlargement (bilateral in 75%) and symptoms of dry mouth [45]. Various pathological entities of the parotid gland have been described in HIV-infected and AIDS patients [46]. Submandibular glands are mostly not involved [47]. Parotid enlargement is associated with benign lesions (e.g., lymphoepithelial cysts), but also with malignant tumors (squamous cell carcinoma, Kaposi's sarcoma or malignant lymphoma) [46]. Fine-needle aspiration for cytology should be performed. Treatment includes radiotherapy, antiviral therapy (zidovudine), cyst aspiration, and/or surgery, varying from local excision to superficial or even total parotidectomy [47].

Esophageal manifestations

Esophagitis with dysphagia or pain upon swallowing is generally caused by infection with *Candida albicans* [48]. Other causes of dysphagia with esophageal ulcerations are CMV and herpes infection [49]. Surgery is only indicated in the case of perforation. Optimal management of esophageal perforation requires prompt diagnosis and treatment. Several factors influence the ultimate outcome in these patients, including factors such as cause of perforation, site (cervical, thoracic, or abdominal), and presence or absence of an intact pleura. Most important is the time interval between the actual perforation and its diagnosis. Mortality increases when a delay of more than 24 hours takes place, owing to the onset of sepsis and related complications [50–52]. Primary care should consist of starvation, introduction of nasogastric suction, and antimicrobial therapy. If primary care is not successful, optimal treatment requires esophageal resection without primary reconstruction, end-cervical esophago-stomy, and feeding gastrostomy [53]. In AIDS patients, the general condition and life expectancy should be taken into account. Often, the general condition of the patient does not allow such extensive surgical therapy and under these circumstances abstinence should be considered.

Kaposi's sarcoma may cause obstruction, perforation, and massive hemorrhage in the esophagus. Only in these situations should surgical management be considered. Radiation therapy may be useful in shrinking the tumor and thus in controlling local symptoms [53].

Stomach and small bowel

Cytomegalovirus can cause severe gastritis with abdominal pain and antral obstruction [13,54–56]. Duodenitis with deep ulceration can result in massive bleeding and gastric as well as small bowel perforations can be caused by CMV infection, often demanding surgical intervention [57,58].

Cryptosporidiosis, microsporidiosis, and isosporiasis may cause infection through the entire GI tract [24,59]. Owing to dissemination, surgical treatment is generally not indicated.

Kaposi's sarcoma and lymphomas have become increasingly important as a cause of morbidity and mortality in AIDS patients (Figures 9.2 and 9.3) [60]. Involvement of the stomach and small bowel may be suspected in cases of nausea, vomiting, hematemesis, and early satiety. Intussusception of the small bowel has also been associated with Kaposi's sarcoma lesions or lymphoid hyperplasia [58]. Aggressive polychemotherapy may be indicated. Perforation can occur inherently in this treatment.

Liver and biliary tract

Intraabdominal opportunistic infections can also affect the liver and biliary tract [61]. The surgeon should be

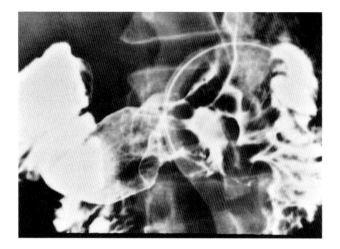

Figure 9.2. Barium examination of the stomach: large, ovoid, deep-penetrating ulceration at the posterior side of the antrum of the stomach, due to AIDS-related B-cell lymphoma.

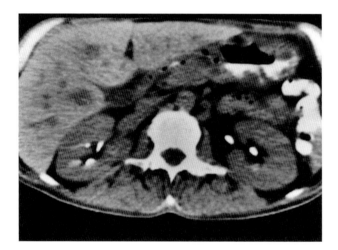

Figure 9.3. CT of the abdomen. CT demonstrates clearly the gastric wall thickening and the ulcer base lining.

consulted for AIDS patients with pain in the right upper quadrant, fever, and jaundice [62]. The diagnosis is difficult since these patients are also at high risk of hepatitis type B. It should be borne in mind that AIDS patients may also present with HIV-unrelated hepatobiliary pathology, e.g. calculous cholecystitis.

In HIV-infected patients, hepatitis may be caused by CMV, MAI or *Pneumocystis carinii* [61,63,64]. Sometimes, cryptosporidiosis, microsporidiosis, and certain drugs (e.g. 2′,3′-dideoxyinosine or ddI) can affect the liver [65–68]. The diagnosis is based on percutaneous or laparoscopic liver biopsy [69,70].

Visceral abscesses that may involve the liver are uncommon in AIDS patients and, if present, they generally originate from a lesion elsewhere, such as the appendix. Treatment consists of percutaneous drainage and antimicrobial therapy [61].

CMV and *Cryptosporidium* infection have been associated with a sclerosing cholangitis-like syndrome [71,72]. Lymphoma and Kaposi's sarcoma can also be associated with cholecystitis or cholangitis due to obstruction of the cystic and/or common bile duct. [61]. Endoscopic retrograde cholangio-pancreatography (ERCP) is the diagnostic procedure of choice. Single or multiple areas of narrowing and dilatation of the intrahepatic or extrahepatic ducts with mucosal ulcerations can be demonstrated. Papillary stenosis and strictures of the distal common bile duct often respond to endoscopic sphincterotomy [73]. Sometimes, a more proximal stricture requires balloon dilatation and/or insertion of an endoprosthetic stent. Surgical intervention is rarely indicated [73].

Patients can develop acalculous cholecystitis due to *Cryptosporidium* or CMV infection, lymphoma and Kaposi's sarcoma, as well as during total parenteral nutrition [61,73–79]. Progressive infection may lead to gallbladder empyema, or gallbladder necrosis and perforation [80]. Management of acalculous cholecystitis with or without perforation includes cholecystectomy, percutaneous cholecystostomy, or transhepatic percutaneous drainage [73].

Pancreas

The pancreas is rarely involved in HIV-infected patients, but pancreatitis can occur in association with opportunistic infections caused by CMV, *Cryptosporidium*, toxoplasmosis, *Mycobacterium tuberculosis* and *Candida albicans* [81]. Moreover, pancreatitis can be a side effect of therapeutic agents (dideoxynucleosides), and more in particular of ddI [82–85], ddI is a purine analog that after intracellular metabolic conversion suppresses the replication of HIV [84]. Approximately 3–6% of the patients treated with ddI develop pancreatitis [86]. This form of pancreatitis can be life-threatening (mortality 0–5% in patients treated with ddI) [79–81]. AIDS-unrelated pancreatitis should be reminded.

Treatment of drug-induced pancreatitis includes cessation of drug therapy. If conservative therapy fails, operative treatment may be indicted, which should not be different from that in non-AIDS patients. Again, pros and cons must be considered with regard to morbidity, mortality, prognosis, and quality of life of the AIDS patient.

Appendix vermiformis

Early diagnosis of acute appendicitis is especially difficult in patients with AIDS, particularly in the presence of chronic abdominal pain often owing to concomitant intestinal infections. Therefore, many patients are not referred for surgical consultation until the disease has advanced to perforation. The presence or absence of leukocytosis is not reliable. The morbidity of a 'negative' appendectomy can be high in these patients. Ultrasonography and diagnostic laparoscopy can be of value to limit a negative exploration [87]. In the diagnostic work-up of acute appendicitis, the surgeon should not be misguided by recent positive stool cultures with enteric pathogens, because cultures will be positive in a majority of the patients [88,89].

Laparoscopic intervention in HIV-infected patients has become an important diagnostic as well as a therapeutic tool. As diagnosis of abdominal pathology in these patients is often complicated, laparoscopy may reveal the actual underlying problem [90]. Laparoscopic biopsies may also establish definite pathology. Furthermore, a number of surgical interventions, such as appendectomy and cholecystectomy, may be performed laparoscopically decreasing the risk of acquiring HIV infection for the surgeon as well as decreasing morbidity for the patient.

Colon

CMV, MAI, and *Cryptosporidium* are the most common causal agents and Kaposi's sarcoma is the commonest tumor in the diseased colon of the AIDS patient [91].

CMV is a frequent cause of colitis and characteristically presents as intractable diarrhea, weight loss, fever, and sometimes melena, or hematochezia [37]. The cause of colitis is difficult to determine as more than 70% of the male homosexual AIDS patients with CMV infection of the GI tract have coexisting alimentary pathogens, e.g. *Shigella* and *Salmonella* [92,93]. Most common indications for urgent surgical intervention are bleeding and perforation of ulcers [94–96]. The bleeding is in general massive, may be multifocal, and often does not respond to medical intervention. If multifocality is restricted to a segment of the colon, segmental resection may be performed. Disseminated bleeding in the entire colon may require a procto-

colectomy. Again, pros and cons must be considered concerning stage and prognosis of the underlying disease [97]. Acute surgical intervention is required for perforation, generally leading to segmental resection. In the literature it is suggested that primary anastomoses should not be made as anastomotic healing in these immunocompromised patients is probably severely disturbed, especially in the presence of generalized intestinal infection. Therefore, an ileostomy or colostomy is advocated [3,95]. When AIDS patients develop a severe CMV colitis for which surgery is indicated, they are generally in an advanced stage of their disease. The direct mortality is 28% and the postoperative mortality ranges from 37% to 71% and increases after 6 months to 86% [3,98].

MAI is another opportunistic infection of the colon [99]. Some patients remain asymptomatic carriers, whereas others develop profuse watery diarrhea with dehydration, malabsorption, and severe abdominal pain [19]. Surgery is only required in patients with obstruction, fistulas, perforation, and bleeding [100].

Kaposi's sarcomas in the colon are less frequent than in the upper part of the GI tract. Surgical resection is rarely indicated [100].

Anorectum

The anorectum is the most common port of entry for HIV and other pathogens in homosexual men, and is commonly involved in AIDS [101]. Intravenous drug abusers who have AIDS seem to have a lower incidence of anorectal disease than male homosexuals with AIDS [102,103]. Biopsy and culture of all anorectal lesions must be carried out [104,105].

Anal fistulas are more common in homosexual men than in heterosexual men and are more prevalent in anoreceptive HIV-positive individuals than in non-anoreceptive ones. The combination of a generally decreased immune status and anal mucosal lesions makes the patients vulnerable to infection from a variety of pathogens [105]. Anal fistulas can be treated with conventional fistulotomy. Surgical treatment must be kept to a minimum in more complicated anal fistulas [100]. Care should be taken to avoid large open wounds and to preserve as much of the anal sphincters as possible, since these patients often already suffer from diarrhea and incontinence [105].

Anal condylomata acuminata are benign viral infections with a high prevalence (57%) in the HIV-positive population (Figure 9.4) [106]. The infections are associated with human papilloma virus and can be

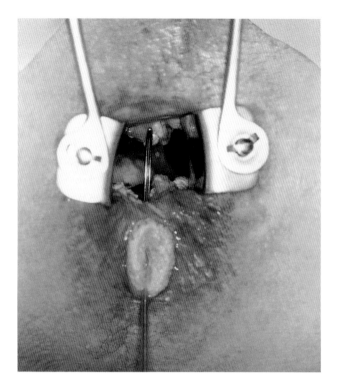

Figure 9.4. Condylomata of the perianal skin with a central fistula tract.

found on the perianal skin, and in the anal canal and lower rectum. Malignant transformation of condylomata into squamous carcinoma has frequently been reported [35,107–109]. Treatment usually consists of local therapy with podophyllin, coagulation, or excision [105]. Local excision has the advantage of a histological diagnosis to exclude carcinoma.

Anorectal ulcers are common in male HIV-positive homosexuals because of the combination of traumatic anoreceptive intercourse and several sexually transmittable microorganisms. The ulcers cause severe pain and are difficult to cure. Anorectal ulcers should be preoperatively cultured and/or biopsied as the subsequent therapy may depend on the result. *Herpes simplex* virus, CMV, HIV, *Chlamydia*, *Treponema pallidum*, *Hemophilus ducrey*, as well as neoplasia, such as squamous cell carcinoma, non-Hodgkin lymphoma, and Kaposi's sarcoma have been encountered (Figure 9.5) [105]. It seems difficult to reach a consensus as to the surgical management of anorectal ulcers in AIDS patients [100]. For previously mentioned reasons, surgery should be minor and elective; excision is a simple procedure and generally without complications. Anorectal ulcers in HIV-infected patients are treated by excision of the ulcer base and margin. Concurrent mucosal advancement improves healing.

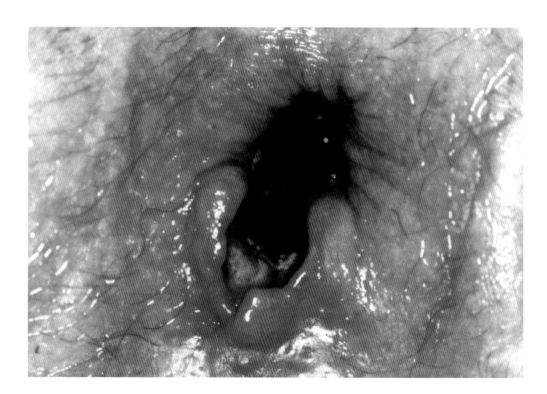

Figure 9.5. Anorectal ulceration due to a non-Hodgkin lymphoma.

Squamous cell carcinoma and cloacogenic carcinoma or transitional cell carcinoma of the anal canal are rare but appear to occur with increased frequency in AIDS patients [35,110–114]. Squamous cell carcinoma is reported with increasing frequency in homosexual men, often in combination with condylomata acuminata [35,115,116]. The increased prevalence of this anal carcinoma was known to be increased in homosexual men before the recognition of AIDS [107,117]. Biopsy is advised for all anorectal lesions in patients with AIDS. Histopathologic evaluation should be performed to define the lesion so specified therapy may be applied [100]. In non-HIV-infected patients therapy usually consists of radiotherapy and chemotherapy. In view of the relatively poor short-term prognosis, a limited local sphincter-saving excision is the treatment of choice for AIDS patients with an anal squamous cell carcinoma not infiltrating the anal sphincter [118].

There is an increase in the incidence of malignant non-Hodgkin lymphoma and Kaposi's sarcoma in the anorectal region of patients with AIDS [119]. Anorectal lymphoma usually presents as a large extraluminal mass [120]. The typical lymphoma is diffuse and deeply seated. The patient usually complains of fever, tenesmus, and perirectal pain. Perianal lymphoma is often misdiagnosed as perianal abscess. Management after diagnostic biopsies includes aggressive chemotherapy, which generally results in a substantial, but short lasting, regression [121]. No indication for excision exists.

Kaposi's sarcoma of the anorectum can cause severe proctalgia, blood loss and diarrhea. Most patients have additional anorectal diseases such as anal condylomata, proctitis, and anal fistulas. Treatment should be directed to the relief of anorectal symptoms. Chemotherapy or local laser-therapy have been reported to be an effective treatment for symptomatic Kaposi's sarcoma lesions [122–124]. Surgical excision is rarely indicated [122-124].

Acute abdomen

An increasing number of AIDS patients are admitted to the hospital with an acute abdomen. The abdominal pain is often associated with opportunistic infection or neoplasm [10]. The incidence of acute intraabdominal interventions in AIDS patients ranges from 2% to 5% [8,10]. The nature of the lesions do markedly differ from those in the non-AIDS population [8]. Acalculous cholecystitis, pancreatitis,

intussusception, and bowel ulcerations with perforations, most frequently due to CMV infection and Kaposi's sarcoma, can be labelled as part of the AIDS syndrome [3,8]. It should be kept in mind that AIDS patients can also have common diseases, such as appendicitis or calculous cholecystitis requiring surgical intervention. Thus, besides the normal surgical indications, more specific conditions that require emergency laparotomy in AIDS patients are: hemorrhage, perforation, obstruction, or ischemia. It is essential to distinguish between the surgical and the non-surgical causes of abdominal pain in order to avoid unnecessary laparotomy. As usual, carefully reviewing the patient's history and repeated physical examination are the best methods of evaluation.

Presence or absence of fever may not be particularly helpful in evaluating the acute abdomen, because many AIDS patients have chronic fever. Hepatosplenomegaly is often a non-surgical cause of pain. Chronic diarrhea mixed with blood and mucus may indicate colitis. Patients with colitis often have abdominal pain and cramps, and usually do not require surgery.

Diagnostic procedures consist of laboratory tests, such as white blood cell counts and plain X-ray examinations. Many AIDS patients with an acute surgical condition have a relatively low number of white blood cells, as a result of immunusuppression and/or drug treatment. A chest X-ray may reveal pulmonary infections or neoplasia, which can cause abdominal signs and symptoms. Obviously, free air under the diaphragm is a definite indication for exploratory laparotomy.

In patients without definite signs of peritonitis, hemorrhage, or free air under the diaphragm, ultrasonography and/or abdominal computed tomography (CT) scanning should be considered before laparotomy. These methods can reveal a non-surgical cause of the abdominal pain (such as liver cysts, pancreatic pseudocysts, splenic infarction) and thus prevent unnecessary laparotomy. A diagnostic laparoscopy may be performed in case of doubt.

Cutaneous and subcutaneous manifestations

Skin lesions in AIDS patients mainly concern Kaposi's sarcoma and a variety of opportunistic infections [125,126]. Diagnosis of opportunistic infections can be obtained by culture. Generally these lesions do not require surgical treatment, with the exception of subcutaneous abscesses. Infections with, e.g. mycobacteria, *Staphylococcus aureus*, *Streptococcus pyogenes* or *Pneumocystis carinii* may cause abscess formation for which incision and drainage is indicated.

The surgeon may be asked to perform cutaneous biopsies to diagnose Kaposi's sarcoma. The tumor consists of a proliferation of endothelial-like cells. Capillary-like structures are formed and, although they usually are filled with erythrocytes, biopsy seldom results in excessive bleeding. Treatment of cutaneous lesions comprises either local therapy (intralesional injection of cytostatic agents, radiation therapy, cryotherapy, or laser therapy) or systemic therapy (zidovudine, alpha-interferon or polychemotherapy) [127–129].

Supportive surgery

Implantation of central venous catheters seems to be the most common surgical procedure in AIDS patients. Central venous catheters are increasingly useful for repeated or permanent management of patients with AIDS. Venous access is needed for prolonged intravenous treatment with antimicrobial agents and supportive parentral nutrition.

Various authors have reported the complications associated with indwelling central venous catheters, such as Port-a-Cath systems and Hickman catheters, in AIDS patients [130–132]. Non-infectious complications consist of catheter occlusion and venous clotting. Infectious complications like infection at the infection site, tunnel infection, septic phlebitis, or septicemia can occur in both systems [133–138]. The prevalence of infections is 30% and the mean catheter life is approximately 90 days [131]. The risk of infection and the mean catheter life are similar for the Hickman and the Porth-a-Cath catheters [131]. Percutaneous multiuse of central venous catheters appears to be safe and is well tolerated by AIDS patients, despite the many possible complications.

Lymph node biopsy

About 10 years ago, diagnostic lymph node biopsy was the most common invasive procedure in AIDS patients. At present, fine-needle aspiration cytology has replaced the open lymph node biopsy as the initial diagnostic tool in the case of a suspicious or enlarged lymph node [106]. In a series of 121 fine-needle aspirations of lymph nodes, no false-positive results were identified. In patients who subsequently underwent lymph-node biopsy, five false-negative results were found [106]. Lymph node biopsy is only indicated in case of a negative fine-needle aspiration, or in the case of suspected lymphoma or extrapulmonary tuberculosis.

As laparoscopy has recently become an accepted and frequently used method, lymph node biopsies may now be taken by this less invasive means.

Thrombocytopenia

Thrombocytopenia is encountered in 3–30% of the HIV-infected patients [138–140]. The possible causes include, apart from immune-mediated destruction, thrombotic thrombocytopenic purpura, impaired hematopoiesis, and toxic effects of medications [141].

Patients with severe thrombocytopenia may be treated with corticosteroids, alpha-interferon, high-dose intravenous immunoglobulin and plasmapheresis. If medical treatment fails, splenectomy may be indicated [142–146]. The postoperative mortality is low even in patients with HIV infection and AIDS [146].

Non-HIV- and non-AIDS-related surgery

Besides the HIV-related and AIDS-related surgical interventions mentioned above, the surgeon may also be involved in the management of pathological conditions not related to HIV infection. As we are dealing with HIV-infected and AIDS patients, surgical options must be weighed against the prognosis of the underlying disease at that moment. In this context, it is essential to realize that the rate of postoperative complications correlates with the general state of health of the patient. A high degree of immunosuppression, for example, may cause problems with wound healing and infection [94,100,147]. If it is not a life-threatening or otherwise serious pathologic condition, the patient's symptoms, the prognosis of his or her disease, and his or her personal attitude should be taken into account.

HIV transmission during invasive procedures

Surgical teams operating on HIV-infected patients run an unquestionable but probably low risk. The risk of HIV infection depends, in general, on three variables: (1) the prevalence of HIV-infected patients to which the surgical personnel is exposed; (2) the frequency of exposure (accidental injuries) to infected blood or body fluids; and (3) the risk of seroconversion after exposure. The cumulated risk of seroconversion due to parenteral blood exposures can be calculated as [148]:

$$I - (I - fp)^{ny}$$

where f is the seroprevalence in the population, p the chance of transmission per incident, n the number of parenteral exposures per year, and y the years of practice.

The seroprevalence among patients to which the surgical personnel is exposed obviously differs per region and per surgical specialism (0.8–25%) [149–155]. Accidental injuries occur in about 2–16% of the operations [148,156–162]. The seroconversion rate after an accidental percutaneous inoculation of seropositive blood is calculated to be 0.5% [163–168]. Based on these data, the risk of contracting HIV infection for a surgeon working during 30 years can be estimated at 0.6–10%.

Until January 1993, a total of 31 cases of confirmed occupational HIV transmission to health care workers exposed to blood or other body fluids of HIV-infected patients have been reported to the CDC [165,168,169]. The CDC has released recommendations, known as universal precautions, intended to prevent transmission in the health care setting [170]. These precautions include in essence:

1. Use of appropriate barriers to prevent skin or mucous membranes from contact with patient's blood or other body fluids. These barriers include (double) gloves, gowns, and protective eyewear and masks.
2. Hands should be thoroughly washed every time after removal of (double) gloves and any skin contacting the patient's blood or other body fluids should also be washed immediately every time.
3. Great care should be taken to avoid injury by needles or other sharp objects that have been used on patients.
4. Members of the surgical team with open skin lesions should avoid direct patient contact.

The basis for the Centers for Disease Control and Prevention recommendations is that surgeons should regard blood and other body fluids from all patients as potentially capable of transmitting blood-borne infection. Moreover, universal precautions should be observed. In this manner, the surgical team can avoid unnecessary contamination or skin punctures/lacerations. This will greatly reduce the chance of transmission of HIV from the patient to the surgeon and his or her personnel. However, although none of the precautions will reduce the risk of contamination to zero, they will greatly decrease incidence. Nevertheless, in practice, these precautions are frequently partly ignored. Reasons for this common attitude could be inaccuracy, thought of invulnerability of the surgical team and/or inconvenience, e.g. loss of sensibility with double gloves.

References

1 Meyer AA. AIDS: the disease and its relevance to the surgeon. *Bull Am Coll Surg* 1986; **71**: 11–17.
2 Davis JM, Mouradian J, Fernandez RD, Cunningham-Rundles S, Metroka CE. Acquired immune deficiency syndrome: a surgical perspective. *Arch Surg* 1984; **119**: 90–95.
3 Wexner SD, Smithy WB, Milsom JW, Dailey TH. The surgical management of anorectal disease in AIDS and pre-AIDS patients. *Dis Colon Rectum* 1986; **29**: 719–723.
4 Wilson SE, Robinson G, Williams RA et al. Acquired immune deficiency syndrome (AIDS): indications for abdominal surgery, pathology and outcome. *Ann Surg* 1989; **210**: 428–434.
5 Dietrich NA, Cacioppo JC, Kaplan G, Cohen SM. A growing spectrum of surgical disease in patients with human immunodeficiency virus/acquired immunodeficiency syndrome. Experience with 120 major cases. *Arch Surg* 1991; **126**: 860–866.
6 Nugent P, O'Donnell TX. The surgeon's role in treating AIDS. *Arch Surg* 1986; **121**: 1117–1120.

7   Cone LA, Woodard DR, Potts BE, Byrd RG, Alexander RM, Last MD. An update on the acquired immunodeficiency syndrome (AIDS): associated disorders of the alimentary tract. *Dis Colon Rectum* 1986; **29**: 60–64.

8   LaRaja RD, Rothenberg RE, Odom JW, Mueller SC. The incidence of intra-abdominal surgery in acquired immunodeficiency syndrome: a statistical review of 904 patients. *Surgery* 1989; **105**: 175–179.

9   Smith PD, Quinn TC, Strober W, Janoff EN, Masur H. Gastrointestinal infections in AIDS. *Ann Intern Med* 1992; **116**: 63–77.

10 Barone JE, Gingold BS, Nealon TF, Arvanitis ML. Abdominal pain in patients with the acquired immune deficiency syndrome. *Ann Surg* 1986; **204**: 619–623.

11 Jacobson MA, Mills J. Serious cytomegalovirus disease in the acquired immune deficiency syndrome (AIDS). *Ann Intern Med* 1988; **108**: 585–594.

12 Knap AB, Horts DA, Eliopoulos G et al. Widespread cytomegalovirus gastroenterocolitis in a patient with acquired immunodeficiency syndrome. *Gastroenterology* 1983; **85**: 1399–1405.

13 Schooley RT. Cytomegalovirus infection in the setting of infection with human immunodeficiency virus. *Rev Infect Dis* 1990; **17**: S811–S819.

14 Braun J, Schumpelick V. Chirurgische probleme bei AIDS. *Zent Bl Chir* 1990; **115**: 65–76.

15 Schumpelick V, Braun J. AIDS aus der sicht des chirurgen. *Chirurg* 1987; **58**: 814–822.

16 Drew WL. Diagnosis of cytomegalovirus infection. *Rev Infect Dis* 1988; **10**: S468–S476.

17 Theise ND, Rotterdam H, Dieterich D. Cytomegalovirus esophagitis in AIDS: diagnosis by endoscopic biopsy. *Am J Gastroenterol* 1991; **86**: 1123–1126.

18 Consten ECJ, Brummelkamp WH, Henny ChP. Cytomegalovirus infection in the pregnant woman. *Eur J Obstet Gynecol Reprod Biol* 1993; **52**: 139–142.

19 Rosengart TK, Coppa GF. Abdominal mycobacterial infections in immunocompromised patients. *Am J Surg* 1990; **159**: 125–131.

20 Schneebaum CW, Novick DM, Chabon AB, Strutinsky N, Yancovitz SR, Freund S. Terminal ileitis associated with MAI infection in a homosexual man with acquired immune deficiency syndrome. *Gastroenterology* 1987; **92**: 1127–1132.

21 Iralu JV, Sritharen VK, Pieciak WS, Wirth DF, Maguire JH, Barker RH Jr. Diagnosis of mycobacterium avium bacteremia by polymerase chain reaction. *J Clin Microbiol* 1993; **31**: 1811–1814.

22 Chiu J, Nussbaum J, Bozzette S et al. Treatment of disseminated mycobacterium avium complex infection in AIDS with amikacin, ethambutol, rifampicin and ciprofloxacin. *Ann Intern Med* 1990; **113**: 358–361.

23 Bach MC. Treating disseminated mycobacterium avium intracellulare infection. *Am Intern Med* 1989; **110**: 169.

24 Rene E, Marche C, Regnier B et al. Intestinal infections in patients with acquired immunodeficiency syndrome. *Dig Dis Sci* 1989; **3-4**: 773–780.

25 Davidson T, Allen-Mersh TG, Miles AJ et al. Emergency laparotomy in patient TOETSENBORDO with AIDS. *Br J Surg* 1991; **78**: 924–926.

26 Petersen C. Cryptosporidiosis in patients infected with human immunodeficiency virus. *Clin Infect Dis* 1992; **15**: 903–909.

27 Gross TL, Wheat J, Bartlett M, O'Connor KW. AIDS and multiple system involvement with cryptosporidium. *Am J Gastroenterol* 1986; **81**: 456–458.

28 Shadduck JA. Human microsporidiosis and AIDS. *Rev Infect Dis* 1989; **11**: 203–207.

29 DeHovitz JA, Pape JW, Boncy M et al. Clinical manifestations and therapy of Isospora belli infection in patients with the acquired immunodeficiency syndrome. *N Engl J Med* 1987; **315**: 87–90.

30 Penn J. Kaposi's sarcoma in immunosuppressed patients. *J Clin Lab Immunol* 1983; **12**: 1–10.

31 Ziegler JL, Templeton AC, Vogel CL. Kaposi's sarcoma: a comparison of classical, endemic, and epidemic forms. *Semin Oncol* 1984; **11**: 47–52.

32 Beral V, Peterman TA, Berkelman RL, Jaffe HW. Kaposi's sarcoma among persons with AIDS: a sexually transmitted infection? *Lancet* 1990; **335**: 123–128.

33 Friedman SL, Wright TL, Altman DF. Gastrointestinal Kaposi's sarcoma in patients with AIDS: endoscopic and autopsy findings. *Gastroenterology* 1985; **89**: 102–108.

34 Hoover DR, Black C, Jacobson LP et al. Epidemiologic analysis of Kaposi's sarcoma as an early and later AIDS outcome in homosexual men. *Am J Epidemiol* 1993; **138**: 266–278.

35 Kotler DP. Gastrointestinal manifestations of HIV infection and AIDS. In : DeVita VT, Hellman S, Rosenberg SA (eds) *AIDS, Etiology, Diagnosis, Treatment and Prevention*, 3rd edn. Philadelphia: JB Lippincott Company, 1992: 259–283.

36 Cosnes J, Darmoni SJ, Evard D, Le Quintrec Y. Interet des explorations endoscopiques digestives au cours du syndrome d'immunodepression acquise (45 cas). *Am Gastroenterol Hepatol* 1986; **22**: 123–127 (English abstract).

37 Quinn TC. Gastrointestinal manifestations of AIDS. *Pract Gastroenterol* 1985; **9**: 23–34.

38 Klein RS, Harris CA, Small CB, Moll B, Lesser M, Friedland GH. Oral candidiasis in high risk patients as the initial manifestation of the acquired immunodeficiency syndrome. *N Engl J Med* 1984; **311**: 354–358.

39 Greenspan D, Greenspan JS, Conant M, Petersen V, Silverman S Jr, DeSouza Y. Oral hairy leukoplakia in male homosexuals: evidence of association with both papilloma virus and a herpes group virus. *Lancet* 1984; **ii**: 831–834.

40 De Souza YG, Greenspan D, Felton JR, Hartog GA, Hammer M, Greenspan JS. Localization of Epstein–Barr virus DNA in the epithelial cells of oral leukoplakia by in situ hybridization of tissue sections. *N Engl J Med* 1989; **320**: 1559–1560.

41 De Wit S, Weerts D, Gossens H, Clumeck N. Comparison of flucanozole and ketoconazole for oropharyngeal candidiasis in AIDS. *Lancet* 1989; **i**: 746–748.

42 Kanas RJ, Jensen JL, Abrams AM, Wuerker RB. Oral mucosal cytomegalovirus as a manifestation of the acquired immune deficiency syndrome. *Oral Surg Oral Med Pathol* 1987; **64**: 183–189.

43 Siegel FP, Lopez C, Hammer GS et al. Severe acquired immunodeficiency syndrome in male homosexuals manifested

by chronic perianal ulcerative herpes simplex lesions. *N Engl J Med* 1981; **305**: 1439–1444.

44 Lipsett P, Allo MD. AIDS and the surgeon. *Surg Clin North Am* 1988; **68**: 73–88.

45 Huang RD, Pearlman S, Friedman WH, Loree T. Benign cystic versus solid lesions of the parotid gland in HIV-patients. *Head Neck* 1991; **13**: 522–527.

46 Zeitlen S, Shaha A. Parotid manifestations of HIV infection. *J Surg Oncol* 1991; **47**: 230–232.

47 Terry JH, Loree TR, Thomas MD, Marti JR. Major salivary gland lymphoepithelial lesions and the acquired immunodeficiency syndrome. *Am J Surg* 1991; **162**: 324–329.

48 Porro GB, Parente F, Cernuschi M. The diagnosis of oesophageal candidiasis in patients with acquired immune deficiency syndrome: is endoscopy always necessary? *Am J Gastroenterol* 1989; **84**: 143–146.

49 Freedman PG, Weiner BC, Balthazar EJ. Cytomegalovirus oesophagogastritis in a patient with the acquired immunodeficiency syndrome. *Am J Gastroenterol* 1985; **80**: 434–437.

50 Nesbitt JC, Sawyers JL. Surgical management of oesophageal perforation. *Am Surg* 1987; **53**: 183–191.

51 Bladergroen MR, Lowe JE, Postlethwait RW. Diagnosis and recommended management of oesophageal perforation and rupture. *Am J Thorac Surg* 1986; **42**: 235–239.

52 DeMeester T. Perforation of the oesophagus. *Am J Thorac Surg*, 1986; **42**: 321–322.

53 Adkins MS, Raccuia JS, Acinapura AJ. Oesophageal perforation in a patient with acquired immunodeficiency syndrome. *Am Thorac Surg* 1990; **50**: 299–300.

54 Elta G, Turnage R, Eckhauser FE, Agha F, Ross S. A submucosal antral mass caused by cytomegalovirus infection in a patient with acquired immunodeficiency syndrome. *Am J Gastroenterol* 1986; **81**: 714–717.

55 Victoria MS, Nangia BS, Jindrak K. Cytomegalovirus pyloric obstruction in a child with AIDS. *Pedriat Infect Dis* 1985; 550–552.

56 Kram HB, Shoemaker WC. Intestinal perforation due to cytomegalovirus infection in patients with AIDS. *Dis Colon Rectum* 1990; **33**: 1037–1040.

57 Burke G, Nichols L, Balogh K. Perforation of the terminal ileum with cytomegalovirus vasculitis and Kaposi's sarcoma in a patient with acquired immunodeficiency syndrome. *Surgery* 1987; **102**: 540–545.

58 Macho JR. Gastrointestinal surgery in the AIDS patient. *Gastroenterol Clin North Am*, 1988; **17**: 563–571.

59 Heller TD, Tierney AR, Kotler DP. Variable localization of intestinal cryptosporidiosis in AIDS. *Proceedings of the Vth international conference on AIDS*, Montreal, Canada, 1989, p. 358A (abstract). Cited in reference 35.

60 Steinberg JJ, Bridges N, Feiner HD, Valensi Q. Small intestinal lymphoma in three patients with acquired immune deficiency syndrome. *Am J Gastroenterol* 1985; **80**: 21–26.

61 Cappell MS. Hepatobiliary manifestations of the acquired immune deficiency syndrome. *Am J Gastroenterol* 1991; **86**: 1–15.

62 Dworkin BM, Stahl RE, Giardina MA et al. The liver in AIDS: emphasis on patients with intravenous drug abuse. *Am J Gastroenterol* 1987; **82**: 231–236.

63 Merkel IS, Good CB, Nalesnik M, Roseman SR. Chronic pneumocystis carinii infection of the liver. A case report and review of the literature. *J Clin Gastroenterol* 1992; **15**: 55–58.

64 Wilkins MJ, Lindley R, Dourakis SP, Goldin RD. Surgical pathology of the liver in HIV infection. *Histopathology* 1991; **18**: 459–464.

65 Terada S, Reddy R, Jeffers LJ, Cali A, Schiff ER. Microsporidian hepatitis in the acquired immunodeficiency syndrome. *Ann Intern Med* 1987; **107**: 61–62.

66 Lai KK, Gang DL, Zawacki CK, Cooley TP. Fulminate hepatic failure associated with 2′,3′-dideoxyinosine (ddI). *Ann Intern Med* 1991; **115**: 283–286.

67 Shriner K, Goetz MB. Severe hepatotoxicity in a patient receiving both acetaminophen and zidovudine. *Am J Med* 1992; **93**: 94–96.

68 Munoz P, Moreno S, Berenguer J, Bernaldo de Quiros JC, Bouza E. Fluconazole-related hepatoxicity in patients with acquired immunodeficiency syndrome. *Arch Intern Med* 1991; **151**: 1020–1221.

69 Cappell MS, Schwartz MS, Biempica L. Clinical utility of liver biopsy in patients with serum antibodies to the human immunodeficiency virus. *Am J Med* 1990; **88**: 123–130.

70 Bach N, Theise ND, Schaffner F. Hepatic histopathology in the acquired immunodeficiency syndrome. *Semin Liver Dis* 1992; **12**: 205–212.

71 Burt AD, Scott G, Shiach CR, Isles CG. AIDS in a patient with no known risk factors: a pathological study. *J Clin Pathol* 1984; **37**: 471–474.

72 Hollman AS, Morley P, Burt AD, Davidson JK. Biliary tract dilatation in AIDS. *Eur J Radiol* 1986; **6**: 309–310.

73 Schneiderman DJ. Hepatobiliary abnormalities in the acquired immunodeficiency syndrome. *Gastroenterol Clin North Am* 1998; **17**: 615–630.

74 Blumberg PS, Kelsey P, Perrone T, Dickersin R, Laquaglia M, Ferruci J. Cytomegalovirus and cryptosporidium associated acalculous gangrenous cholecystitis. *Am J Med* 1984; **76**: 1118–1123.

75 Margulis SJ, Honig CL, Soave R, Govoni AF, Mouradian JA, Jacobson IM. Biliary tract obstruction in the acquired immunodeficiency syndrome. *Ann Intern Med* 1986; **105**: 207–210.

76 Hinnant K, Rotterdam K. Acalculous cholecystitis in the acquired immunodeficiency syndrome. *Prog AIDS Pathol* 1990; **2**: 51–62.

77 Ianuzzi C, Belghiti J, Erlinger S, Menu Y, Fekete F. Cholangitis associated with cholecystitis in patients with acquired immunodeficiency syndrome. *Arch Surg* 1990; **125**: 1211–1213.

78 Ong EL, Ellis ME, Tweedle DE, Ferguson G, Haboubi NY, Knox WF. Cytomegalovirus cholecystitis and colitis associated with the acquired immunodeficiency syndrome. *J Infect Dis* 1989; **18**: 73–75.

79 Kevin H, Jonas RB, Choudhary L, Kabins S. Acalculous cholecystitis and cytomegalovirus infection in the acquired immunodeficiency syndrome. *Ann Intern Med* 1986; **104**: 53–54.

80 Prufer-Kramer L. Gallenwege bei erworbenen AIDS. *Verdauungskrankheiten* 1988; **6**: 141–147.

81 Schwartz MS, Brandt LJ. The spectrum of pancreatic disease in patients with AIDS. *Am J Gastroenterol* 1989; **84**: 459–462.

82   Yarchoean R, Pluda JM, Perno CF et al. Initial clinical experience with ddI as single agents and in combination therapy. *Ann N York Acad Sci* 1990; **616**: 328–343.

83   Cooley TP, Kunchies LM, Saunders CA et al. Once-daily administration of 2′,3′-dideoxyinosine (ddI) in patients with the acquired immunodeficiency syndrome or AIDS-related complex. *N Engl J Med* 1990; **322**: 1340–1345.

84   Lambert JS, Seidlin M, Reichman RC et al. 2′,3′-Dideoxyinosine (ddI) in patients with the acquired immunodeficiency syndrome or AIDS related-complex. *N Engl J Med* 1990; **322**: 1333–1340.

85   Connolly KJ, Allan JD, Fitch H et al. Phase I study of ddI administered orally twice daily to patients with AIDS or AIDS-related complex and haematologic intolerance to zidovudine. *Ann J Med* 1991; **91**: 471–478.

86   Richman DR. Antiretroviral therapy. In: DeVita VT, Hellman S, Rosenberg SA (eds) *AIDS, Etiology, Diagnosis, Treatment and Prevention,* 3rd edn. Philadelphia: JB Lippincott Company, 1992: 373–395.

87   Jeffrey RB Jr, Laing FC, Lewis FR. Acute appendicitis: high resolution real-time ultrasound findings. *Radiology* 1987; **163**: 11–14.

88   Binderow SR, Shaked AA. Acute appendicitis in patients with AIDS/HIV infection. *Am J Surg* 1991; **162**: 9–12.

89   Whitney TM, Macho JR, Russell TR, Bossart KJ, Heer TW, Schecter WP. Appendicitis in AIDS. *Am J Surg* 1992; **164**: 467–470.

90   Lowy AM, Barie PS. Laparotomy in patients infected with human immunodeficiency virus: indications and outcome. *Br J Surg* 1994; **81**: 942–945.

91   Smith L. Sexually transmitted diseases. In: Gordon PH, Nivatvongs S. *Principles and Practice of Surgery for the Colon, Rectum and Anus.* St Louis: Quality Medical Pub., 1992: 317–335.

92   Hinnant KL, Rotterdam HZ, Bell ET, Tapper ML. Cytomegalovirus infection of the alimentary tract: a clinicopathological correlation. *Am J Gastroenterol* 1986; **81**: 944–950.

93   Nelson MR, Shanson DC, Hawkins DA, Gazzard BG. Salmonella, Campylobacter and Shigella in HIV-seropositive patients. *AIDS* 1992; **6**: 1495–1498.

94   Wexner SD, Smithy WB, Trillo C, Smith Hopkins B, Dailey TH. Emergency colectomy for cytomegalovirus ileocolitis in patients with the acquired immune deficiency syndrome. *Dis Colon Rectum* 1988; **31**: 755–761.

95   Meiselman MS, Cello JR, Margretten W. Cytomegalovirus colitis. Report of the clinical, endoscopic and pathological findings in two patients with the acquired immunodeficiency syndrome. *Gastroenterology* 1985; **88**: 171–175.

96   Kram HB, Hino ST, Cohen RE, DeSantis SA, Shoemaker WC. Spontaneous colonic perforation secondary to cytomegalovirus in a patient with acquired immune deficiency syndrome. *Crit Care Med* 1984; **12**: 469–471.

97   Burack JH, Mandel MS, Bizer LS. Emergency abdominal operations in the patient with acquired immunodeficiency syndrome. *Arch Surg* 1989; **124**: 285–286.

98   Williams RA, Wilson SE. Gastrointestinal disorders requiring surgical treatment in patients with AIDS. *Comprehen Ther* 1992; **18**: 9–12.

99   Desforges JF. Mycobacterium avium complex infection in the acquired immunodeficiency syndrome. *N Engl J Med* 1991; **324**: 1332–1338.

100   Wexner SD. Sexually transmitted disease of the colon, rectum and anus. *Dis Colon Rectum* 1990; **33**: 1048–1062.

101   Scholefield JH, Northover JM, Carr ND. Male homosexuality, HIV infection and colorectal surgery. *Br J Surg* 1990; **77**: 493–496.

102   Wolkomir AF, Barone JE, Hardy HW, Cotton JF. Abdominal and anorectal surgery and the acquired immune deficiency syndrome in heterosexual drug users. *Dis Colon Rectum* 1990; **33**: 267–270.

103   Sim A. Anorectal HIV infections and AIDS: diagnosis and management. *Baillieres Clin Gastroenterol* 1992; **6**: 95–103.

104   Miles AJ, Mellor CH, Gazzard B, Allen-Mersh TG, Wastell C. Surgical management of anorectal disease in HIV-positive homosexuals. *Br J Surg* 1990; **77**: 869–871.

105   Safavi A, Gottesman L, Dailey TH. Anorectal surgery in the HIV positive patient: update. *Dis Colon Rectum* 1991; **34**: 299–304.

106   Macho JR, Schecter WP. Surgical care of HIV-infected patients. *Infect Dis Clin North Am* 1992; **6**: 745–761.

107   Kovi J, Tillman RL, Lee SM. Malignant transformation of condylomata acuminata: a light microscopic and ultrastructural study. *Am J Clin Pathol* 1974; **61**: 702–710.

108   Longo WE, Ballantyne GH, Gerald WL, Modlin JM. Squamous cell carcinoma in situ in condylomata acuminata. *Dis Colon Rectum* 1986; **29**: 503–506.

109   Wexner SD, Milsom JW, Dailey TH. The demographics of anal cancers are changing: identification of a high-risk population. *Dis Colon Rectum* 1987; **30**: 942–946.

110   Golden GT, Horsley JS. Surgical management of epidermoid carcinoma of the anus. *Am J Surg* 1976; **131**: 275–280.

111   Sischy B. The use of radiation therapy combined with chemotherapy in the management of squamous cell carcinoma of the anus and marginally resectable adenocarcinoma of the rectum. *Int J Radiat Oncol* 1985; **11**: 1587–1593.

112   Slors JFM, Taat CW, Eeftinck Schattenkerk JK, Brummelkamp WH. Komt anus carcinoom vaker voor bij homosexuele mannen met antistoffen tegen HIV? *Ned Tijdschr Geneeskd* 1987; **131**: 473–475.

113   Hickey RC, Martin RG, Kheir S, MacKay B, Gallager HS. Anal cancer with special reference to the cloacogenic variety. *Surg Clin North Am* 1972; **52**: 943–950.

114   Klotz RG, Pamukcogly T, Souillard DH. Transitional cloacogenic carcinoma of the anal canal: clinicopathologic study of three hundred seventy three cases. *Cancer* 1967; **20**: 1727–1745.

115   Croxson T, Chabon AB, Rorat E, Barash IM. Intraepithelial carcinoma of the anus in homosexual men. *Dis Colon Rectum* 1984; **27**: 325–330.

116   Nash G, Allan W, Nash S. Atypical lesions of the anal mucosa in homosexual men. *JAMA* 19867; **256**: 873–876.

117   Cooper HS, Patchefsky AJ, Marks G. Cloacogenic carcinoma of the anorectum in homosexual men: an observation of four cases. *Dis Colon Rectum* 1979; **22**: 557–558.

118   Beahrs OH. Management of squamous cell carcinoma of the anus and adenocarcinoma of the low rectum. *Int J Radiat Oncol* 1985; **11**: 1741–1742.

119 Ziegler JL. Non-Hodgkin's lymphoma in 90 homosexual men; relationship to generalized lymphadenopathy and acquired immune deficiency syndrome. *N Engl J Med* 1984; **311**: 565–571.

120 Morrison JG, Scharfenberg JC, Timmcke AE. Perianal lymphoma as a manifestation of the acquired immune deficiency syndrome. *Dis Colon Rectum* 1989; **32**: 521–523.

121 Kwak LW, Halpern J, Olshen RA, Horning SJ. Prognostic significance of actual dose intensity in diffuse large cell lymphoma. *J Clin Oncol* 1990; **8**: 963–977.

122 Wexner SD. What the colorectal surgeon needs to know. In: T Schrock (ed.) *Perspectives in Colon and Rectal Surgery.* St Louis: Quality Medical Pub, 1989: 19–54.

123 Steis RG, Longo DL. Clinical, biological, and therapeutic aspects of malignancies associated with the acquired immunodeficiency syndrome: part I. *Ann Allergy* 1988; **60**: 310–323.

124 Lorenz HP, Wilson W, Leigh B, Schecter WP. Kaposi's sarcoma of the rectum in patients with the acquired immunodeficiency syndrome. *Am J Surg* 1990; **160**: 681–682.

125 Coldiron BM, Bergstresser PR. Prevalence and clinical spectrum of skin disease in patients infected with human immunodeficiency virus. *Arch Dermatol* 1989; **125**: 357–361.

126 Cockerell CJ. The dermatopathologist and human immunodeficiency virus infection. *Arch Dermatol* 1989; **125**: 1565–1567.

127 Mistuyasu RT, Groppman JE. Biology and therapy of Kaposi's sarcoma. *Semin Oncol* 1984; **11**: 53–59.

128 DeWit R, Danner SA, Bakker PJ, Lange JM, Eeftinck Schattenkerk JK, Veehof CH. Combined zidovudine and interferon-alpha treatment in patients with AIDS-associated Kaposi's sarcoma. *J Intern Med* 1991; **229**: 35–40.

129 DeWit R, Bakker PJ, Veenhoff KH, Danner SA. Continued zidovudine and interferon-alpha therapy in Kaposi's sarcoma and the acquired immunodeficiency syndrome. *Ann Intern Med* 1990; **112**: 306–307.

130 Prichard JG, Nelson MJ, Burns L. Infections caused by central venous catheters in patients with acquired immunodeficiency syndrome. *South Med J* 1988; **81**: 1496–1498.

131 Skoutelis AT, Murphy RL, MacDonell KB, VonRoenn JH, Sterkel CD, Phair JP. Indwelling central venous catheter infections in patients with acquired immune deficiency syndrome. *J Acquir Immune Defic Syndr* 1990; **3**: 335–342.

132 Raviglione MC, Battan R, Pablos-Mendez A, Aceves-Casillas P, Mullen MP, Taranta A. Infections with Hickman catheters in patients with acquired immunodeficiency syndrome. *Am J Med* 1989; **86**: 780–786.

133 Moosa HH, Julian TB, Rosenfeld CS, Shadduck RK. Complications of indwelling central venous catheters in bone marrow transplant recipients. *Surg Gynecol Obstet* 1991; **172**: 275–279.

134 Presant CA. Tunnelled central venous catheter complications and the iatrogenic superior vena cava syndrome. *N York St J Med* 1992; **92:** 43–44.

135 Strum S, McDermed J, Korn A, Joseph C. Improved methods for venous access; the Port-a-Cath system, a totally implanted catheter. *J Clin Oncol* 1986; **4**: 596–603.

136 Brun-Buisson C, Fekri Abrouk, Legrand P, Huet Y, Larabi S, Rapin M. Diagnosis of central venous catheter related sepsis. Critical level of quantitative tip cultures. *Arch Int Med* 1987; **147**: 873–877.

137 Sitzmann JV, Towsend TR, Siler MC, Bartlet JG. Septic and technical complications of central venous cathetgerization. *Ann Surg* 1985; **202**: 766–770.

138 Kaslow RA, Phair JP, Friedman HB et al. Infection with the human immunodeficiency virus: clinical manifestations and their relationship to immune deficiency. A report from the multicenter AIDS-Cohort Study. *Ann Intern Med* 1987; **107**: 474–480.

139 Jost J, Tauber MG, Luthy R, Siegenthaler W. HIV-assozierte thrombozytopenie. *Schweiz Med Wochenschr* 1988; **118**: 206.

140 Murphy MF, Metcalfe P, Waters AH et al. Incidence and mechanism of neutropenia and thrombocytopenia in patients with human immunodeficiency virus infection. *Br J Haematol* 1987; **66**: 337–340.

141 Schneider PA, Abrams DI, Rayner AA, Hohn DC. Immunodeficiency-associated thrombocytopenic purpura (IDTP). Response to splenectomy. *Arch Surg* 1987; **122**: 1175–1178.

142 Ferguson CM. Splenectomy for immune thrombocytopenia related to HIV. *Surg Gynecol Obstet* 1988; **167**: 300–302.

143 Barbui T, Cortelazzo S, Minette B, Galli M, Buelli M. Does splenectomy enhance risk of AIDS in HIV-positive patients with chronic thrombocytopenia? *Lancet* 1987; **i**: 342–343.

144 Tyler DS, Shaunuk S, Iglehart ID. HIV-1 associated thrombocytopenia. The role of splenectomy. *Ann Surg* 1990; **211**: 211–217.

145 Ravikumar TS, Allan JD, Bothe A Jr, Steele G Jr. Splenectomy. The treatment of choice for human immunodeficiency virus-related immune thrombocytopenia? *Arch Surg* 1989; **124**: 625–628.

146 Alonso M, Gossot D, Bourstyn E, Galera MJ, Oksenhendler E, Celerier M, Clot P. Splenectomy in human immunodeficiency virus-related thrombocytopenia. *Br J Surg* 1993; **80**: 330–333.

147 Robinson G, Wilson SE, Williams RA. Surgery in patients with acquired immunodeficiency syndrome. *Arch Surg* 1987; **122**: 170–175.

148 Schiff SJ. A surgeon's risk of AIDS. *J Neurosurg* 1990; **73**: 651–660.

149 Evrard S, Meyer P, van Haaften K, Christmann D, Marescaux J. Occupational risk to surgeons of unrecognized HIV infection in a low-prevalence area. *World J Surg* 1993; **17**: 232–236.

150 Kelen GD, DiGiovanni T, Bisson L. HIV infection in emergency department patients. *JAMA* 1989; **262**: 516–522.

151 Kelen GD, Fritz S, Qaqish B. Unrecognized HIV infection in emergency department patients. *N Engl J Med* 1988; **318**: 1645–1650.

152 Janssen RS, St. Louis ME, Scatten GA, Critchley SE, Petersen LR, Stafford RS. HIV infection among patients in US acute care hospitals − strategies for the counselling and testing of hospital patients. The hospital HIV surveillance group. *N Engl J Med* 1992; **327**: 445–452.

153 Watters DAK, Sinclair JR, Luo N, Verma R. HIV seroprevalence in critically ill patients in Zambia. *AIDS* 1988; **2**: 142–143.

154 Van der Hoek W. AIDS in een Zambiaans district. *Ned Tijdschr Geneeskd* 1992; **136**: 2432–2435 (English abstract).

155   Quarterly report to the domestic policy council on the prevalence and rate of spread of HIV and AIDS – US. *MMWR* 1988; **37**: 551–559.

156   Hussain SA, Latif ABA, Choudhary AAAA. Risk to surgeons: a survey of accidental injuries during operations. *Br J Surg* 1988; **75**: 314–316.

157   Houweling H, Coutinho RA. Risk of HIV infection among Dutch expatriates in sub-Saharan Africa. *Int J STD AIDS* 1991; **2**: 252–257.

158   Lowenfels AB, Wormser GP, Jain R. Frequency of puncture injuries in surgeons and estimated risk of HIV infection. *Arch Surg* 1989; **124**: 1284–1286.

159   Bird AG, Gore SM, Leigh-Brown AJ, Carter DC. Escape from collective denial: HIV transmission during surgery. *Br Med J* 1991; **303**: 351–352.

160   Veeken H, Verbeek J, Houweling H, Cobelens F. Occupational HIV infection and HCW in the tropics. *Trop Doct* 199; **21**: 28–31.

161   Quebbeman JE, Telford GL, Hubbard S et al. Risk of blood contamination and injury to operating room personnel. *Ann Surg* 1991; **126**: 614–620.

162   Gerberding JL, Littell C, Tarkington A, Brown A, Schecter WP. Risk of exposure of surgical personnel to patient's blood during surgery at San Francisco General Hospital. *N Engl J Med* 1990; **322**: 1788–1793.

163   Centers for Disease Control. Update: AIDS and HIV infection among HCW. *MMWR* 1988; **37**: 229–234.

164   Marcus R. Centers for Disease Control Cooperative Needlestick Surveillance Group: Surveillance of HCW exposed to blood from patients infected with HIV. *N Engl J Med* 1988; **319**: 1118–1123.

165   Henderson DK, Fahey BJ, Willy M et al. Risk for occupational transmission of HIV-1 associated with clinical exposures: a prospective evaluation. *Ann Intern Med* 1990; **113**: 740–746.

166   Berglund O. HIV transmission by blood transfusions in Stockholm 1979–1985: nearly uniform transmission from infected donors. *AIDS* 1988; 2: 51–54.

167   Centers for Disease Control. Apparent transmission of HTLV-III/lymphadenopathy-associated virus from a child to a mother providing health care. *MMWR* 1986; **35**: 76–79.

168   Centers for Disease Control. Update: HIV infection in HCW exposed to blood of infected patients. *MMWR* 1987; **36**: 285–289.

169   Houweling H. AIDS en HIV-infectie als beroepsziekte. *Ned Tijdschr Geneeskd* 1993; **137**: 696–700.

170   Centers for Disease Control. Recommendation for preventing transmission of infection with HTLV-III/LAV during invasive procedure. *MMWR* 1986; **35**: 221–223.

Part II Organ Systems

CLINICAL NEUROLOGY

Peter Portegies
Roelien H. Enting

Introduction

Neurological complications occur in at least 70% of all human immune deficiency virus (HIV)-infected individuals and in 10% of patients neurologic disease is the presenting manifestation of HIV infection [1,2]. The stage of HIV infection is important in differential diagnosis. Some of these complications occur in early HIV infection: examples are HIV-myopathy and inflammatory polyneuropathies. However, most complications occur during severe immunosuppression, with CD4+ cell counts below $0.2 \times 10^9/1$ (normal is $>0.5 \times 10^9/1$).

Several clinical syndromes occur in HIV infection: meningitis, focal neurological symptoms, diffuse encephalopathy, dementia, myelopathy, and neuromuscular disorders. A specific diagnosis based on the clinical examination may be virtually impossible because of the overlap in clinical presentations. Ancillary investigation may not always distinguish between the different specific causes of disease. It is important to keep in mind that only a limited set of causes leads to a specific therapy. A rigorous search for these diagnoses is always necessary. Invasive diagnostic procedures, such as brain biopsy, should be reserved for patients in reasonable clinical condition. It is also important to realize that multiple, neurological complications may coexist, which further complicates that diagnosis.

In this chapter, the description of the neurological disorders will be classified according to their etiologies. Opportunistic infections, HIV-1-related complications, other central nervous system (CNS) complications, neuro-oncological complications, and neuromuscular complication will be described.

Opportunistic infections of the CNS

Cerebral toxoplasmosis

Toxoplasmic encephalitis is almost always due to reactivation of a latent infection caused by the parasite *Toxoplasma gondii*. The simultaneous development of multifocal brain lesions strongly suggest a hematogenous spread of the parasite [3]. About 25% of patients with low CD4+ cell counts and a positive toxoplasma serology develop toxoplasmic encephalitis within a 1-year period [4]. The incidence of toxoplasmic encephalitis is directly proportional to the prevalence of antibodies to *Toxoplasma*, which differs among various regions in the world. It is the most frequent cause of focal CNS infection complicating acquired immune deficiency syndrome (AIDS) [5]. Clinical features consist of focal neurologic deficits (hemiparesis, aphasia, hemanopia), a diffuse encephalopathy, characterized by confusion and lethargy, or seizures. Fifty per cent of the patients have headache or fever. Because toxoplasmic encephalitis causes predominantly encephalitis with little or no meningeal involvement, meningismus is rare. The duration of symptoms ranges from days to weeks. Computed tomography (CT) scans (after contrast administration) typically show multiple ring-enhancing lesions surrounded by cerebral edema. The basal ganglia and corticomedullary junction are most involved [6]. A single lesion on CT scan may be seen; a single lesion on magnetic resonance imaging (MRI) scan favors a diagnosis of cerebral lymphoma [7]. A rapidly progressive diffuse encephalopathy without focal signs caused by toxoplasmosis and without focal CT scan abnormalities has been described [8]. The cerebrospinal fluid (CSF) may be normal, or show non-specific abnormalities [3]. However, lumbar puncture is often contraindicated because of the risk of cerebral herniation.

Treatment is initiated upon a presumptive diagnosis based on clinical and radiographic findings, and supported by positive serology and ultimately by response to therapy. In patients who are treated empirically, a clear clinical response should be evident within 14 days, and there should be a clear radiographic response within 3 weeks. If not, another cause of the lesions is probable, and brain biopsy should be seriously considered [3]. The combination of pyrimethamine (50–75 mg/day with a loading dose of 100 mg) and sulfadiazine (4–6 g/day) orally represents the standard therapy. Folinic acid is commonly given at a dosage of 10 mg/day to prevent the hematologic toxic effects of pyrimethamine. Experimental therapy consists of clarithromycin (2 g/day), or azithromycin (500 mg/day) in combination with pyrimethamine or atovaquone (3 g/day) as monotherapy. Because of the high rate of relapse, life-long suppressive therapy is necessary. Pyrimethamine (25 mg/day) combined with sulfadiazine (2 g/day) is the standard therapy, with a 5–10% relapse rate [9]. Trimethoprim–sulfamethoxazole given as prophylaxis against *P. carinii* pneumonia also appears to be an effective prophylaxis against toxoplasmic encephalitis [10]. Additional prophylaxis with pyrimethamine in this population appears unnecessary [11].

Progressive multifocal leukoencephalopathy

Progressive multifocal leukoencephalopathy (PML) is a demyelinating disease of the CNS caused by a papovavirus, the JC virus. The seroprevalence in the population is about 60% [12]. JC virus typically remains latent, possibly in the CNS or in the kidneys, until reactivation by a depressed cellular immune function [13]. It occurs in 3.8% of patients with AIDS. Patients present with focal neurological symptoms, most frequently spastic hemiparesis, visual field loss, and altered mentation. Headache and seizures are infrequent [14]. CT scan demonstrates regions of low attenuation in the white matter. MRI is more sensitive and shows patchy or confluent areas of increased signal intensity in the white matter on proton-density and T_2-weighted images, without substantial mass effect [15]. Contrast enhancement is an exception. Results of CSF examination are often normal or show non-specific abnormalities. Detection of JC virus DNA

by the polymerase chain reaction (PCR) in the CSF has become an alternative for more invasive diagnostic procedures [16]. In CSF PCR negative cases, brain biopsy remains the definitive diagnostic procedure: characteristic histological changes can be observed, and viral antigen or genome or DNA detected [12]. The mean survival is only 4 months, although occasionally prolonged survival and improvement in neurologic function have been described [14]. Favorable response to cytarabine or zidovudine have been reported, but these successes have not been confirmed by others. In an open trial of alpha-2a interferon, no clinical improvement was seen [12].

Cryptococcal meningitis

About 6–10% of patients with AIDS will develop cryptococcal meningitis, caused by the fungus *Cryptococcus neoformans*. The organism is assumed to gain access to the host via the respiratory route, and, in the presence of immunodeficiency, disseminates widely, especially to the CNS [17]. About two-thirds of patients present with a subacute meningitis; symptoms often exist for 2–4 weeks and consist of fever, headache and malaise, often with nausea or vomiting. However, fever and malaise may be the only symptoms. On physical examination, meningismus is found in only one-fourth of patients, and altered mentation in one-sixth. On CSF examination a high opening pressure is often found. CSF samples frequently show minimal lymphocytic inflammatory response with mild elevation of protein and a normal level of glucose. Direct staining of the CSF often shows the organisms. Cultures will become positive after a few days to weeks. Cryptococcal antigen is found in 98% of serum samples and 91% of CSF samples [18]. Testing for antigen in the serum may be useful as initial screening for febrile patients [17]. CT or MRI may show parenchymal cryptococcoma, dilated Virchow–Robin spaces, non-enhancing lesions (gelatinous pseudocysts) or meningeal enhancement [19].

Treatment of acute infection consists of amphotericin B (0.7 mg/kg intravenously) plus flucytosine (100 mg/kg in four divided doses orally) for 2–3 weeks. This is followed by 'consolidation' therapy for 8–10 weeks with fluconazole (400 mg daily). Lifelong suppressive treatment with fluconazole (200 mg daily) is necessary to prevent relapses. Symptomatic intracranial hypertension must be treated by daily lumbar punctures or a lumbar drain. The acute mortality may be as high as 10–25%. Predictors are abnormal mental status, high CSF cryptococcal antigen titer, and a low CSF leukocyte count. Preliminary data on the use of liposomal amphotericin B or higher doses of fluconazole as initial therapy and itraconazole as suppressive therapy are promising [17].

Acute lumbosacral polyradiculopathy

Acute lumbosacral polyradiculopathy is uncommon, seen in fewer than 3% of AIDS patients [1]. Cytomegalovirus (CMV) infection is the most frequent causative agent; others are neurosyphilis, toxoplasmosis, and lymphoma. Patients present with a subacute ascending hypotonic lower extremity weakness, often accompanied by pain and paresthesias in the legs and perineum, with areflexia, urinary retention, and loss of sphincter control. In the case of CMV polyradiculopathy, the CSF shows moderate to severe pleocytosis, with a significant percentage of polymorphonuclear cells. CMV is cultured from the CSF in about half of the patients. In other instances, the CSF may be normal or reveal a low-grade mononuclear pleocytosis or lymphoma cells. Nerve conduction studies and electromyography show findings typical of motor axonal loss and acute denervation. MRI and myelographic studies are of no clinical significance. Patients with polymorphonuclear pleocytosis or a rapid progression of weakness should receive empiric treatment with ganciclovir (or in case of suspected resistance with foscarnet). Clinical improvement or stabilization occur in about half of treated patients; recovery may take months [20,21].

Neurosyphilis

Early neurosyphilis in HIV infection may be present as asymptomatic infection, meningitis, cranial nerve abnormalities, or strokes. It may occur in early HIV infection. Abnormalities in the CSF are non-specific, and the CSF VDRL reaction may be negative. Radiologic findings are non-specific. Treatment for early syphilis consists of three courses of benzathine penicillin. In the case of neurosyphilis a 10-day course of high-dose intravenous penicillin is given; failures have been reported [22].

CNS tuberculosis

Infection with *Mycobacterium tuberculosis* is a common complication of HIV infection and is often seen in the early stages. About 10% of patients with culture-proved tuberculosis have the organism isolated from the CSF. Fever, headache, and altered consciousness are the most frequent presenting symptoms. Meningeal signs may be absent. In the majority, analysis of the CSF shows an increased white cell count and decreased glucose. CT or MRI may reveal meningeal enhancement, hydrocephalus, enhancing lesions, or ischaemic lesions. The overall mortality in patients treated in conventional antituberculosis therapy is 20% [23,24].

Cytomegalovirus encephalitis

CMV encephalitis has been found at necropsy in 30% of patients with AIDS [25]. Neurological symptoms are non-specific and may include meningeal signs, a diffuse encephalopathy, seizures, or brainstem signs such as oculomotor abnormalities [26,27]. CT findings are also non-specific, including diffuse subependymal contrast enhancement, and white matter hypodensities [27]. CSF examination is often normal. CMV is rarely cultured from the CSF. There is no good correlation between presence of CMV antigen detection in CSF and CMV infection of brain parenchyma. If CMV is detected in the CSF by PCR, there is a 50% chance of a false-positive result. However, a negative PCR practically rules out CMV encephalitis [28]. Ganciclovir maintenance treatment for other CMV infections does not necessarily prevent CNS disease [29]. The prognosis is, even with antiviral treatment, poor.

Unusual opportunistic infections

Intracerebral lesions owing to *Nocardia asteroides*, *Candida albicans*, *Aspergillus fumigatus*, *Mycobacterium avium*, *Coccidioides immitis*, *Herpes simplex* virus and *Listeria monocytogenes* have been described, but are uncommon. *Listeria* meningitis is important as it may be prevented by refraining from consumption of raw milk products, soft cheeses, and raw meat [30.31].

HIV-1-related complications

AIDS dementia complex

AIDS dementia complex (ADC) is a complication of advanced HIV-1 infection, which is caused by the direct effect of the virus on the brain, although its pathogenesis is not well understood [32]. The annual incidence of ADC in AIDS patients is approximately 7% [33]. Impaired memory and concentration with psychomotor slowing are the early features of AIDS dementia complex. Motor deficits, such as ataxia, leg weakness, and loss of fine-motor coordination, and behavioral changes, most commonly apathy or social withdrawal, are other symptoms. In the most advanced stage, patients are severely demented, mutistic, incontinent, and paraplegic. The onset is usually insidious, although many experience either an abrupt onset or an abrupt acceleration [34]. The neuropathologic entity is HIV encephalitis, which is defined by the presence of HIV-infected multinucleated giant cells and diffuse myelin pallor. It is present in only half of patients [35]. The diagnosis is one of exclusion; opportunistic infections or tumors should have been excluded. MRI may show diffuse high signal intensity in the periventricular white matter [36]. CSF examination shows HIV-1 p24 antigen in about 40% [37]. Neuropsychological testing shows features of a so-called subcortical dementia. The incidence of ADC has declined after the introduction of zidovudine [38]. Zidovudine treatment is effective in many patients with mild to end-stage ADC, albeit sometimes only transiently [39]. Mean survival is 6 months [37].

Vacuolar myelopathy

A vacuolar myelopathy is found in 20% of autopsies performed in AIDS patients. Vacuolation is most prominent in the lateral and posterior columns of middle to lower thoracic levels. Clinical symptoms may be non-existent or consist of a steadily progressive spastic–ataxic gait, minor sensory impairment, and urinary incontinence. The cause of the myelopathy is unknown. The similarity between this disorder and subacute combined degeneration of the spinal cord associated with vitamin B_{12} deficiency is evident, but serum vitamin B_{12} and folic acid levels are normal [40]. HIV infection may play an etiological role, although a direct spinal cord infection is not found [41]. Myelography or MRI of the spinal cord may be helpful to exclude other causes of spinal cord pathology. No treatment is available.

HIV meningitis

An aseptic meningitis may occur at the time of sero-conversion or in later stages of HIV infection. Patients present with headache, fever, and meningeal signs. A cranial neuropathy may occur. The CSF reveals a mild mononuclear pleocytosis and increased protein. HIV can be cultured from the CSF. Spontaneous remission is the rule, but chronicity and recurrences have been described [42]. So-called HIV-related headache, which occurs in late HIV-infection, has the same clinical features, except for the absence of a mononuclear pleocytosis. This probably reflects the more advanced state of HIV infection with a general CSF cell count decline [43].

Other CNS complications
Seizures

New-onset seizures occur in more than 10% of patients with HIV infections. Focal brain lesions are the most common cause, followed by meningitis and metabolic disturbances. In about half of patients, extensive work-up (including laboratory investigation, CT or MRI, and lumbar puncture) fails to identify an obvious cause [44]. Focal seizures do not necessarily imply the presence of focal cerebral lesions. Because recurrence of seizures is high without treatment, anticonclusive treatment is generally recommended even after a single seizure [45].

Cerebrovascular complications

AIDS patients appear to be at increased risk for cerebrovascular complications, in spite of their young age. Cerebral infarction and transient neurologic deficits are most frequent. Certain infections, such as tuberculosis, syphilis, CMV, and *Herpes zoster* are known for their ability to produce CNS vasculitis and infarction. Because specific therapy for the underlying opportunistic process may be useful in preventing further neurological deterioration, evidence for a treatable disease should be sought. The etiology in many cases remains unknown [46].

Neuro-oncological complications
Primary CNS lymphoma

Primary CNS lymphoma is the second most common cause of diffuse or focal CNS symptoms [5]. Duration of symptoms rarely exceeds 2–3 months. They consist of neurologic focal deficits (hemiparesis, visual field defects), mental status changes, seizures, or signs suggestive of increased intracranial pressure (headache or vomiting) [47]. CT scans show single or multiple lesions that are ring-shaped or enhance homogeneously, and show mass effect. CT scan is unable to distinguish mass lesions caused by toxoplasmosis from those caused by lymphoma. Solitary lesions on magnetic resonance (MR) images most often are lymphomas [7]. CSF cytologic examination, if not contraindicated because of the danger of cerebral herniation, should be performed. Polymerase chain reaction (PCR) for Epstein–Barr virus DNA may be useful as a diagnostic tumor marker [48]. Slit-lamp examination of the eyes may reveal a cellular infiltrate in the vitreous; in these cases vitrectomy may lead to pathologic confirmation. Brain biopsy should be reserved for patients with early AIDS who wish to be treated [49]. Treatment with curative intent consists of standard whole-brain radiation. Radiation may also be used to alleviate symptoms in patients with major morbidity to increase quality of life, even if survival is not prolonged. The efficacy of added chemotherapy is unclear. Steroids may be used to cause transient amelioration of symptoms. Mean survival without treatment is 1 month, and with treatment is 3 months [47].

Lymphomatous meningitis

Systemic non-Hodgkin lymphomas occur in 2.3% of AIDS patients. Most HIV-associated lymphomas are disseminated high-grade B-cell lymphomas [50]. Meningeal involvement occurs in more than 20%. Clinical symptoms consist of cranial nerve palsies, radiculopathy, headache, or diffuse encephalopathy. CSF examination reveals pathological cells. Treatment with intraventricular methotrexate is administered by an Ommaya reservoir. Results are disappointing in symptomatic patients: mean survival is only 5 weeks [51]. In the case of systemic lymphoma, intensive combination chemotherapy together with CNS prophylaxis may result in higher response rates [52].

Neuromuscular complications

Peripheral neuropathies

A distal symmetrical peripheral neuropathy is found in about 10% of AIDS patients. HIV or CMV may play a role in the pathogenesis. Pain is the most prominent finding, often described as burning or 'pins and needles', almost made worse by contact. Most patients also complain of numbness. On neurological examination, distal sensory abnormalities, or weakness and progressive loss of ankle reflexes may be found. Nerve conduction studies may show reduction in (sensory) nerve action potentials and conduction velocities or signs of denervation. Symptomatic relief may be obtained with carbamazepine or amitriptyline [53].

Some antiretroviral drugs – didanosine, zalcitabine and d4T (stavudine) – cause a dose-dependent painful peripheral neuropathy [54–56].

Other forms of peripheral neuropathies are rare [53,57].

Table 10.1. Treatment for neurological complications in AIDS.

Complication	Treatment
Cerebral toxoplasmosis	Sulfadiazine and pyrimethamine
	Clindamycine and pyrimethamine
	Experimental: clarithromycin, azithromycin, atovaquone
Cryptococcal meningitis	Amphotericin and flucytosine
	Maintenance treatment: fluconazole
	Experimental: itroconazole, liposomal amphotericine
PML	Experimental: cytarabine
CMV encephalitis	Ganciclovir (with or without foscarnet)
Primary CNS lymphoma	Radiotherapy (with dexamethason)
Meningitis lymphomatosa	Methotrexate intrathecally
AIDS dementia complex	Zidovudine
Vacuolar myelopathy	No treatment
Peripheral neuropathy	Carbamazepine, amitriptyline

Myopathies

A myopathy may occur as a complication at various stages of HIV infection or as a result of treatment with zidovudine. Complaints are myalgia and proximal muscle weakness. Ancillary investigation may show elevated creatinine kinase levels, myopathic changes during needle electromyography, and muscle biopsy abnormalities. If muscle biopsy shows an inflammatory myopathy, symptoms may improve in response to steroids.

Zidovudine-associated myopathy (which generally occurs after 9 months or more of therapy) usually responds to stopping the drug [57,58].

A summary of the treatments for neurological complications in AIDS is given in Table 10.1.

References

1 DeGans J, Portegies P. Neurological complications of infection with HIV type 1. *Clin Neurol Neurosurg* 1989; **91**: 197–217.

2 Levy RM, Janssen RS, Bush TJ, Rosenblum ML. Neuroepidemiology of acquired immunodeficiency syndrome. In: Rosenblum ML, Levy RM, Bredesen DE (eds) *AIDS and the Nervous System*. New York: Raven Press, 1988: 13–27.

3 Luft BJ, Remington JS. Toxoplasmic encephalitis in AIDS. *Clin Infect Dis* 1992; **15**: 211–222.

4 Oksenhendler E, Charreau I, Tournerie C, Azihary M, Carbon C, Aboulker JP. Toxoplasma gondii infection in advanced HIV infection. *AIDS* 1994; **8**: 483–487.

5 De la Paz R, Enzmann D. Neuroradiology of acquired immunodeficiency syndrome. In: Rosenblum ML, Levy RM, Bredesen DE (eds) *AIDS and the Nervous System*. New York: Raven Press, 1988: 121–153.

6 Porter SB, Sande MA. Toxoplasmosis of the central nervous system in the acquired immunodeficiency syndrome. *N Engl Med* 1992; **327**: 1643–1648.

7 Ciricillo SF, Rosenblum M. Use of CT and MR imaging to distinguish intracranial lesions and to define the need for biopsy in AIDS patients. *J Neurosurg* 1990; **73**: 720–724.

8 Gray F, Gherardi R, Wingate E. Diffuse 'encephalitic' cerebral toxoplasmosis in AIDS. *J Neurol* 1989; **236**: 273–277.

9 Katlama C. New perspectives on the treatment and prophylaxis of toxoplasma gondii infection. *Curr Opin Infect Dis* 1992; **5**: 833–839.

10 Carr A, Tindall B, Brew BJ et al. Low-dose trimethoprim-sulfamethoxazole prophylaxis for toxoplasmic encephalitis in patients with AIDS. *Ann Intern Med* 1992; **117**: 106–111.

11 Jacobson MA, Besch CL, Child C et al. Primary prophylaxis with pyrimethamine for toxoplasmic encephalitis in patients with advanced human immunodeficiency virus disease: results of a randomized trial. *J Infect Dis* 1994; **169**: 384–394.

12 Editorial. PML: more neurologic bad news for AIDS patients. *Lancet* 1992; **340**: 943–944.

13 Quinlivan EB, Norris M, Bouldin TW et al. Subclinical central nervous system infection with JC virus in patients with AIDS. *J Infect Dis* 1992; **166**: 80–85.

14 Berger JR, Kaszovitz B, Post JD, Dickinson G. Progressive multifocal leukoencephalopathy associated with HIV infection. *Ann Intern Med* 1987; **107**: 78–87.

15 Hansman-Whiteman ML, Donovan Post MJ, Berger JR, Tate LG, Bell MD, Limonte LP. Progressive multifocal leukoencephalopathy in 47 HIV-seropositive patients: neuroimaging with clinical and pathologic correlation. *Radiology* 1993; **187**: 233–240.

16 Weber T, Turner RW, Frye S et al. Progressive multifocal leukoencephalopathy diagnosed by amplification of JC virus-specific DNA from cerebrospinal fluid. *AIDS* 1994; **8**: 49–57.

17 Powderly WG. Cryptococcal meningitis and AIDS. *Clin Infect Dis* 1993; **17**: 837–842.

18 Chuck SL, Sande MA. Infections with cryptococcus neoformans in the acquired immunodeficiency syndrome. *N Engl Med* 1989; **321**: 794–799.

19 Tien RD, Chu PK, Hesselink JR, Duberg A, Wiley C. Intracranial cryptococcosis in immunocompromised patients: CT and MR findings in 29 cases. *Am J Neuro-Radiology* 1991; **12**: 283–289.

20 Cohen BA, McArthur JC, Grohmans S, Patterson B, Glass JD. Neurologic prognosis of cytomegalovirus polyradiculomyelopathy in AIDS. *Neurology* 1993; **43**: 493–499.

21 So YT, Olney RK. Acute lumbosacral polyradiculopathy in acquired immunodeficiency syndrome: Experience in 23 patients. *Ann Neurol* 1994; **35**: 53–58.

22 Musher DM. Syphilis, neurosyphilis, penicillin, and AIDS. *J Infect Dis* 1991; **163**: 1201–1206.

23 Berenguer J, Moreno S, Launa F et al. Tuberculous meningitis in patients infected with the human immunodeficiency virus. *N Engl J Med* 1992; **326**: 668–672.

24 Villoria MF, de la Torre J, Fortea F, Munoz L, Hernandez T, Alarcon JJ. Intracranial tuberculosis in AIDS: CT and MRI findings. *Neuroradiology* 1992; **34**: 11–14.

25 Morgello S, Cho ES, Nielsen S, Devinsky O, Petito CK. CMV encephalitis in patients with AIDS: an autopsy study of 30 cases and a review of the literature. *Hum Pathol* 1987; **18**: 289–297.

26 Fuller GN, Guiloff RM, Scaravilli F, Harcourt-Webster JN. Combined HIV-CMV encephalitis presenting with brainstem signs. *J Neurol Neurosurg Psychiatry* 1989; **52**: 975–979.

27 Post MJD, Hensley GT, Moskowitz LB, Fischl M. Cytomegalic inclusion virus encephalitis in patients with AIDS: CT, clinical and pathologic correlation. *AJR* 1986; **146**: 1229–1234.

28 Achim CL, Nagra RM, Wang R, Nelson JA, Wiley CA. Detection of cytomegalovirus in cerebrospinal fluid autopsy specimens from AIDS patients. *J Infect Dis* 1994; **169**: 623–627.

29 Berman S, Kim R, Hook B et al. CMV encephalitis in patients receiving ganciclovir for CMV retinitis. *VII International Conference on AIDS*, Florence, 1991, abstract WB 2366.

30 Gradon JD, Timpone JG, Schnittman SM. Emergence of unusual opportunistic pathogens in AIDS: a review. *Clin Infect Dis* 1992; **15**: 134–157.

31 Jurado RL, Farley MM, Pereira E et al. Increased risk of meningitis and bacteremia due to Listeria monocytogenes in patients with HIV infection. *Clin Infect Dis* 1993; **17**: 224–227.

32 Price RW, Brew B, Sidtis J et al. The brain in AIDS: central nervous system HIV-1 infection and AIDS dementia complex. *Science* 1988; **239**: 586–592.

33 McArthur JC, Hoover DR, Bacellar H et al. Dementia in AIDS patients: incidence and risk factors. *Neurology* 1993; **43**: 2245–2252.

34 Navia BA, Jordan BD, Price RW et al. The AIDS dementia complex: I. Clinical features. *Ann Neurol* 1986; **19**: 517–524.

35 Glass JD, Wesselingh SL, Selnes OA, McArthur JC. Clinical-neuropathologic correlation in HIV-associated dementia. *Neurology* 1993; **43**: 2230–2237.

36 Olson WL, Longo FM, Mills CM, Norman D. White matter disease in AIDS: findings at MR imaging. *Radiology* 1988; **169**: 445–448.

37 Portegies P, Enting RH, De Gans J et al. Presentation and course of AIDS dementia complex: 10 years of follow-up in Amsterdam, The Netherlands. *AIDS* 1993; **7**: 669–675.

38 Portegies P, De Gans J, Lange JMA et al. Declining incidence of AIDS dementia complex after introduction of zidovudine treatment. *Br Med J* 1989; **299**: 819–821.

39 Tozzi V, Narciso P, Galgani S et al. Effects of zidovudine in 30 patients with mild to end-stage AIDS dementia complex. *AIDS* 1993; **7**: 683–692.

40 Petito CK, Navia BA, Cho ES. Vacuolar myelopathy pathologically resembling subacute combined degeneration in patients with acquired immunodeficiency syndrome. *N Engl J Med* 1985; **312**: 874–879.

41 Bergmann M, Gullotta F, Kuchelmeister K, Masini T, Angeli G. AIDS-myelopathy: a neuropathological study. *Path Res Pract* 1993; **189**: 58–65.

42 Hollander H, Stringari S. Human immunodeficiency virus-associated meningitis: clinical course and correlations. *Am J Med* 1987; **83**: 813–816.

43 Brew BJ, Miller J. Human immunodeficiency virus-related headache. *Neurology* 1993; **43**: 1098–1100.

44 Wong MC, Suite NA, Labar DR. Seizures in human immunodeficiency virus infection. *Arch Neurol* 1990; **47**: 640–642.

45 Holtzman DM, Kaku DA, So YT. New onset seizures associated with human immunodeficiency virus infection: causation and clinical features in 100 cases. *Am J Med* 1989; **87**: 173–177.

46 Engstrom JW, Lowenstein DH, Bredesen DE. Cerebral infarctions and transient neurologic deficits associated with acquired immunodeficiency syndrome. *Am J Med* 1989; **86**: 528–532.

47 Fine HA, Mayer RJ. Primary central nervous system lymphoma. *Ann Intern Med* 1993; **199**: 1093–1104.

48 Cinque P, Bryting M, Vago L et al. Epstein–Barr virus DNA in cerebrospinal fluid from patients with AIDS-related primary lymphoma of the central nervous system. *Lancet* 1993; **342**: 398–401.

49 Editorial. Brain biopsy for intracranial mass lesion in AIDS. *Lancet* 1992; **340**: 1135.

50 Beral V, Peterman T, Berkelman R, Jaffe H. AIDS-associated non-Hodgkin lymphoma. *Lancet* 1991; **337**: 805–809.

51 Enting RH, Esselink RAJ, Portegies P. Lymphomatous meningitis in AIDS-related system non-Hodgkin's lymphoma: a report of eight cases. *J Neurosurg Psychiatry* 1994; **57**: 150–153.

52 Gisselbrecht C, Oksenhendler E, Tirelli U et al. Human immunodeficiency virus-related lymphoma treatment with intensive combination chemotherapy. *Am J Med* 1993; **95**: 188–196.

53 Fuller GN, Jacobs JM, Guiloff RM. Nature and incidence of peripheral nerve syndromes in HIV infection. *J Neurol Neurosurg Psychiatry* 1993; **56**: 372–381.

54 Berger AR, Arezzo JC, Schaumburg HH et al. 2′,3′-Dideoxycytidine (ddC) toxic neuropathy: a study of 52 patients. *Neurology* 1993; **43**: 358–362.

55 Browne MJ, Mayer KH, Chafee SBD et al. 2′,3′-Didehydro-3′-deoxythymidine (d4T) in patients with AIDS or AIDS-related complex: a phase I trial. *J Infect Dis* 1993; **167**: 21–29.

56 Lambert JS, Seidlin M, Reichman RC et al. 2′3′-Dideoxyinosine (ddI) in patients with the acquired immunodeficiency syndrome or AIDS-related complex: a phase I trial. *N Engl J Med* 1990; **322**: 1333–1340.

57 Lange D. AAEM minimonograph #4: neuromuscular diseases associated with HIV-1 infection. *Muscle Nerve* 1994; **17**: 16–30.

58 Simpson DM, Citak KA, Godfrey E, Godbold J, Wolfe DE. Myopathies associated with human immunodeficiency virus and zidovudine: can their effects be distinguished? *Neurology* 1993; **43**: 971–976.

11 NEUROLOGICAL IMAGING: CT AND MRI

Philip B. Harrison

Introduction

Neurological involvement in AIDS is common. A total of 10–20% of patients with acquired immune deficiency sydrome (AIDS) will present with neurologic disease and up to 39% will have neurological involvement clinically at some point in their illness. Seventy-nine per cent of patients dying with AIDS will show central nervous system (CNS) disease. Of this group, one-third die with a profound subcortical dementia secondary to human immune deficiency virus (HIV) brain infection. This represents a major cause of morbidity in these patients [1].

The greatest benefit of cranial imaging in AIDS patients is the identification of a lesion for which effective treatment is available. Unfortunately, this group represents a minority of HIV-positive patients who present with neurological disease. CNS signs and symptoms, particularly dementia, usually herald accelerated overall clinical deterioration. Even when untreatable disease is suspected, imaging may be helpful in establishing a prognosis, at least in the short term. In a review of 41 AIDS patients with computed tomography (CT) or magnetic resonance imaging (MRI) brain scans, Mundinger described a correlation between the grade of intracranial disease at imaging and shortening of survival times. The mean survival in AIDS patients with normal scans was 700 days, but this decreased dramatically when atrophy (326 days) or focal disease (202 days) was shown. When both were present survival dropped to 78 days [2].

The brain may be involved by a variety of disease processes when immunity is suppressed as a result of HIV infection. HIV itself has been implicated in acute meningoencephalitis, a more indolent leukoencephalopathy associated with atrophy, and in the increased frequency of cortical infarction demonstrated in these patients. Parasitic opportunistic infections (toxoplasmosis, amebiasis), and mycobacterial and spirochete

infections occur with increased frequency as do infections with papovavirus, cytomegalovirus, and other herpes infections. Of the neoplastic complications of AIDS, the commonest by far is primary CNS lymphoma. Its imaging features bear both significant differences from primary brain lymphoma in immune competent individuals, and similarities to the parasitic and mycobacterial infections often encountered in AIDS. In addition, the clinical presentation with most of these illnesses is protean, and laboratory analysis may offer little help in arriving at an accurate diagnosis. As a result, frequent disagreement occurs between the diagnoses reached after biopsy or autopsy, and those suspected based on clinical and laboratory grounds alone. In a series of 56 patients with AIDS, Anson showed that in patients undergoing biopsy, only 70% of preoperative diagnoses were confirmed, and that less than 50% of antemortem diagnoses were supported at autopsy. Even those brains from neurologically asymptomatic patients harbored significant abnormalities 50% of the time [3]. Since an accurate diagnosis often follows tissue analysis, imaging also becomes helpful when it lends strength to the argument for early biopsy, particularly when the clinical and scan features implicate a treatable lesion.

A history of HIV positivity and the identification of an imaging abnormality brings to mind a short list of the unusual infectious and neoplastic complications which are seen with increased frequency in these patients (*Table 11.1*). It is important to remember that some of these complications only occur when the patient is both infected with HIV and is immune suppressed. When an imaging abnormality is found, knowledge of the CD4 count as a measure of immunosuppression is helpful in developing a rational differential diagnosis. Many patients who contract Kaposi's sarcoma or systemic lymphoma have normal CD4 counts. Patients who develop *Pneumocystis carinii* pneumonia and toxoplasmosis usually show quite

Table 11.1 Common causes of abnormal cranial imaging in AIDS.

Mass effect present	Mass effect absent
Toxoplasmosis	PML
Primary CNS lymphoma	HIV encephalitis
Cryptococcal disease	CMV encephalitis
Other infections	
Herpes simplex/zoster	
M. tuberculosis	
M. avium intracellulare	
T. pallidum	
Fungi	
Aspergillosis	
Candidiasis	
Nocardiosis	
Coccidioidomycosis	
Amebiasis	
Infarction (acute)	

marked immune suppression, with counts less than 200. Patients who develop *Mycobacterium avium intracellulare* and primary brain lymphoma usually are severely immunosuppressed with counts less than 50.

Imaging findings

Cranial CT and MRI are the most sensitive and specific modalities for imaging the intracranial complications of AIDS. With a few exceptions, these diagnoses can be grouped into those conditions with, and those without mass effect at imaging. Those showing mass effect frequently have a specific treatment available.

Intracranial lesions with mass effect

1. Toxoplasmosis

Toxoplasma gondii is a parasitic intracellular protozoan for whom the cat is the final host. Oocysts are released by the feline gut and transformed in the soil to sporozoites which are ingested by birds, mice, sheep, and pigs. Cats are reinfected through predation on small animals. Transmission to humans occurs through the ingestion of undercooked pork and mutton, or through direct fecal-oral contamination from soil. In humans, toxoplasma tissue cysts are found in skeletal muscle, heart, and brain, and contain viable tachyzoites

which are periodically released and destroyed by the immunologically intact host. Individuals with suppressed immunity are unable to kill *Toxoplasma* tachyzoites, and reactivation infection ensues [4]. Typically reactivation foci in the brain do not encapsulate. The lesions show a hypovascular center, a vascular rim of subacute inflammatory tissue, and an outer zone with less marked vascularity. The viable organisms tend to be clustered around small vessels [5].

Patients with reactivation toxoplasmosis frequently have no focal clinical findings, and usually present with fever, headache, and behavioral disturbances. The median CD4 count is 48, and these patients are almost always seropositive [6]. Treatment with pyrimethamine and sulfadiazine produce clinical and radiological improvement in 1–2 weeks in 75–89% of patients. However, organisms remain viable within tissue cysts, and therapy must be maintained for life. Relapse occurs in 25–80% of patients, often at the site of previously documented infection [8].

The imaging features of reactivation toxoplasmosis in AIDS patients are non-specific. Since the initial, usually subclinical, dissemination to brain is hematogenous, the distribution of intracranial foci in reactivation disease is similar to other infectious and neoplastic diseases which seed the brain through the circulation. The cerebral hemispheres are more frequently affected than the cerebellum and brainstem, and tend to be involved close to the corticomedullary junctions and within the basal ganglia, where small end arteries were embolized during the primary infection.

CT or MRI is the mainstay of lesion detection. On cranial CT, 82% of lesions are hypodense prior to contrast medium administration. On these examinations, the inflammatory focus lesion cannot be distinguished from the surrounding edema. While most lesions will eventually show contrast-medium enhancement, this feature may be absent in up to 20% of lesions. When lesion enhancement does occur, it is usually well defined and annular, or less commonly nodular and may rarely be subependymal, mimicking a more infiltrative disorder, for example, primary lymphoma [7]. Localization of contrast in the lesion is due to a combination of the inflammation-related neovascularity present in the margins of the lesion and to disruption of the blood brain barrier. The number of lesions and the intensity of their contrast enhancement is, in part, technique dependent. When a double-dose delayed technique is employed, more nodules are seen and the lesions are more frequently

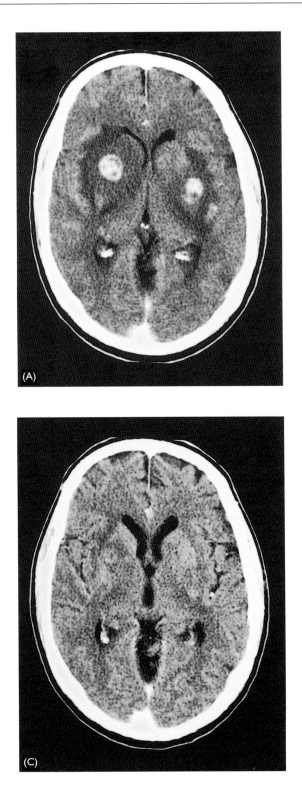

(A)

(C)

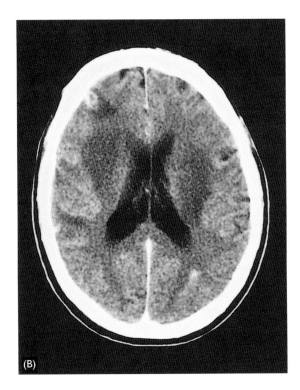

(B)

Figure 11.1   Toxoplasmosis: enhanced CT shows bilateral ganglionic mixed density lesions surrounded by vasogenic edema and signs of mass effect (A), with other nodules located at the corticomedullary junctions (B). After 17 days of antitoxoplasmosis therapy, the lesions have regressed (C).

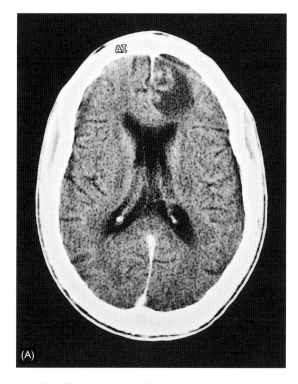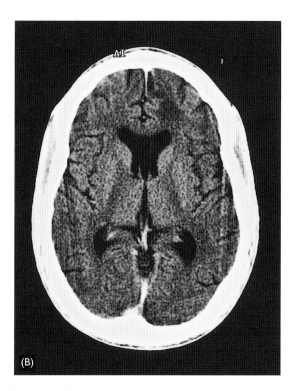

Figure 11.2. Toxoplasmosis: (A) a solitary superficially located ring lesion with surrounding vasogenic edema and central hyperdensity decreases in size and density over 13 days of treatment (B). Brain size also has decreased.

nodular due to uptake of contrast in the less vascular center of the lesion [8]. The vasogenic edema associated with toxoplasmosis is characteristically seen in the centrum semiovale and in diencephalic white matter tracts (Figure 11.1). Calcification can occur following treatment and is more readily seen with CT than with MRI.

MRI demonstrates more lesions than does CT. The foci are usually of increased signal on long repetition time images, occasionally with isointense or hypointense centers. On short TR images they are hypointense and show enhancement characteristics similar to CT. The hemorrhage that occasionally occurs in these lesions is more readily appreciated with MRI (Figure 11.3) [9]. While contrast administration is essential in identifying and characterizing lesions demonstrated with CT, MRI can reliably detect toxoplasmosis foci without the use of contrast enhancement owing to its superior ability to resolve differences in tissue contrast [10]. However, gadolinium compounds are helpful in further characterizing these lesions and aid in establishing a more accurate diagnosis.

Following treatment with pyrimethamine and sulfadiazine or clindamycin, both radiological and clinical improvement occurs in the majority of patients (Figure 11.2). Resolution of lesions on CT is not diagnostic of toxoplasmosis, and spontaneous regression of primary CNS lymphoma may be coincidentally seen during a course of antitoxoplasmosis therapy (Figure 11.5) [11].

Acute dissemination of the organism to the brain with abrupt neurologic decline may occur and show little or no evidence of the infection at imaging [12]. These patients present with diffuse encephalopathy which often is rapidly progressive and characteristically associated with fever, helping differentiate it from the other causes of acute encephalopathy seen in AIDS patients. In the four cases reported by Gray [12], only one focal CT abnormality was demonstrated, a small enhancing nodule in the internal capsule. As imaging contributes little, the institution of appropriate therapy rests on clinical suspicion in a patient with abrupt global neurological decline and fever.

Toxoplasmosis may mimic primary brain lymphoma, the second most frequent cause of a focal CNS lesion in AIDS patients. Differentiation of the two is in part statistical, and reflects the local seroprevalence of *T. gondii* infection. Within the USA toxoplasmosis

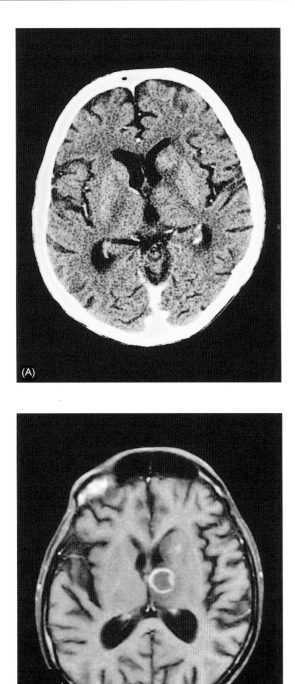

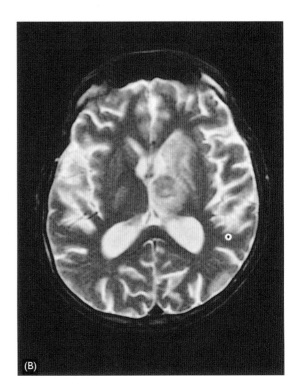

Figure 11.3. Toxoplasmosis: a mildly enhancing mass surrounded by vasogenic edema is located in the left caudate head. (A) On MRI scans the caudate lesion is mildly hyperintense on long TR sequences. (B) A second mass barely perceptible on CT lies in the anterior left thalamus. (C) Following gadolinium administration, both lesions show enhancement.

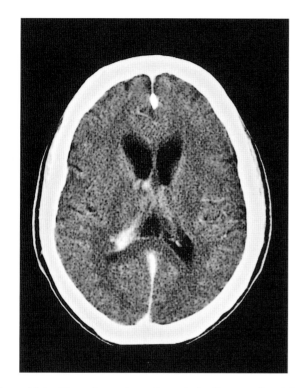

Figure 11.4. Toxoplasmosis: periventricular linear and nodular enhancement. The peritrigonal lesion was confirmed as toxoplasmosis following biopsy. There was no evidence of lymphoma in the specimen.

prevalence estimates range from 3% (western regions) to 70% (southeast coast), and undoubtedly influences the relative proportions of AIDS patients encountered with toxoplasmosis and lymphoma. In North America, published ratios of toxoplasmosis to brain lymphoma in AIDS patients vary from 1:1 to 15:1 [8]. Toxoplasmosis is a commonly seen CNS complication in AIDS populations in France and Germany, and in the Caribbean where seroprevalence for the organism approaches 90%. Geographic variation in seroprevalence has been attributed to cultural variations in diet, particularly the practice of ingesting undercooked meat, and to poor standards of public health [4].

2. Primary brain lymphoma

Primary CNS lymphoma in the immunocompetent patient is an uncommon disease, accounting for 1–1.5% of all primary brain tumors, but has been reported with increased frequency in transplant patients treated with immunosuppressives. The spread of the HIV in the last 15 years has also seen a dramatic increase in the incidence of this tumor, with estimates of its prevalence in the AIDS population approaching 2.5% [13,14]. After toxoplasmosis, focal intracranial lymphomatous masses are now the second most

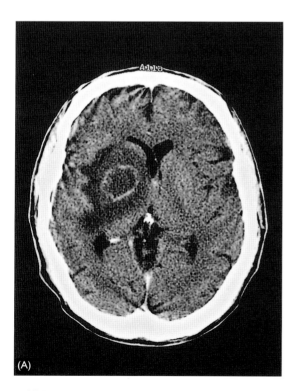

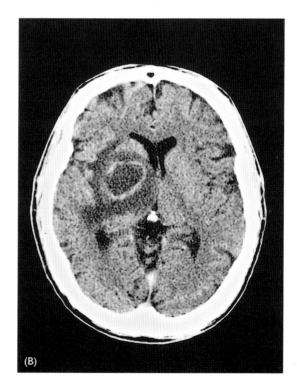

Figure 11.5. Toxoplasmosis: a ring of enhancement enclosing low-density change with surrounding vasogenic edema demonstrates little response to 2 weeks of antitoxoplasmosis therapy in hospital (A,B).

common focal brain lesions encountered in adults with AIDS in most published series. In North American young men this neoplasm is now more common than low-grade astrocytoma, and is almost as common as meningioma. Pathologically, it is typically a large-cell immunoblastic tumor, and is usually both monoclonal and Epstein-Barr virus (EBV) positive. In contrast, only half of systemic lymphomas are monoclonal, and the rate of EBV positivity is much lower. Since intracranial lymphoma in AIDS patients is often multifocal, this neoplasm may develop as a result of failure of the immune system to limit the normal lymphoproliferative response following infection of the brain with EBV [13,15].

Similar to that seen in toxoplasmosis, the clinical presentation of lymphoma patients is non-specific, most presenting with headache and behavioral disturbance. A focal deficit is uncommon. Once imaging has confirmed intracranial disease in AIDS patients with lymphoma, the course is an aggressive one, with 75% of untreated patients being dead in 4–6 weeks. Radiotherapy offers some hope as these tumors are radiosensitive. Irradiation stabilizes disease progression or offers improvement in 85%, and increases mean survival time from 1.5 to 4.5 months. As a rule,

responders die not of tumor progression, but of opportunistic infection [13,16]. Patients with lymphoma benefit most from early biopsy and radiation.

AIDS patients with primary CNS lymphoma demonstrate lesions which are well seen with CT and MRI, although both modalities underestimate the true extent of disease. On CT, lymphomatous masses are typically multiple and are isodense or less commonly, hyperdense prior to contrast administration. They are well seen in the striatum, where mass effect on adjacent ventricular walls may be visible (Figure 11.8). Involvement of the hemispheric white matter and periventricular supratentorial brain is usual with imaging evidence of infratentorial involvement occurring less commonly (Figures 11.6 and 11.10). Most parenchymal deposits in the brains of AIDS patients are shown to best advantage on CT following contrast-medium administration, after which up to 80% will enhance strongly in a rounded or oval nodular fashion [17]. When deposits are large, ring enhancement is seen, and this may be due to delayed penetration of contrast into the center of the lesion or to central necrosis. Linear and nodular subpial and subependymal enhancement is characteristic of this disease (Figure 11.7), and such involvement helps differentiate these

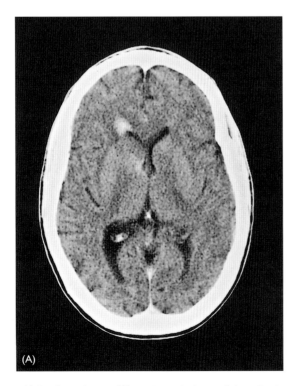

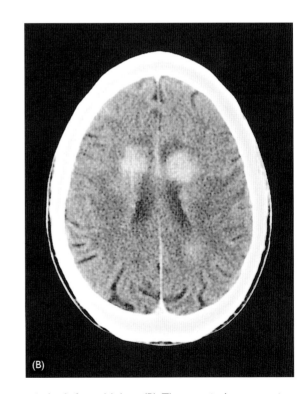

Figure 11.6. Lymphoma: (A) periventricular nodules of enhancement are seen in both frontal lobes. (B) The ventricular system is compressed, but little edema is seen.

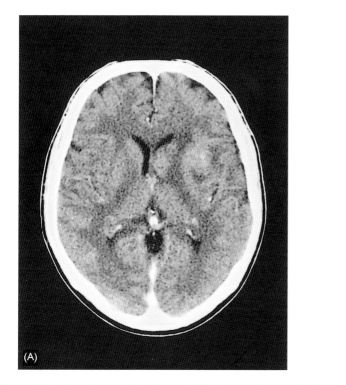
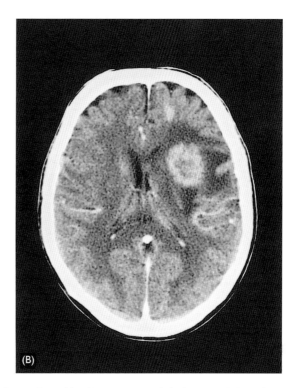

Figure 11.7.   Lymphoma: (A) enhanced CT shows edema in the left internal capsule, mild enhancement and thickening of the left caudate head and distortion of the left subinsular white-gray pattern. (B) Twenty-four days later, faint subependymal enhancement has developed, a discrete mass has formed in the left basal ganglia, and a second nodular becomes apparent in the left frontal pole.

lesions from other AIDS-related CNS complications which show mass effect [8]. The propensity to involve regions close to the brain surface is probably related to the perivascular pattern of brain infiltration characteristically identified at autopsy. The amount of surrounding vasogenic edema is quite variable, ranging from none at all to a marked degree. Typically, the amount of edema is less than is found with toxoplasmosis.

In comparison with enhanced CT, unenhanced MRI is more sensitive in detecting lymphomatous deposits and may be advantageous over CT in demonstrating imaging features more typical of lymphoma. Lymphoma is more likely to present with a single intracranial mass than toxoplasmosis. In patients in whom only one mass lesion is seen on MRI, the probability of lymphoma is 71% [16]. In addition to weighting the diagnosis in favor of lymphoma, MRI is also of value in identifying surgically accessible lesions when biopsy is being considered [10]. Prior to contrast administration the lesions are usually hypointense on T_1-weighted images and are indistinguishable from surrounding vasogenic edema. In a minority of lesions the isointense deposit may become visible on MRI when its margins are defined by

abnormal signal changes in surrounding edematous brain. The T_2-weighted image appearance is more variable. Relative to gray matter, areas of increased, isointense and decreased signal may be seen in the masses (Figure 11.9). Following contrast administration, lesions visible on unenhanced scans are almost always contrast avid. Typically, the center of the lesions remains hypointense while the margins enhance in a smooth or irregular ring-like fashion [17]. As is also seen in patients with toxoplasmosis, contrast administration appears to confer no advantage in the detection of lesions with MRI, but is of help in characterizing them.

AIDS-related primary CNS lymphoma shows imaging features which differentiate it from primary CNS lymphoma identified in patients with normal immune function. AIDS patients with CNS lymphoma will usually have more lesions than non-AIDS patients, and the lesions are more likely to show inhomogenous enhancement, or even ring enhancement, owing to the higher incidence of central necrosis in AIDS-related lymphoma. Also, infratentorial involvement is less common in AIDS than non-AIDS lymphoma patients [18].

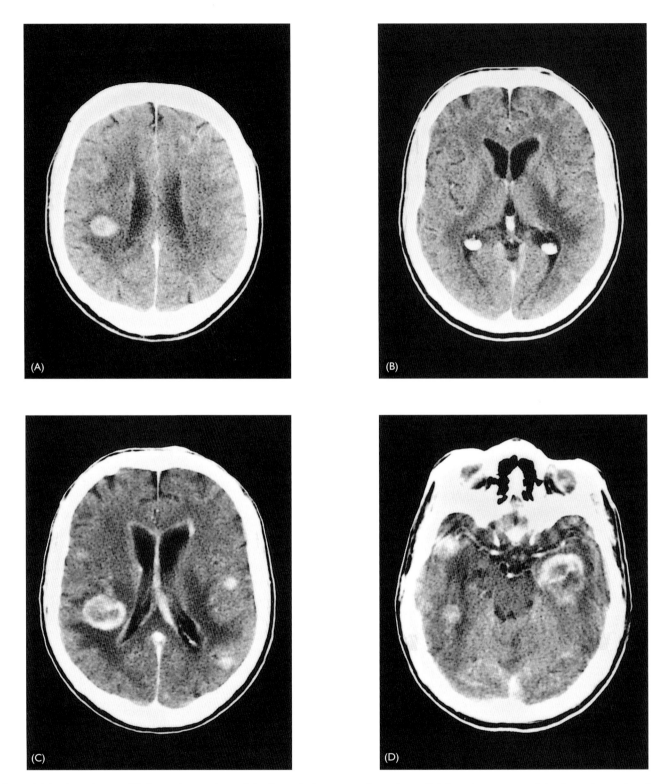

Figure 11.8. Lymphoma: (A) 2–cm deep right nodule shows little surrounding edema. Subtle enhancement of the frontal ependymal margins bilaterally is also seen (B) as well as edema in the left temporal lobe and subinsular brain. After 15 days of antitoxoplasmosis therapy, the right hemisphere lesion has increased in size, the ependymal enhancement has thickened, and multiple new lesions have become apparent (C,D).

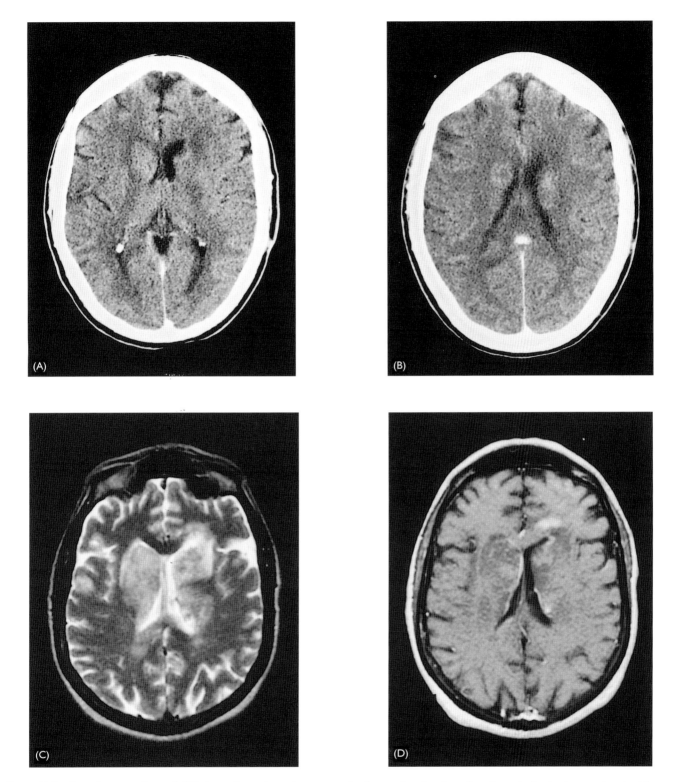

Figure 11.9. Lymphoma: enhanced CT shows irregular enhancement in the caudate heads and periventricular brain associated with ventricular compression and mild adjacent edema (A,B). MRI demonstrates mildly hyperintense heterogeneous lesions in the periventricular brain (C) which show linear and nodular areas of enhancement (D).

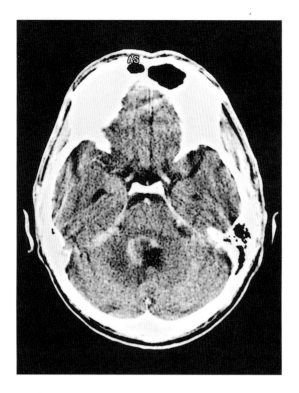

Figure 11.10. Lymphoma: enhanced CT demonstrates a ring lesion associated with surrounding edema adjacent to the fourth ventricle.

The imaging features of primary CNS lymphoma are not pathognomonic and accurate differentiation of toxoplasmosis from lymphoma based on CT and MR imaging appearances is presently not possible (Figure 11.4), but scintigraphy may be of help. In a review of 37 AIDS patients with intracranial masses reported by Ruiz, 12 patients with primary CNS lymphoma could be differentiated from 24 patients with toxoplasmosis and 1 with tuberculosis based on uptake of thallium-201 [19]. Given scintigraphic and imaging characteristics appropriate for lymphoma, a strong argument can be made for early biopsy and irradiation.

3. Cryptococcal disease

Cryptococcus neoformans is the most common fungus to infect the brain, and represents the third commonest intracranial pathogen identified in patients with AIDS, following HIV and *Toxoplasma gondii*. Up to 7% of patients with AIDS will have intracranial infection at autopsy, but as many as 20% of these patients may have no signs or symptoms of neurologic disease. When symptomatic, infected patients usually present with fever, headache, and other non-specific clinical findings which fail to differentiate cryptococcosis from

other complications of AIDS. The diagnosis in the majority of cases rests with the determination of cryptococcal antigen titers in the blood or spinal fluid [20]. Treatment involves a course of amphotericin B, with or without flucytosine.

Brain infection follows inhalation of the organism, and hematogenous dissemination from the lungs to the brain. The majority of patients who present with symptoms of cryptococcal disease show clinical evidence of meningitis. Once the meninges are involved, the organism may seed the Virchow-Robin spaces, where they proliferate, dilating the perivascular spaces and eventually rupturing into adjacent brain to form cryptococcomas or gelatinous pseudocysts [21]. Little inflammatory reaction surrounds these dilated perivascular spaces filled with organisms. Imaging with CT and MRI in patients with meningitis usually demonstrates no abnormalities related to the fungal infection. Occasional reports of meningeal enhancement with MRI, but not with CT, may be related to the high incidence of multiple intracranial pathogens often found in these patients.

Cryptococcomas are most frequently seen in those portions of the brain where perivascular spaces are commonly seen at MRI, such as the basal ganglia, the thalami, and the midbrain. They may also be seen in the corpus callosum and cerebral cortex, as well as other posterior fossa sites. On CT images, cryptococcomas are spherical, well defined, and are isodense or hypodense. The corresponding lesions on MR images demonstrate high signal on long TR images and decreased signal on short TR images. In addition, perivascular spaces dilated to 3 mm or greater are frequently visible at MRI but may not be seen on CT images. Contrast enhancement and surrounding vasogenic edema are not seen on either CT or MRI, in AIDS-related cryptococcomas. The host's altered inflammatory response secondary to AIDS undoubtedly plays a role in the lack of enhancement seen with intracranial cryptococcosis. In addition, the organism's polysaccharide coat, which gives the gelatinous appearance to the pseudocysts, may also play a role in suppressing inflammation. CNS cryptococcal infections in immunocompetent patients more commonly show enhancement on both CT and MRI [21] (Figure 11.11).

4. Other lesions with mass effect

A variety of other disorders can involve the brain, and may be identified by the presence of mass effect. These

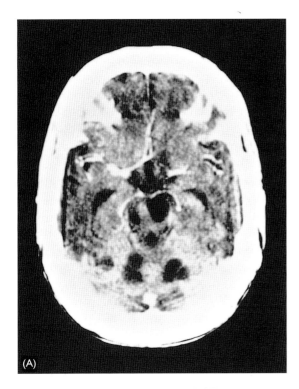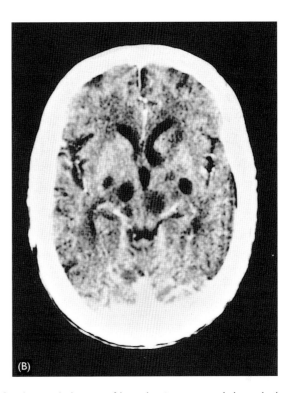

Figure 11.11.   Cryptococcosis: enhanced CT demonstrates multiple well-defined, rounded areas of hypodensity scattered through the cerebellum, midbrain (A) and basal ganglia (B).

are usually viral, bacterial, or fungal infections, but can be due to acute ischemia or to spread from Kaposi's sarcoma or other malignancies.

Intracranial *Herpes simplex* and *Herpes zoster* are infrequent complications of AIDS. Both organisms may produce an encephalitis or ventriculitis which can spread caudally to cause a necrotizing vasculitis of the entire cord and spinal roots. The intracranial changes at pathology may mimic those seen with cytomegalovirus (CMV) ventriculo-ependymitis, and as with CMV, these infections are not usually diagnosed before death. Herpes encephalitis in AIDS patients is distinguished from the predominantly frontotemporal distribution seen in immunocompetent patients by more diffusely involving the brain [22]. Imaging may demonstrate generalized swelling, abnormal density or signal changes in white matter, and rarely cortical enhancement.

Disseminated infection by *Mycobacterium tuberculosis* or *M. avium intracellulare* both occur with increased frequency in AIDS patients and are similarly indistinguishable from the more common infections and neoplasms seen in the brains of AIDS patients. Tuberculosis in particular may pursue a more fulminant course in AIDS patients owing to the host's impaired ability to form the epithelioid granulomata necessary to combat the infection. This disease is reportedly more common in AIDS which has occurred secondary to intravenous drug use. These patients frequently present with hydrocephalus, meningeal enhancement, and less commonly with parenchymal involvement. Deep zones of infarction are particularly common in this disease, and lie in the distribution of the perforating end arteries at the base of the brain. When parenchymal enhancement occurs, it is most commonly ring-like or nodular, and indistinguishable from toxoplasmosis or lymphoma, but may be gyral. MRI will demonstrate a greater number of lesions than CT [23].

Syphilis also occurs with increased frequency and similarly pursues a more rapid course in AIDS patients [24]. Gummata are poorly formed in AIDS patients and as these are a marker for the cell-mediated immune response to the organism and serve to help limit the infection, neurosyphilis in the HIV-infected patient can progress rapidly to tertiary and quaternary forms. AIDS patients with syphilis more frequently present with its meningovascular form and, as with tuberculosis, develop infarction owing to occlusion of basal vessels [25].

In addition to cryptococcosis, other fungal brain infections occur with increased frequency in the setting of immune suppression, including coccidioidomycosis, histoplasmosis, and mucormycosis. Unlike crypto-coccal disease, these diseases will often show ring or nodular enhancement indistinguishable from the more common causes of focal brain masses in AIDS. Candidiasis and aspergillosis may be suspected when hemorrhage is identified. These organisms produce an arteritis which causes infarction and bleeding since an intracranial enhancing focus. Although both CT and MRI may be used to demonstrate bleeding, since the clinical course is usually a rapid one and the hemorrhage is acute, and CT scanning is often adequate to prompt early biopsy.

HIV infection is a risk factor for brain infarction. The reason for its increased prevalence in AIDS patients is presently unknown. It has been postulated that inanition, the perivascular localization of CMV and HIV recovered from the brains of patients with AIDS, and the angiocentric nature of lymphomatous infiltration partly explain this propensity to stroke [26]. There are no distinguishing features of the cortical or deep infarcts seen in adults with AIDS. In children with AIDS, symmetrical calcification of the basal ganglia will occasionally be seen and may be associated with enhancement. At autopsy these changes are due to small-vessel inflammation possibly with infarction, and likely reflect the deep and perivascular localization of HIV [27]. Such calcification and enhancement is a rare observation in adults.

Intracranial lesions without mass effect

Those disorders involving the brain with increased frequency in AIDS and which produce abnormal changes without mass effect at imaging can be grouped into complications producing focal abnormalities, and those which produce diffuse and symmetrical abnormal changes in the brain. In general, effective treatment for these latter conditions is not presently available.

1. Atrophy

Generalized brain atrophy is the most common post-mortem finding in the brains of patients who die with AIDS, with reported series estimating an incidence of 31–84% of autopsies. Atrophy is observed more commonly as patients develop more of the complications of AIDS. Signs of cerebral tissue loss are visible on the scans of 31% asymptomatic HIV-

positive patients, in 59% of patients with AIDS-related complex, and in 70% of patients who fulfill the diagnostic criteria for AIDS [25]. The presence of atrophy correlates with cognitive impairment, including memory difficulties, problem-solving errors, motor control, and, ultimately, dementia. The correlation between the severity of imaging abnormality and the degree of cognitive impairment is generally poor, and depends on the method chosen to measure atrophy, and the sensitivity of the neuropsychological testing [28]. Overtly demented patients, on the other hand, almost always shows signs of atrophy, which is predominately seen in the deep regions and spares the cortex. The atrophy visible on CT and MR images is supra-tentorial in almost all patients but may be seen infratentorially in up to 70%. The changes may progress rapidly (Figure 11.13), with serial scanning in one study demonstrating worsening at 1 year in 60% of patients [29]. Such a rapid course is more typical of patients who have begun to show cognitive decline. When neurological symptoms are lacking, progression is more indolent [30].

The tissue loss appears to develop in specific regions of the deep brain. In a sample of 139 AIDS patients,

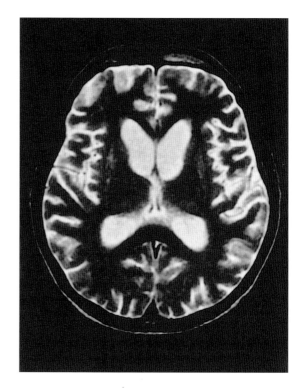

Figure 11.12. Central atrophy: 34-year-old demented male with disproportionate ventricular enlargement compared to the degree of sulcal widening. The caudate heads are particularly atrophic.

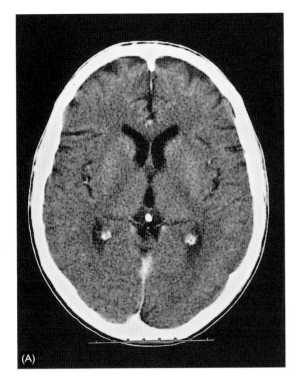

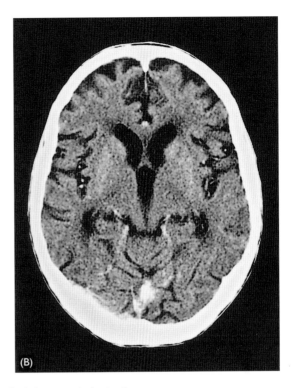

Figure 11.13. Progressive atrophy: (A,B) scans 18 months apart show a marked decrease in brain size.

Dal Pan demonstrated that the bicaudate ratio (BCR) was significantly higher in demented patients when compared with otherwise normal patients or with those with mild cognitive deficits. Caudate head atrophy (or atrophy of the adjacent white matter as measured by the BCR) appears to be strongly correlated with HIV dementia, and supports the clinical impression that the dementia seen in AIDS is predominately subcortical (Figure 11.12). The so-called 'cortical atrophy' on CT and MRI brain scans of AIDS patients probably represents widened sulci secondary to tissue loss in the deeper regions of the brain, and not primarily to cellular loss in the cortical layers [31] (Figure 11.13). This is supported by the observation that, in autopsied patients with HIV encephalitis, HIV glycoproteins are more abundantly recovered from deep parts of the brain, and are scant in the cortex [26].

2. Progressive multifocal leuko-encephalopathy

Progressive multifocal leukoencephalopathy (PML) or Richardson's disease occurs as a result of brain infection with the JC virus, a member of the papova virus group. The organism is ubiquitous and the infection is common, with 80% of the normal adult population being seropositive. The virus appears to reside in the kidney in the asymptomatic adult, and can pass to the brain within infected lymphocytes. Suppression of host immunity allows the organism to proliferate unchecked, and brain infection is incited. Such evidence of brain infection is frequent in the immune suppressed population and can be recovered from the brains of up to 7% of AIDS patients at autopsy [32]. As a rule, HIV-positive patients with clinical evidence of this infection show quite marked immune suppression, and have CD4 counts of less than 100. Unlike those who present with many other infectious and neoplastic complications of AIDS, patients with PML classically present with a focal neurologic deficit, rather than a general decline in mental faculties. No current treatment has proven effective for these patients, and death usually ensues within 9 months.

The CT and MRI appearance reflects the underlying pathophysiology. Once 'trojan horse' lymphocytes bearing the organism enter the brain, the virus enters and destroys oligodendrocytes, cells which normally maintain and produce myelin. The resultant demyelination involves primarily subcortical 'U' or arcuate fibers which lie in the white matter at the corticomedullary junctions, particularly those in the

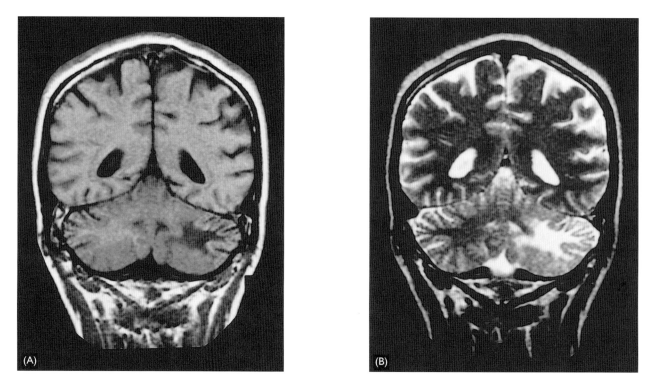

Figure 11.14. PML: (A,B) T_1 and T_2-weighted (TR, 500; TE, 20/Fr) (TR, 4116; TE, 102/Ef) MR images demonstrate prolonged relaxation in the immediately subcortical cerebellar white matter. The cortex is uninvolved and no mass effect is shown.

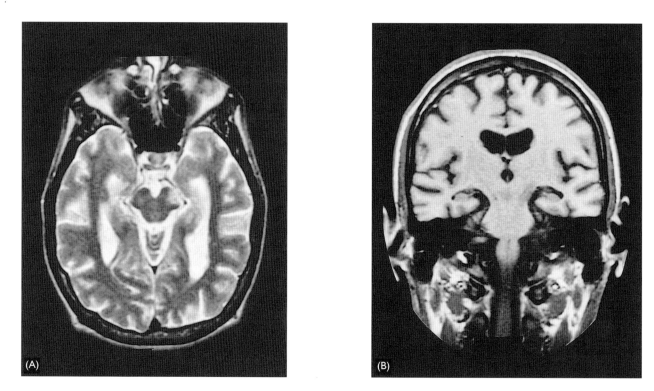

Figure 11.15. PML: (A,B) using MRI, the left crus cerebri shows a zone of high signal change on the long TR sequence (TR, 4000; TE, 102/Ef) (A), and diminished signal on the short TR sequence (TR, 450; TE, 20/Fr). (B) The changes are more easily discernible on T_2-weighted images.

frontal, parietal, and occipital lobes. CT reveals areas of diminished density which correspond with zones of increased signal on long TR images and decreased signal on short TR images on MRI scans (Figures 11.14 and 11.15). The lesions classically lie against the corticomedullary junction and, as the overlying cortical mantle shows little change, the junction appears abnormally accentuated on both CT and MRI scans (Figure 11.16). Uncommonly, the lesions of PML may also be found in gray matter, particularly deep gray matter, probably owing to involvement of white matter fiber tracts passing through deep nuclei (Figure 11.17). Posterior fossa involvement is common, and may be the only site of involvement visible at imaging in up to 10% of patients (Figure 11.19) [32]. Cervical cord involvement is uncommon [33]. Despite its name, the disease may only involve one site at imaging in as many as 23% of patients. The identification of a single lesion on MRI does not exclude the diagnosis. MRI is more sensitive than CT in demonstrating foci of demyelination with 44% more lesions being seen with MRI [34], particularly when short and long TR images in the coronal plane are obtained (Figure 11.18).

3. Focal white matter hyperintensities

Unlike the atrophy observed in HIV-positive patients, particularly those patients who fulfill the diagnostic criteria for AIDS, the demonstration of focal white matter hyperintensities (FWMH) is not significantly correlated with AIDS-related dementia [35]. There appears to be no significant difference between the frequency of small focal white matter abnormalities in HIV-infected individuals compared with their seronegative controls as demonstrated on long repetition time MRI. While most of both groups show no focal white matter abnormalities, a small proportion demonstrate between one and five hyperintensities [36]. Series examining white matter hyperintensities on the MRI scans of healthy older patients indicate that these likely represent zones of perivascular demyelination or are dilated perivascular spaces secondary to atrophy. It is probable that the same explanation holds true for younger patients regardless of seropositivity for the AIDS virus. The presence of these abnormalities does not predict HIV positivity and does not herald clinical decline in AIDS patients.

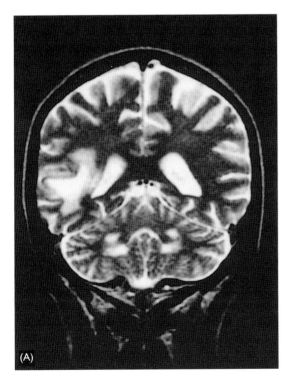

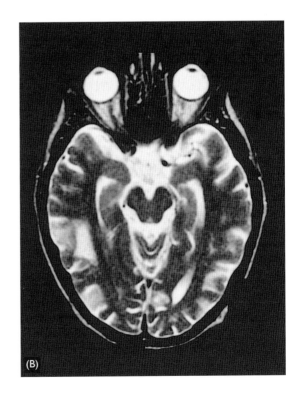

Figure 11.16. PML: using MRI, high signal change on long TR images involving the subcortical 'U' fibers is more graphically demonstrated with coronal (A) (TR, 4166; TE, 102/Ef) rather than axial imaging (TR, 4000; TE, 102/Ef) (B).

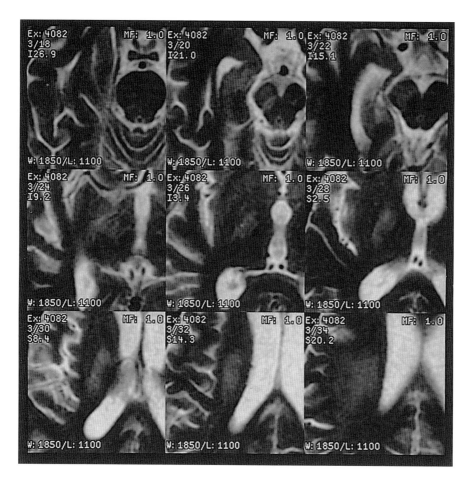

Figure 11.17.   PML: using MRI, an abnormal signal can be followed from the centrum semiovale through corticospinal fibrous tracts to the pons.

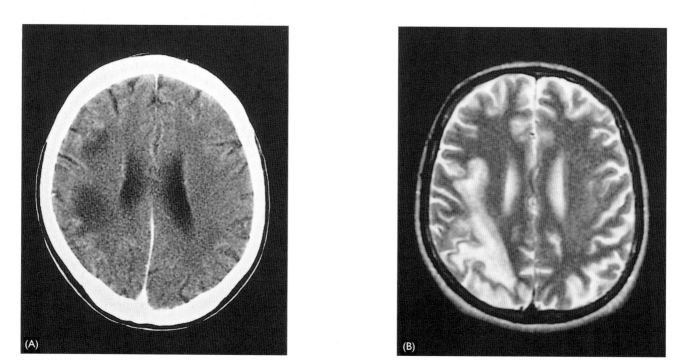

Figure 11.18.   PML: (A) enhanced CT shows two areas of low-density change in the immediately subcortical brain without enhancement or mass effect. (B) Long TR MR images confirm maximum involvement in the region of the subcortical arcuate fibers.

4. HIV encephalitis

Clinical and laboratory evidence of acute meningitis often accompanies HIV seroconversion, indicating that the brain is involved early in HIV infection [37]. Encephalitis is a common sequela of HIV infection and seroconversion, with histopathological evidence of the infection found in up to 30% of AIDS autopsies. If more sophisticated viral identification techniques are used, the true incidence of HIV infection at autopsy appears to be considerably higher, as 80% of patients will show immunocytological evidence of HIV in the brain. The microscopic diagnosis rests on the demonstration of the histological hallmarks of HIV encephalitis: angiocentric microglial nodules containing multinucleated giant cells, vacuolar myelin damage and diffuse myelin pallor owing to blood-brain barrier disruption [38–40].

The imaging features of HIV encephalitis are nonspecific, and consist of atrophy with deep white matter changes. Microglial nodules remain undetectable by CT but may rarely be seen by MRI when these microscopic lesions coalesce to form aggregate masses of greater than 3 mm. In a series of 24 patients with autopsy-proven HIV encephalitis, Chrysikopoulos found that, in patients with HIV encephalitis as the only abnormality at autopsy, 71% of patients demonstrated moderate to severe atrophy and 60% of these showed symmetrical diffuse or periventricular white matter disease without mass effect, manifested as areas of low attenuation on CT and high signal on long TR MR images [29]. Diffuse abnormal signal change without atrophy is rare. The combined imaging features of global atrophy and diffuse symmetrical white matter hyperintensity on T_2-weighted images, which respects the immediately subcortical brain, help differentiate HIV encephalitis from PML and from other disorders associated with mass effect (Figures 11.20 and 11.21).

Isolated HIV involvement of the brain is uncommon in autopsy series. In 70% of patients with HIV encephalitis identified at autopsy, other coexistent AIDS-related complications can be seen in the CNS. The commonest is CMV (38%) but less frequently toxoplasmosis, PML, lymphoma, or cryptococcal disease may also be present. The classic diffuse symmetrical imaging findings of HIV encephalitis may be obscured by these, and features atypical for encephalitis or focality suggest an alternative or second pathogen, or lymphoma [29].

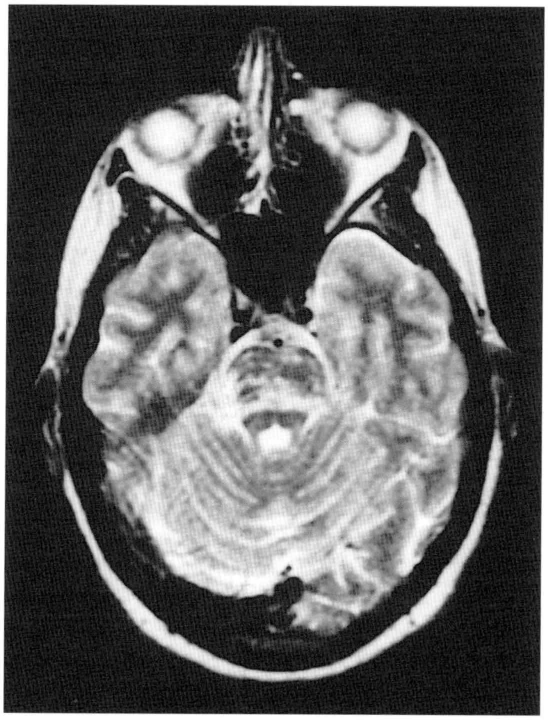

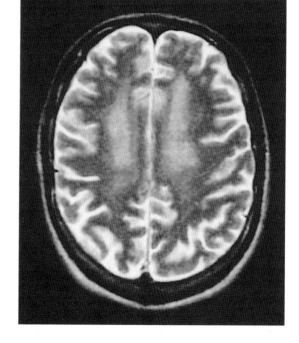

Figure 11.19. PML: using MRI, an abnormal T_2 prolongation (TR, 4000; TE, 102/Ef) outlines fiber tracts in the pons.

Figure 11.20. HIV encephalitis: using MRI, symmetrical areas of T_2 prolongation (TR, 4116; TE, 102/Ef) lie centrally in the corona radiata. Unlike PML, the changes do not extend to the corticomedullary junction.

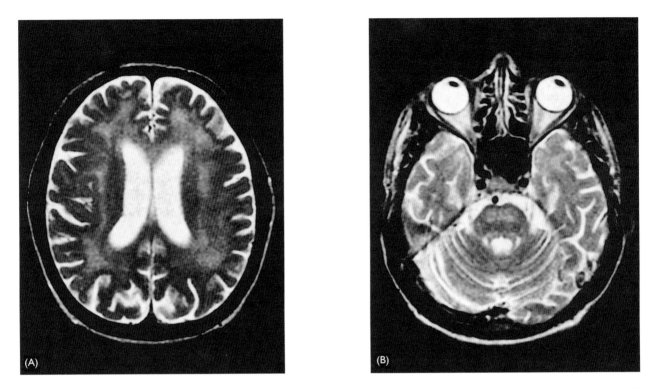

Figure 11.21. HIV encephalitis: using MRI, diffuse symmetrical T_2 hyperintensity in the centrum semiovale is shown (TR, 3733; TE, 96/Ef) (A). An increased signal extends caudally through the brainstem and into the pons (TR, 3733; TE, 96/Ef) (B).

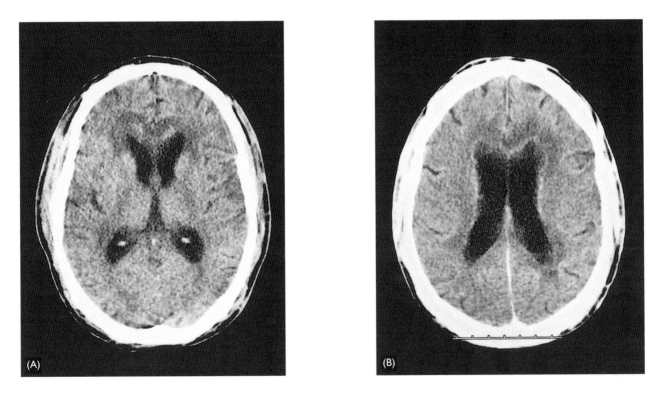

Figure 11.22. CMV ventriculo-ependymitis: bifrontal and periventricular mixed density change indicating hemorrhage with necrosis and edema. The scalp soft tissues are thickened from widespread Kaposi's sarcoma involvement (A). Faint enhancement outlining the ependymal margins with low-density change in the adjacent centrum semiovale likely representing edema and necrosis (B).

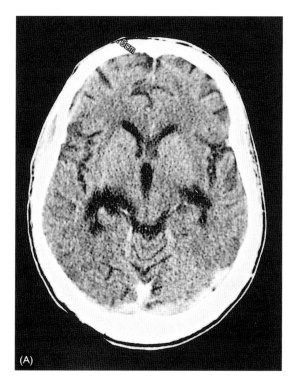

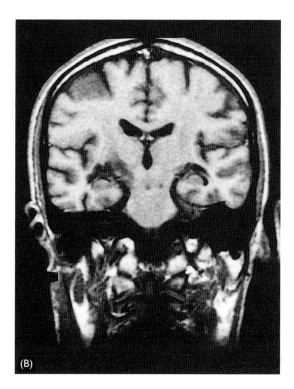

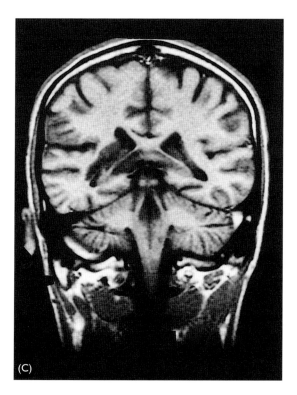

Figure 11.23. CMV ventriculo-ependymitis: the wings of both ambient cisterns are widened, and low-density change extends into the surrounding brain (A). Coronal MRI (TR, 383; TE, 16/Fr) shows prolonged T_1 relaxation in the posterior thalamus (B) and periventricular white matter (TR, 383; TE, 16/FR) (C).

Similar to the progression seen in patients with brain atrophy, progression of white matter disease on CT and MR images showing HIV encephalitis is usually seen only in those patients who are encephalopathic. The initial MR images in patients with rapid neurological decline frequently demonstrate more severe atrophy, and more extensive and confluent high signal than is seen in asymptomatic patients, and are more commonly associated with posterior fossa atrophy as opposed to isolated supratentorial atrophy [30].

5. Cytomegalovirus encephalitis

CMV CNS infection is most commonly seen in newborns as a congenitally acquired infection, or in immunocompromised patients [41]. In the neonate, CMV causes ependymal necrosis followed by calcification. CMV encephalitis also occurs in patients who are immunosuppressed as a result of organ transplantation or AIDS. It is most commonly manifested pathologically as microglial nodules which predominantly involve cortex, and is seen in up to 48% of autopsied cases. Of these 40% will also show an ependymitis which is similar to that seen in neonates [42]. The infected cells at both sites contain inclusion bodies classic for CMV. As a rule, no surrounding inflammation is seen. In AIDS patients the distribution of the pathologic changes contrasts with those of HIV encephalitis in which involvement of the deep brain is more characteristic. Unfortunately, the severity of CMV encephalitis demonstrated at autopsy correlates poorly with clinical findings and dementia. Therefore, the role that CMV encephalitis plays in the patient's neurological symptoms and clinical decline is often unclear, and may be difficult to separate from the effects of other coexistent diseases [43].

Clinically, patients with CMV ependymitis frequently present with ocular motor palsies and nystagmus, uncommon findings in the majority of AIDS patients. The diagnosis of CMV ependymitis can be suspected in the face of non-specific MRI findings when appropriate neuro-ophthalmologic abnormalities are elicited, and particularly when manifest evidence of an associated peripheral neuropathy or of radiculomyelitis. At autopsy, the commonest brain abnormalities due to CMV are vasculitis and, more commonly,

a necrotizing ependymitis. Patients with ventriculitis pursue a rapid downhill course, with time from presentation to death averaging 6 weeks.

Brain scanning with CT in these patients is usually normal, but may show progressive ventriculomegaly, and rarely may show smooth periventricular enhancement with compression of the ventricular margins (Figure 11.22). MRI is more sensitive in demonstrating evidence of a ventriculo-ependymitis. MRI demonstrated abnormal high signal change in the periventricular brain in five of six patients with CMV ependymitis at autopsy (Figure 11.23). This finding, however, is nonspecific and can also be seen with lymphoma [41].

Antiviral therapy with gancyclovir may be somewhat helpful, but the outlook is usually dismal for these patients.

Summary

Since the most easily treatable intracranial lesions are those with mass effect, and since imaging alone cannot reliably distinguish between them, an intracranial mass visible on CT or MRI should receive an antemortem diagnosis. The two commonest causes, lymphoma and toxoplasmosis, cannot usually be differentiated by imaging findings alone, as the individual lesions may appear identical in up to 80% of cases. The diagnosis of toxoplasmosis usually rests on the diagnosis of compatible lesions on CT or MRI, and both a clinical and an imaging response following an appropriate course of antitoxoplasmosis therapy. However, as primary CNS lymphoma in AIDS is aggressive, and the lesions may increase in number and size rapidly, the decision to biopsy mass lesions should be made as early as possible, determined both by the shortest effective antitoxoplasmosis therapeutic trial and the lack of conformity of the imaging with appearances typical for toxoplasmosis. Since toxoplasmosis shows features of a hematogenously borne inflammatory disease, which tends to seed the corticomedullary junctions, early biopsy should be considered when a single lesion is visible on MRI, when subependymal involvement is identified, or when enhancement is scant.

References

1   Levy RM, Rosenblum S, Perrett LV. Neuroradiologic findings in AIDS: review of 200 cases. *AJNR* 1986; **7**: 833–839.

2   Mundinger A, Adam T, Ott D et al. CT and MRI: prognostic tools in patients with AIDS and neurological deficits. *Neuroradiology* 1992; **35**: 75–78.

3   Anson, JA, Glick RP, Reyes M. Diagnostic accuracy of AIDS-related CNS lesions. *Surgi Neurol* 1992; **37**: 432–440.

4   Frenkel JK. Toxoplasmosis. In: Strickland GT (ed.) *Hunter's Tropical Medicine*, 7th edn. Philadelphia: WB Saunders, 1991: 658–662.

5   Donovan Post MJ, Chan JC, Hensley GT et al. Toxoplasma encephalitis in Haitian adults with acquired immunodeficiency syndrome: a clinical-pathologic-CT correlation. *AJNR* 1983; **4**: 155–162.

6   Reynold C, Sugar A, Chave J-P et al. Toxoplasma encephalitis in patients with the acquired immunodeficiency syndrome. *Medicine* 1992; **71**: 224–239.

7   Cohen W, Koslow M. An unusual presentation of cerebral toxoplasmosis. *J Comput Assist Tomogr* 1985; **9**: 384–385.

8   Harrison PB, Clarke SD, Silver SF. Focal brain lesions on computed tomography in patients with acquired immune deficiency syndrome. *J Can Assoc Radiol* 1990; **41**: 83–86.

9   Donovan Post MJ, Kursunoglu DJ, Hensley GT et al. Cranial CT in acquired immunodeficiency syndrome: spectrum of diseases and optimal contrast enhancement technique. *AJNR* 1985; **6**: 743–754.

10 Jensen MC, Brant-Zawadski M. MR Imaging of the brain in patients with AIDS: value of routine use of IV gadopentetate dimeglumine. *AJR* 1993; **160**: 153–157.

11 Terriff B, Harrison P, Holden JK. Apparent spontaneous regression of AIDS-related primary CNS lymphoma mimicking resolving toxoplasmosis. *J of Acquir Immune Defici Syndr* 1992; **5**: 953–954.

12 Gray F, Gherardi R, Wingate E et al. Diffuse 'encephalitic' cerebral toxoplasmosis in AIDS. *J Neurol* 1989; **236**: 273–277.

13 Baumgartner JE, Rachlin JR, Beckstead JH et al. Primary central nervous system lymphomas: natural history and response to radiation therapy in 55 patients with acquired immunodeficiency syndrome. *J Neurosurg* 1990; **73**: 201–211.

14 Levy RM, Janssen RS, Bush TJ et al. Neuroepidemiology of acquired immunodeficiency syndrome. In: Rosenblum ML, Levy RM, Bredesen DE (eds) *AIDS and the Nervous System*. New York: Raven Press, 1988: 13–27.

15 Morgello S, Laufer H. Quaternary neurosyphilis in a haitian man with human immunodeficiency virus infection. *Hum Pathol* 1989; **20**: 808–811.

16 Ciricillo SF, Rosenblum ML. Use of CT and MR imaging to distinguish intracranial lesion and to define the need for biopsy in AIDS patients. *J Neurosurg* 1990; **73**: 720–724.

17 Dina TS. Primary central nervous system lymphoma versus toxoplasmosis in AIDS. *Radiology* 1991; **179**: 823–828.

18 Lee Y-Y, Bruner JM, VanTassel P et al. Primary central nervous system lymphoma: CT and pathologic correlation. *AJR* 1986; **147**: 747–752.

19 Ruiz A, Ganz WI, Donovan Post J et al. Use of thallium-201 brain SPECT to differentiate cerebral lymphoma for toxoplasma encephalitis in AIDS patients. *AJNR* 1994; **15**: 1885–1894.

20 Chuck SL, Sande MA. Infections with Cryptococcus neoformans in the acquired immunodeficiency syndrome. *N Engl J Med* 1989; **321**: 794–799.

21 Matthews VP, Alo PL, Glass JD et al. AIDS-related CNS cryptococcosis: radiologic-pathologic correlation. *AJNR* 1992; **13**: 1477–1486.

22 Chretien F, Gray F, Lescs MC et al. Acute varicella-zoster virus ventriculitis and meningo-myelo-radiculitis in acquired immunodeficiency syndrome. *Acta Neuropath* 1993; **86**: 659–665.

23 Villoria MF, de la Torre J, Forgea F et al. Intracranial tuberculosis in AIDS: CT and MRI findings. *Neuroradiology* 1992; **34**: 11–14.

24 Nash G, Said JW. *Pathology of AIDS and HIV Infection*. Philadelphia; WB Saunders, 1992.

25 Raininko R, Elovaara I, Virta A et al. Radiological study of the brain at various stages of human immunodeficiency virus infection: early development of brain atrophy. *Neuroradiology* 1992; **33**: 190–196.

26 Smith, T, DeGirolami U, Henin D et al. Human immunodeficiency virus (HIV) leukoencephalopathy and the microcirculation. *J Neuropathol Exp Neurol* 1990; **49**: 357–370.

27 Epstein LG, Berman CZ, Sharer LR et al. Unilateral calcification and contrast enhancement of the basal ganglia in a child with AIDS encephalopathy. *AJNR* 1987; **8**: 163–165.

28 Levin HS, Williams DH, Borucki MJ et al. Magnetic resonance imaging and neuropsychological findings in human immunodeficiency virus infection. *J of Acquir Immune Defici Syndr* 1990; **3**: 757–762.

29 Chrysikopoulos HS, Press, GA, Grafe MR et al. Encephalitis caused by human immunodefiency virus: CT and MR imaging manifestations with clinical and pathologic correlation. *Radiology* 1990; **175**: 185–191.

30 Donovan Post MJ, Levin BE, Berger JR et al . Sequential cranial MR findings of asymptomatic and neurologically symptomatic HIV+ patients. *AJNR* 1992; **13**: 359–370.

31 Dal Pan G, McArthur J, Aylward E et al. Patterns of the cerebral atrophy in HIV-1–infected individuals: results of a quantitative MRI analysis. *Neurology* 1992; **42**: 2125–2130.

32 Hansman Whiteman ML, Donovan Post MJ, Berger JR et al. Progressive multifocal leukoencephalopathy in 47 HIV-seropositive patients: neuroimaging with clinical and pathologic correlation. *Radiology* 1993; **187**: 233–240.

33 von Einsiedel RW, Fife TD, Aksamit AJ et al. Progressive multifocal leukoencephalopathy in AIDS: a clinicopathologic study and review of the literature. *J Neurol* 1993; **240**: 391–406.

34 Karahalios D, Breit R, Dal Canto MC et al. Progressive multifocal leukoencephalopathy in patients with HIV infection: lack of impact of early diagnosis by stereotactic brain biopsy. *J of Acquir Immune Defici Syndr* 1992; **5**: 1030–1038.

35 Broderick D, Wippold F, Clifford D et al. White matter lesions and cerebral atrophy on MR images in patients with and without AIDS dementia complex. *AJR* 1993; **161**: 171–181.

36   McArthur J, Kumar A, Johnson D et al. Incidental white matter hyperintensities on magnetic resonance imaging in HIV-1 infection. *J of Acquir Immune Defici Syndr* 1990; **3**: 252–259.

37   Hollander H, Levy J. Neurologic abnormalities and recovery of human immunodeficiency virus from cerebral spinal fluid. *Ann Intern Med* 1987; **106**: 692–695.

38   Schmidbauer M, Huemer M, Cristina S et al. Morphological spectrum, distribution and clinical correlation of white matter lesions in AIDS brains. *Neuropath and Appl Neurobiol* 1992; **18**: 489–501.

39   Power C, Kong PA, Crawford TO et al. Cerebral white matter changes in acquired immunodeficiency syndrome dementia. *Ann Neurol* 1993; **34**: 339–350.

40   Masliah E, Achim CL, Ge N et al. Spectrum of human immunodeficiency virus-associated neocortical damage. *Ann Neurol* 1992; **32**: 321–329.

41   Kalayjian RC, Cohen ML, Bonomo RA et al. Cytomegalovirus ventriculoencephalitis in AIDS. A syndrome with distinct clinical and pathologic features. *Medicine* 1993; **72**: 67–77.

42   Wiley CA, Nelson JA. Role of human immunodefiecency virus and cytomegalovirus in AIDS encephalitis. *Am J Pathol* 1988; **133**: 73–81.

43   Navia BA, Cho ES, Petito CK et al. The AIDS dementia complex: II. neuropathology. *Ann Neurol* 1986; **19**: 525–535.

12 IMAGING OF CARDIAC INVOLVEMENT IN HIV DISEASE

Christopher R. Thompson
Marla C. Kiess

Introduction

Cardiovascular system involvement is common in patients with human immune deficiency virus (HIV) infection, particularly in those with advanced disease. Despite the high prevalence of cardiac involvement in acquired immune deficiency syndrome (AIDS), it is relatively uncommon for cardiovascular dysfunction to be responsible for the major symptoms of patients with AIDS or for hospital admission. Indeed, it has been estimated that less than 7% of HIV patients have symptomatic heart disease and that cardiac disease can be an expected cause of death in only 1–6% of cases [1]. Familiarity with cardiac involvement in AIDS is perhaps most important, then, to be able to distinguish the common, but clinically unimportant, from the uncommon, but clinically very important, disorders. Clinicians face patients with clinical syndromes of unknown etiology in whom it is important to establish the likely etiologies and patients with known infections in whom it is important to identify the organ systems involved. This chapter will first focus on the common forms of cardiac involvement in patients with AIDS, including pericardial effusion, ventricular dysfunction, endocarditis, and cardiac tumours, then explore the cardiac manifestations of various specific infections. Rather than attempting to encompass the potential uses and findings with each imaging modality, we have focused on those most commonly used for specific problems. Thus, echocardiography is emphasized for ventricular dysfunction but any available appropriate cardiac imaging modality such as magnetic resonance imaging (MRI), cine-computed tomography (CT), or radionuclide ventriculography could be substituted.

Clinical scenario

Patients with HIV infection commonly have intercurrent illnesses associated with dyspnea and labored breathing. If the jugular venous pressure is elevated and the cardiac silhouette is enlarged on chest radiograph, the possibility of pericardial effusion and cardiac tamponade should be entertained. Suspicion may be enhanced if the labored breathing causes exaggerated inspiratory and expiratory excursion in intrathoracic pressure, which results in the clinical observation of significant pulsus paradoxus. This clinical scenario is a quite common one, which results in an appropriate request for an echocardiogram. This echocardiogram would commonly reveal a small to moderate pericardial effusion with or without biventricular enlargement and significant ventricular dysfunction. What is the significance of these findings?

Pericardial effusion

The literature suggests that the prevalence of pericardial effusion in HIV-infected patients increases as the disease progresses (Tables 12.1, 12.2). Echocardiograms demonstrate the classic echo-free or echo-poor space separating the parietal pericardium from the epicardium. Levy et al. demonstrated pericardial effusion in 9 out of 60 (15%) HIV patients [2]. The prevalence was 8% in 25 HIV patients without AIDS-defining illness and 20% in those with AIDS. Himelman observed pericardial effusions in 7 out of 25 (28%) hospitalized HIV patients compared with 0 out of 45 ambulatory HIV patients, and 6 out of 20 (30%) hospitalized patients with acute leukemia undergoing baseline echocardiography [3]. Mirri demonstrated an increase in the prevalence of clinical, electrocardiographic, or echocardiographic cardiac abnormalities from 4% of HIV patients with lymphadenopathy through 14% with so-called AIDS-related complex (ARC) to 37% of those with AIDS [4]. There are no particular echocardiographic features of pericardial effusion in HIV patients that would distinguish these effusions from those of non-HIV-infected patients.

The effusions may be secondary to opportunistic infection with agents, such as *Mycobacterium* tuberculosis [5–8], *Mycobacterium avium intracellulare* [9,10], cytomegalovirus [11], Coxsackie, *Herpes simplex* [12–14], *Cryptococcus* [15,16], *Salmonella typhimurium*, *Nocardia* [17], *Listeria monocytogenes* [18], or *Toxoplasma gondii* [19]; to malignancies such as Kaposi's sarcoma [20,50] or non-Hodgkin lymphoma [52]; or to heart failure associated with ventricular dysfunction. Although most commonly relatively asymptomatic and unimportant, pericardial effusion has been associated with tamponade [11,20–22] and death [10,11] in AIDS patients.

Ventricular dysfunction

Overt ventricular dysfunction is relatively uncommon in patients with AIDS. These patients may, however, present with symptoms and signs of either pulmonary or systemic congestion (secondary to left and/or right ventricular dysfunction) or both. Prior to the onset of symptoms it is possible to identify quire subtle ventricular dysfunction by exercise radionuclide ventriculography. Herst and coauthors observed a fall in left ventricular ejection fraction during exercise in 5 out of 15 patients with AIDS and Kaposi's sarcoma compared with 3 out of 12 controls, while 7 out of 21 patients had right ventricular enlargement [23]. The etiology was not established, but they speculated that early myocarditis might play a role. Although myocarditis has been identified in approximately 50% of patients dying with AIDS [24,25] dilated cardiomyopathy is evident pathologically in only approximately 20% of those with myocarditis.

As with pericarditis, it appears that the prevalence of myocarditis increases as HIV disease progresses (Tables 12.1, 12.2). Mirri demonstrated that left ventricular size was larger and left ventricular ejection fraction was lower in patients with AIDS than in those who were HIV positive [4]. In the series of Reilly, 26 out of 58 autopsied patients with AIDS (45%) had myocarditis including all six patients who had congestive heart failure or clinical left ventricular dysfunction.

Left ventricular systolic dysfunction was identified antemortem by radionuclide ventriculography in 4 out of 58 patients (7%) dying with AIDS in this series [25]. Echocardiography revealed left ventricular enlargement or reduced systolic function in 4 out of 25 (16%) of HIV-positive patients compared with 10 out of 35 (29%) of those with AIDS in the series studied by Levy [2], while Himelman found dilated cardiomyopathy in 8 out of 25 (32%) hospitalized HIV patients, seven of whom had AIDS, but in none of 45 ambulatory HIV patients or 20 controls [3]. Similarly, Hecht found reduced systolic function in 8 out of 27 (30%) AIDS patients, but in only 1 out of 21 (5%) controls [26]. It is clear that the prevalence of left ventricular dysfunction increases as HIV disease progresses, but that congestive heart failure becomes manifest clinically in only a small percentage of those with dysfunction.

We have seen several patients who presented with classic signs of myocarditis including dyspnea, electrocardiographic abnormalities and left ventricular dysfunction following a febrile illness with constitutional symptoms compatible with viral illness. Most have demonstrated significant improvement in ventricular function after relief of symptoms with standard supportive therapy including digitalis, diuretics, and angiotensin converting enzyme inhibitors. One of these patients, whose echocardiograms are shown in Figure 12.1, presented with fulminant pulmonary edema which required mechanical ventilation. Over the ensuing 5 days, his ventricular function improved dramatically and he was discharged from hospital feeling well. An organism responsible for this illness was never identified.

Blanchard detected left ventricular dysfunction in 8 out of 70 HIV-positive patients undergoing serial echocardiography. All four patients with AIDS and reduced left ventricular function at two consecutive studies died within 1 year [27].

Occasional patients are seen in whom marked pulmonary hypertension is the sole or first manifestation of cardiovascular involvement in AIDS. Figure 12.2 demonstrates the typical echocardiographic appearance of pulmonary hypertension with both diastolic and systolic flattening of the ventricular septum in response to the markedly abnormal transseptal pressure gradient. This 39–year-old HIV-positive male presented with gradually increasing dyspnea over 30 months culminating in dyspnea at rest. Clinical examination demonstrated findings of severe pulmonary

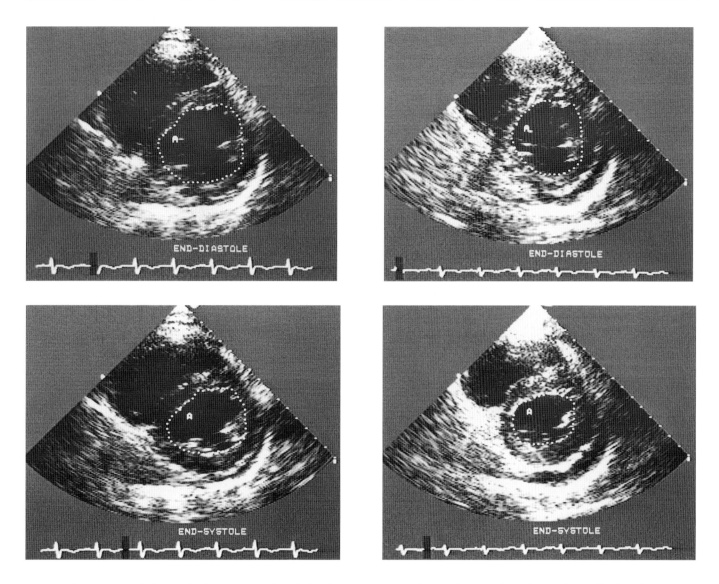

Figure 12.1. Parasternal short axis views at end-diastole (top) and end-systole (bottom) at the time of acute illness (left) and several months later (right). The left ventricular endocardium is outlined and the cavity area is displayed in the upper left corner of each frame. Global systolic dysfunction and inferior marked hypokinesis (left) resolves at follow-up (right).

hypertension with a right ventricular heave; loud, palpable, single-second heart sound; elevated jugular venous pressure with prominent V-waves; and an enlarged, non-tender, pulsatile liver. Echocardiography confirmed the enlarged right ventricle, abnormal septal position and motion, and severe tricuspid regurgitation with an estimated pulmonary artery systolic pressure of 90 mmHg. This patient demonstrated an excellent response to captopril. Himelman initially described six patients who developed subacute onset of moderate or severe pulmonary hypertension associated with right ventricular hypertrophy and failure [28]. Others have since reported larger series.

Dilated cardiomyopathy remains idiopathic in the vast majority of AIDS cases but it is possible that the nutritional deficiencies which result from AIDS may contribute. We described five patients with AIDS with clinical mild to severe cardiac dysfunction which was confirmed by echocardiography or radionuclide angiography [29]. Four of the five patients had necropsies and in none was there evidence of myocarditis, myofibrillar loss or myocyte necrosis. All of the patients were severely malnourished and one had markedly depressed level of selenium. Although no specific cause of the ventricular dysfunction was identified, it is quite possible that malnutrition played a role.

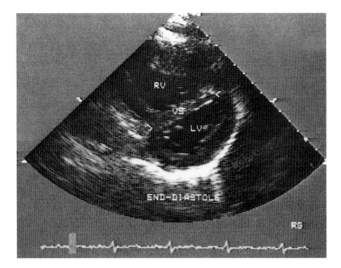

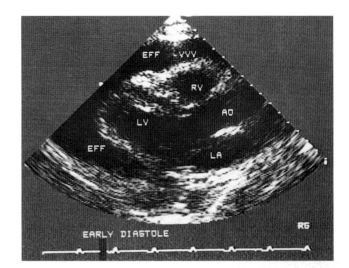

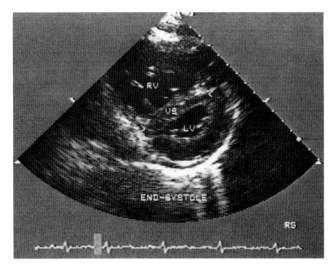

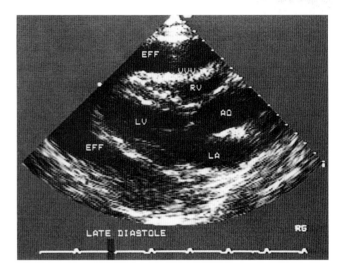

Figure 12.2. Short axis views of a patient with a systolic pulmonary artery pressure of 90 mmHg. The ventricular septum (VS) is markedly flattened both at end-diastole (top) and end-systole (bottom). The right ventricle (RV) is dilated. LV, left ventricle.

Figure 12.3. Parasternal long axis views in early diastole (top) and late diastole (bottom). There is collapse of the free wall of the right ventricle (RV) (arrows) in late diastole but not early diastole. EFF, effusion; LV, left ventricle; LA, left atrium; AO, aorta.

With this background, if we return to the case of the dyspneic patient with AIDS, a pericardial effusion, ventricular dysfunction and pulsus paradoxus, the clinical question becomes: is cardiac tamponade or ventricular dysfunction responsible for the clinical manifestations? If there is a diastolic collapse of the right ventricle (Figure 12.3) or collapse of the right atrium, which is present for more than 33% of the cardiac cycle (the usual echocardiographic indicators of 'tense' pericardial effusion [30–32], it is highly likely that the tamponade is present. If not, it is, in our experience, very rare for pericardial involvement to play a significant role. Rather, therapy of the underlying pulmonary infection or therapy directed at ventricular dysfunction, such as diuretics, digoxin, nitrates, and converting enzyme inhibitors, is usually effective in resolving symptoms and signs. Unless there is clear reason to suspect acute myocarditis or pericarditis, it has not been our practice to perform endomyocardial biopsy, or prescribe specific immunosuppresive or antimicrobial therapy for myocarditis. The observed clinical response suggests that the pericardial effusion observed at the time of presentation was an innocent bystander. In the absence of hemodynamic compromise, the pericardial effusion may play a significant role if it is the source of opportunistic infection.

There remains some controversy about the appropriate role for pericardiocentesis and catheter drainage of the pericardial space in patients with AIDS. Hsia and Ross found that analysis of pericardial fluid from 14 HIV-infected patients (one at autopsy) yielded a diagnosis in five patients (lymphoma 2, *Staphylococcus aureus* 1, *Mycobacterium avium intracellulare* 1, and hyphae 1) [33]. Our practice has been not to perform pericardiocentesis unless the effusion is suspected of causing hemodynamic compromise or it is believed to be the likely source of infection. When pericardiocentesis is performed, we use the Mayo Clinic approach of puncturing where the echocardiogram indicates the distance to the effusion is minimal [34]. This is commonly near the left ventricular apex but occasionally the subxiphoid approach is more suitable. Echo contrast consisting of 9.75 ml of normal saline and 0.25 ml of air agitated through a three-way stopcock is injected through the aspirating needle once fluid has been aspirated to confirm that the needle tip is in the pericardial space. A guidewire and a catheter are then introduced into the pericardial space and corrected to an evacuated drainage container until drainage ceases.

Electrocardiogram

Given the high prevalence of cardiac involvement, albeit asymptomatic, it is not surprising that 30–45% of AIDS patients demonstrate electrocardiographic abnormalities, such as non-specific repolarization changes and conduction disturbances [2]. Electrocardiogram (ECG) abnormalities and underlying myocarditis were associated in the series described by Reilly [25]. The ventricular arrhythmias seen in these patients may be life-threatening or fatal. We described the association of intravenous pentamidine therapy for *Pneumocystis carinii* pneumonia with the unique polymorphic ventricular tachycardia Torsades-de-pointes (Figure 12.4). This patient's recurrent cardiac arrests ceased following administration of isoproterenol and withdrawal of pentamidine. Patients with AIDS also, however, have frequent serious metabolic and electrolyte disturbances, which also result in non-specific ECG changes or, for example, with profound hypokalemia and hypomagnesemia, serious ventricular arrhythmias.

Endocarditis

Endocarditis occurs not infrequently in the total population of AIDS patients. Intravenous drug users are obviously at high risk for both HIV disease and right-sided infective endocarditis. With the exception of this group, infective endocarditis is relatively rare in patients with AIDS. Marantic or non-bacterial thrombotic endocarditis is also seen in AIDS patients [35]. Although this entity is relatively rate, it is important because the echocardiographic appearance is very similar or identical to that of infective endocarditis. It has been associated with clinical neurologic dysfunction and widespread systemic embolization in patients with AIDS [36]. The sterile marantic lesions may also become infected during transient bacteremia associated with opportunistic infections [37].

Mycobacteria

Mycobacterium tuberculosis causes both pericardial and myocardial disease in patients with AIDS [6]. Indeed, tuberculous pericarditis has been the first manifestation of AIDS [5] and *Mycobacterium* tuberculosis is the most common infectious agent responsible for pericarditis in AIDS, accounting for 25–50% of cases [7,8]. *Mycobacterium avium intracellulare* can cause both pericarditis [7,10] and myocarditis [1,24].

Viruses

Viral illness is common in patients with AIDS with CMV being the most prevalent virus affecting multiple organ systems. CMV clearly has caused myocarditis in some patients, but the relationship between the presence of the virus, inclusion bodies, lymphocytic infiltrate, and muscle destruction remains unclear. The high prevalence (almost 90%) of CMV in patients with AIDS makes it difficult to be clear when CMV is a bystander and when it is the agent responsible for myocarditis. Pericarditis can also result from infection with CMV [11,22]. Coxsackie virus [38] may cause myocarditis, and *Herpes simplex* virus has caused pericarditis directly [14] and in association with esophageal ulceration and perforation [13] in immunosuppressed AIDS patients. There continues to be controversy about whether or not HIV itself may cause myocardial inflammation and destruction. HIV has been

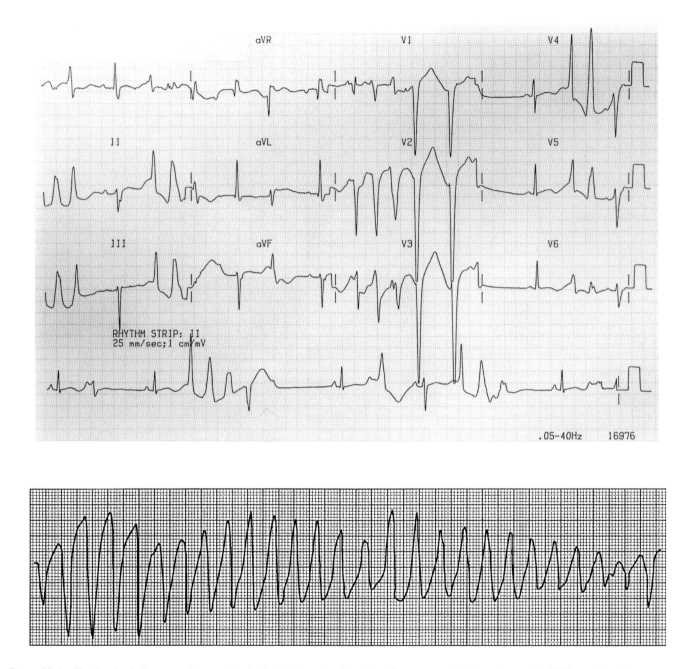

Figure 12.4. Twelve-lead electrocardiogram (top) obtained on the day of cardiac arrests of this patient with AIDS receiving intravenous pentamidine. The QT internal is markedly prolonged (approximately 560 ms) and frequent runs of ventricular ectopy are seen. The rhythm strip (bottom) demonstrates the classic twisting multimorphic ventricular tachycardia of Torsades-de-pointes.

identified in myocardium by investigators including Grody [39] and Calabrese [40], but that this indicates HIV myocarditis has been disputed. For example, in the series described by Grody, there was no myocyte inflammation or death in the cells infected with HIV. Dittrich, responding to Calabrese's report, described a patient with AIDS, congestive cardiomyopathy and an endomyocardial biopsy specimen which grew HIV [38]. Immunocytochemistry and in-situ co-hybridization failed to show HIV antigens or nucleic acid. Coxsackie B2 titers suggested recent infection. He suggested caution in ascribing cardiomyopathy to HIV and concluded that a causative role for HIV in myocarditis had not been established. Thus, there has, to our knowledge, never been direct evidence of myocarditis caused by HIV.

Protozoa

Other pathogens, including protozoa, have played an important role in cardiac disorders in patients with AIDS. *Toxoplasma gondii* causes myocarditis, but the prevalence varies widely in various subpopulations of those with AIDS, for example, *T. gondii* is very common in Haitians and uncommon in non-Haitians. Hofman reported *Toxoplasma myocarditis* causing sudden death without other organ system involvement [41]. He has advocated empiric antimicrobial therapy for toxoplasmosis in patients with sudden heart failure in an area in which toxoplasmosis is endemic [42]. Interestingly, Memel has reported positive gallium-67 citrate myocardial uptake in a patient with positive *Toxoplasma* titers, which resolved following completion of treatment for toxoplasmosis [43]. Positive gallium scintigraphy has been described in two other cases of myopericarditis in patients with AIDS [44]. Although direct infection of the heart and pericardium by *Pneumocystis carinii* has not been reported, the prevalence of pericardial effusions is higher in patients with *P. carinii* infection [3]. In addition, right ventricular dilation has been reported in a patient with *P. carinii* and CMV pneumonia [3].

Fungi

Fungal diseases are responsible for myocarditis, pericarditis, and, very rarely, endocarditis [45] in AIDS. Hofman reviewed eight cases of fungal myocarditis gleaned from autopsies of 118 patients with AIDS. Although two of the patients had symptoms of the cardiac disease responsible for their deaths, intramyocardial pathogens were only identified postmortem. The organism was *Candida albicans* in three, *Cryptococcus neoformans* in three, and *Aspergillus fumigatus* in two [46].

Bacteria

Bacteria are rarely responsible for cardiac disease other than infective endocarditis in patients with AIDS. *Staphylococcus aureus* [47] and *Nocardia asteroides* [17,48] have both caused pericarditis. Karve described two HIV-positive patients who developed bacterial pericarditis and tamponade as a consequence of pneumonia caused by *Streptococcus pneumoniae* [49].

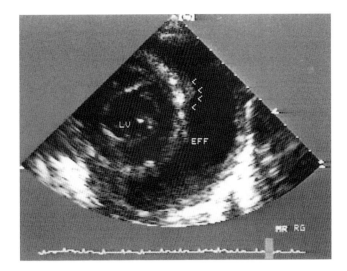

Figure 12.5. Parasternal short axis view of a patient with AIDS and visceral Kaposi's sarcoma demonstrating epicardial studding (arrows) presumed to be Kaposi's sarcoma. LV, left ventricle; EFF, effusion.

Malignancies

Malignancies may also involve the heart and pericardium in patients with AIDS. Kaposi's sarcoma is the most common malignancy seen in patients with AIDS and it is particularly prevalent in homosexual men [37]. Although cardiac involvement may occur in the absence of skin lesions and may result in clinical manifestations, it is usually seen in disseminated disease and is usually clinically silent. Kaposi's sarcoma may be confined to the epicardium or may invade the myocardium, pericardium, or coronary arteries. Large pericardial effusions and cardiac tamponade from hemorrhagic pericardial effusion [20,50] have been reported. The epicardial studding with Kaposi's sarcoma, whether visualized by echocardiography (Figure 12.5) or MRI, has the usual appearance of epicardial tumor deposits. Anderson identified epicardial Kaposi's sarcoma at necropsy in 7 out of 71 HIV patients of whom 53 were homosexual or bisexual [24], while Lewis described cardiac Kaposi's sarcoma in 12% of 115 patients with AIDS [51].

Both myocardial and pericardial involvement with lymphoma have been reported in patients with AIDS. Hodgkin's disease as well as non-Hodgkin lymphoma may involve the endocardium, myocardium or, predominantly, the pericardium manifesting as

Table 12.1. Echocardiographic abnormalities (Abn) in HIV patients by disease stage.

Series	HIV-positive				ARC			AIDS		
	n	n	abn	%	n	abn	%	n	abn	%
DeCastro[53]	114	31	5	16	11	0	0	72	47	65
Hecht[26]	27	-	-	-	-	-	-	27	13	48
Himelman[53]	70	6	0	0	13	1	7	51	15	29
Levy[2]	60	25	7	28	-	-	-	35	14	40
Mirri[4]	138	48	2	4	49	7	14	41	15	37

Table 12.2. Prevalence of pericardial effusion and left ventricular enlargement or dysfunction by disease severity.

Abnormality	Himelman [3]			Levy [2]		De Castro [53]		Hecht [26]	
	Con	Amb	Hosp	HIV	AIDS	HIV	AIDS	Con	AIDS
n	20	45	25	25	35	31	72	21	27
Pericardial effusion	6(30)	0	7(28)	2(8)	7(20)	1(3)	13(18)	(5)	7(26)
LV dilation and/or dysfunction	0	0	8(32)	3(12)	6(17)	5(16)	12(17)	1(5)	8(30)

Con: Control; Amb: Ambulatory; Hosp: Hospitalized

Table 12.3. Etiologic agents for pericardial effusion or ventricular dysfunction.

Agent	Pericarditis	Myocarditis
Bacteria		
Chlamydia trachomatis	+[54]	
Listeria monocytogenes	+[18]	
Mycobacterium tuberculosis	+[5–8]	+[1,24]
Mycobacterium avium complex	+[9,10]	+[1,10,24]
Nocardia asteroides	+[17,48]	
Salmonella typhimurium	+	
Staphylococcus aureus	+[47]	
Streptococcus pneumoniae	+[49]	
Viruses		
CMV	+[11,2]	+
Coxsackie	+	+[38]
Herpes simplex I, II	+[12–24]	+[13]
Protozoa		
Toxoplasma gondii	+[19]	+[41–43,55,56]
Fungi		
Aspergillus fumigatus		+[45,46]
Candida albicans		+[46]
Cryptococcus neoformans	+[15,16]	+[36,46,57]
Tumors		
Kaposi's sarcomaa	+[20,50]	[20,50]
Hodgkin's lymphoma	+	
Non-Hodgkin lymphoma	+[52]	+[52]

pericardial effusion. Again, the cardiac involvement is normally silent. Gill et al. described nine cases of cardiac involvement with lymphoma at the time of initial presentation, a rare phenomenon for lymphoma with only 50 reported cases at that time [52]. Four of the nine patients were homosexual or bisexual men with AIDS. Of the nine patients, eight had echocardiographic abnormalities with pericardial effusion in six, intracardiac (right atrial and left and right ventric-ular) mass lesions in four, regional hypokinesia in three, and markedly thickened pericardium in one.

Clinically important cardiac involvement in HIV disease is relatively rare. This chapter has outlined the most common forms of cardiac involvement, emphasizing the etiologic agents responsible for the various manifestations. It should provide a useful resource to health care providers who utilize cardiac imaging in patients with HIV disease.

References

1 Anderson DW, Virmani R. Emerging patterns of heart disease in human immunodeficiency virus infection [review]. *Hum Pathology* 1990; **21**: 253–259.

2 Levy WS, Simon GL, Rios JC, Ross AM. Prevalence of cardiac abnormalities in human immunodeficiency virus infection. *Am J Cardiol* 1989; **63**: 86–89.

3 Himelman RB, Chung WS, Chernoff DN, Schoiller NB, Hollander H. Cardiac manifestations of human immunodeficiency virus infection: a two-dimensional echocardiographic study. *J Am Coll Cardiol* 1989; **13**: 1030–1036.

4 Mirri A, Rapezzi C, Iacopi F et al. Cardiac involvement in HIV infection: a prospective, multicenter clinical and echocardiographic study [in Italian]. *Cardiologia* 1990; **35**: 203–209.

5 Dalli E, Quesada A, Juan G, Navarro R, Paya R, Tormo V. Tuberculous pericarditis as the first manifestation of acquired immunodeficiency syndrome. *Am Heart J* 1987; **114**: 905–906.

6 D'Cruz IA, Sengupta EE, Abrahams C, Reddy HK, Turlapati RV. Cardiac involvement, including tuberculous pericardial effusion, complicating acquired immune deficiency syndrome. *Am Heart J* 1986; **112**: 1100–1102.

7 Monsuez JJ, Kinney EL, Vittecoq D et al. Comparison among acquired immune deficiency syndrome patients with and without clinical evidence of cardiac disease. *Am J Cardiol* 1988; **62**: 1311–1313.

8 de Miguel J, Pedreira JD, Campos V, Perez Gomez A, Lorenzo Porto JA. Tuberculous pericarditis and AIDS. *Chest* 1990; **97**: 1273.

9 Cohen IS, Anderson DW, Virmani R et al. Congestive cardiomyopathy in association with the acquired immunodeficiency syndrome. *N Engl J Med* 1986; **315**: 628–630.

10 Woods GL, Goldsmith JC. Fatal pericarditis due to Mycobacterium avium-intracellulare in acquired immunodeficiency syndrome. *Chest* 1989; **95**: 1355–1357.

11 Nathan PE, Arsura EL, Zappi M. Pericarditis with tamponade due to cytomegalovirus in the acquired immunodeficiency syndrome. *Chest* 1991; **99**: 765–766.

12 Acierno LJ. Cardiac complications in acquired immunodeficiency syndrome (AIDS): a review. *J Am Coll Cardiol* 1989; **13**: 1144–1154.

13 Cronstedt JL, Bouchama A, Hainau B, Halim M, Khouqeer F, al Darsouny T. Spontaneous esophageal performation in herpes simplex esophagitis. *Am J Gastroenterol* 1992; **87**: 124–127.

14 Freedberg RS, Gindea AJ, Dieterich DT, Greene JB. Herpes simplex pericarditis in AIDS. *N York State J Med* 1987; **87**: 304–306.

15 Zuger A, Louie E, Holzman RS, Simberkoff MS, Rahal JJ. Cryptococcal disease in patients with the acquired immunodeficiency syndrome: diagnostic features and outcome of treatment. *Ann Intem Med* 1986; **104**: 234–240.

16 Brivet F, Livartowski J, Herve P, Rain B, Dormont J. Pericardial Cryptococcal disease in acquired immunodeficiency syndrome. *Am J Med* 1987; **82**: 1273.

17 Poland GA, Jorgensen CR, Sarosi GA. Nocardia asteroides pericarditis: report of a case and review of the literature. *Mayo Clinic Proc* 1990; **65** 819–824.

18 Ferguson R, Yee S, Finkle H, Rose T, Schneider V, Gee G. Listeria-associated pericarditis in an AIDS patient. *J Natl Med Assoc* 1993; **85**: 225–228.

19 Tschirhart D, Klatt KC. Disseminated Toxoplasmosis in the acquired immunodeficiency syndrome. *Arch Pathol Lab Med* 1988; **112**: 1237–1241.

20 Stotka JL, Good CB, Downer WR, Kapoor WN. Pericardial effusion and tamponade due to Kaposi's sarcoma in acquired immunodeficiency syndrome. *Chest* 1989; **95**: 1359–1361.

21 Turco M, Seneff M, McGrath BJ, Hsia J. Cardiac tamponade in the acquired immunodeficiency syndrome. *Am Heart J* 1990; **120**: 1467–1468.

22 Scott PJ, Conway SP, Da Costa P. Cardiac tamponade complicating cytomegalovirus pericarditis in a patient with AID [letter]. *J Infection* 1990; **20**: 92–93.

23 Herst JA, Shepherd FA, Liu P et al. Prospective assessment of cardiac function in patients with Kaposi's sarcoma and the acquired immunodeficiency syndrome. *Clin Invest Med – Med clini Exp* 1991; **14**: 21–27.

24 Anderson DW, Virmani R, Reilly JM et al. Prevalent myocarditis at necropsy in the acquired immunodeficiency syndrome. *J Am Coll Cardiol* 1988; **11**: 792–799.

25 Reilly JM, Cunnion RE, Anderson DW et al. Frequency of myocarditis, left ventricular dysfunction and ventricular tachycardia in the acquired immune deficiency syndrome. *Am J Cardiol* 1988; **62**: 789–793.

26 Hecht SR, Berger M, Van Tosh A, Croxson S. Unsuspected cardiac abnormalities in the acquired immune deficiency syndrome. An echocardiographic study [see comments]. *Chest* 1989; **96**: 805–808.

27 Blanchard DG, Hagenhoff C, Chow LC, McCann HA, Dittrich H. Reversibility of cardiac abnormalities in human immunodeficiency virus (HIV)-infected individuals: a serial echocardiographic study. *J Am Coll Cardiol* 1991; **17**: 1270–1276.

28 Himelman RB, Dohrmann M, Goodman P et al. Severe pulmonary hypertension and cor pulmonale in the acquired immunodeficiency syndrome. *Am J Cardiol* 1989; **64**: 1396–1399.

29 Webb JG, Chan-Yan C, Kiess MC. Cardiac dysfunction associated with the acquired immunodeficiency syndrome (AIDS). *Clin Cardiol* 1988; **11**: 423–426.

30 Gillam LD, Guyer DE, Gibson TC, King ME, Marshall J, Weyman AE. Hydrodynamic compression of the right atrium: a new echocardiographic sign of cardiac tamponade. *Circulation* 1983; **68**: 294–301.

31 Singh S, Wann LS, Klopfenstein HS, Hartz A, Brooks HL. Usefulness of right ventricular diastolic collapse in diagnosing cardiac tamponade and comparison to pulsus paradoxus. *Am J Cardiol* 1986; **57**: 652–671.

32 Eisenberg MJ, Schiller NB. Bayes' theorem and the echocardiographic diagnosis of cardiac tamponade. *Am J Cardiol* 1991; **68**: 1242–1244.

33 Hsia J, Ross AM. Pericardial effusion and pericardiocentesis in human immunodeficiency virus infection. *Am J Cardiol* 1994; **74**: 94–96.

34 Callahan JA, Seward JB, Nishimura RA et al. Two-dimensional echocardiographically guided pericardiocentesis: experience in 117 consecutive patients. *Am J Cardiol* 1985; **55**: 476–469.

35 Fink L, Reichek N, Sutton MG. Cardiac abnormalities in acquired immune deficiency syndrome. *Am J Cardiol* 1984; **54**: 1161–1163.

36 Cammarosano C, Lewis W. Cardiac lesions in acquired immune deficiency syndrome (AIDS). *J Am Coll Cardiol* 1985; **5**: 703–706.

37 Francis CK. Cardiac involvement in AIDS. *Curr Prob Cardiol* 1990; **XV**: 571–639.

38 Dittrich H, Chow L, Denaro F, Spector S. Human immunodeficiency virus, Coxsackie virus, and cardiomyopathy. *Ann Intern Med* 1988; **108**: 308–309.

39 Grody WW, Cheng L, Lewis W. Infection of the heart by the human immunodeficiency virus. *Am J Cardiol* 1990; **66**: 203–206.

40 Calabrese LH, Proffitt, MR, Yen-Lieberman, B, Hobbs RE, Ratliff NB. Congestive cardiomyopathy and illness related to the acquired immunodeficiency syndrome (AIDS) associated with isolation of retrovirus from myocardium. *Ann Intern Med* 1987; **107(5)**: 691–692.

41 Hofman P, Bernard E, Michiels JF, Dellamonica P, Loubiere R. [Acute toxoplasmic myocarditis. A cause of sudden death in a case of acquired immunodeficiency syndrome]. [Review] [French]. *Arch Malad Coeur Vaisseaux* 1990; **83(11)**: 1735–1738.

42 Hofman P, Drici MD, Gibelin P, Michiels JF, Thyss A. Prevalence of toxoplasma myocarditis in patients with the acquired immunodeficiency syndrome. *Brit Heart J* 1993; **70(4)**: 376–381.

43 Memel DS, DeRogatis AJ, William DC. Ga-67 citrate myocardial uptake in a patient with AIDS, toxoplasmosis, and myocarditis. *Clin Nuc Medicine* 1991; **16(5)**: 315–317.

44 Cregler LL, Sosa I, Ducey S, Abbey L. Myopericarditis in acquired immunodeficiency syndrome by gallium scintigraphy. *J Nat Med Assoc* 1990; **82(7)**: 511–513.

45 Cox JA, di Dio F, Pizzolato G-P, Lerch R, Pochon N. Aspergillus endocarditis and myocarditis in a patient with acquired immunodeficiency syndrome (AIDS). *Virchows Archiv – A, Pathol Anat & Histopathol* 1990; **417**: 255–259.

46 Hofman P, Gari-Toussaint M, Bernard E, et al. [Fungal myocarditis in acquired immunodeficiency syndrome]. [Review] [French]. *Archiv Malad Coeur Vaisseaux* 1992; **85(2)**: 203–208.

47 Stechel RP, Cooper DJ, Greenspan J, Pizzarello RA, Tenenbaum MJ. Staphylococcal pericarditis in a homosexual patient with AIDS-related complex. *New York State J Med* 1986; **86**: 592–593.

48 Holtz HA, Lavery DP, Kapila R. Actinomycetales infection in the acquired immunodeficiency syndrome. *Ann Inter Med* 1985; **102**: 203–205.

49 Karve MM, Murali MR, Shah HM, Phelps KR. Rapid evolution of cardiac tamponade due to bacterial pericarditis in two patients with HIV-1 infection. *Chest* 1992; **101(5)**: 1461–1463.

50 Steigman CK, Anderson DW, Macher AM, Sennesh JD, Virmani R. Fatal cardiac tamponade in acquired immunodeficiency syndrome with epicardial Kaposi's sarcoma. *Am Heart J* 1988; **116(4)**: 1105–1107.

51 Lewis W. AIDS: cardiac findings from 115 autopsies. [Review]. *Prog cardiovasc Dis* 1989; **32(3)** 207–215.

52 Gill PS, Chandraratna PA, Meyer PR, Levine AM. Malignant lymphoma: cardiac involvement at initial presentation. *J Clin Onc* 1987; **5(2)**: 216–224.

53 DeCastro S, Migliau G, Silvestri A, et al. Heart involvement in AIDS: a prospective study during various stages of the disease. *Eur Heart J* 1992; **13(11)**: 1452–1459.

54 Kroon FP, van't Wout JW, Weiland HT, van Furth R. Chlamydia trachomatis pneumonia in an HIV-seropositive patient. *New Eng J Med* 1989; **320**: 906–907.

55 Cappell MS, Mikhail N, Ortega A. Toxoplasma myocarditis in AIDS [letter]. *Am H J* 1992; **123(6)**: 1728–1729.

56 Grange F, Kinney EL, Monsuez JJ, et al. Successful therapy for Toxoplasma gondii myocarditis in acquired immunodeficiency syndrome. *Am H J* 1990; **120(2)**: 443–444.

57 Lafont A, Wolff M, Marche C, Clair B, Regnier B. Overwhelming myocarditis due to *Cryptococcus neoformans* in an AIDS patient. *Lancet* 1987; **2**: 1145–1146.

13 CLINICAL ASPECTS OF PULMONARY COMPLICATIONS IN HIV/AIDS

Julio S. G. Montaner
Peter Phillips

Introduction

Pneumocystis carinii pneumonia (PCP) together with Kaposi's sarcoma (KS) were the harbingers of the acquired immune deficiency syndrome (AIDS) epidemic more than 10 years ago. Since then, the spectrum of the pulmonary disease affecting these individuals has become better understood. Although the majority of these conditions remain infectious in nature, neoplastic and inflammatory diseases also occur with increased frequency among individuals infected with the human immunodeficiency virus (HIV), the causative agent of AIDS [1].

The main infectious causes of pulmonary disease among HIV-infected individuals are shown in Table 13.1. PCP, *Mycobacterium* tuberculosis (MTb), and pyogenic bacterial pneumonia secondary to *Streptococcus pneumoniae*, *Hemophilus influenzae*, or *Staphylococcus*

aureus are the most frequent. Less frequently, a variety of fungi, and viruses can give rise to pulmonary disease. Although initially a rare AIDS-related complication, aspergillosis has become the leading pulmonary mycosis in many centers. Cytomegalovirus (CMV) pneumonitis is uncommon. However, CMV is often recovered from bronchial specimens of patients undergoing investigation of other pulmonary infections (e.g. PCP). This represents infection but not disease due to CMV. Although *Mycobacterium avium intracellulare* (MAI or MAC) is a frequent late complication of AIDS. Respiratory disease secondary to MAC is distinctly uncommon [2].

The main non-infectious causes of pulmonary disease among HIV-infected individuals are listed in Table 13.2. Among them, KS is particularly frequent. More recently, an increased frequency of airways hyperreactivity and emphysema has been described in

Table 13.1. Infectious pulmonary diseases in HIV/AIDS

Most common
    Pneumocystis carinii pneumonia
    Pyogenic bacterial pneumonia
    Mycobacterium tuberculosis

Less common
    Aspergillosis
    Cryptococcosis
    Coccidioidomycosis
    Histoplasmosis
    Cytomegalovirus
    Mycobacterium avium intracellulare
    Nocardia
    Cryptosporidium
    Toxoplasmosis

Table 13.2. Non-infectious pulmonary diseases in HIV/AIDS

Common
    Kaposi's sarcoma
    Airways hyperreactivity (asthma)
    Emphysema

Less common
    Lymphocytic interstitial pneumonitis
    Non-specific interstitial pneumonitis
    Lymphoma
    Drug-related pneumonitis
    Radiation-related pneumonitis
    Pulmonary hypertension
    Pneumothorax (usually related to PCP)
    Pulmonary emboli

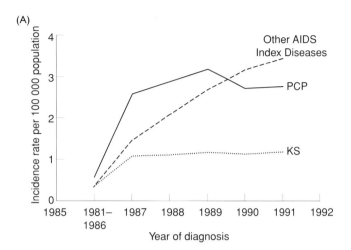

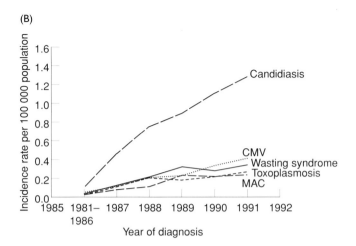

Figure 13.1 (A,B). AIDS index diseases.

these patients [3,4]. Less frequently, lymphocytic interstitial pneumonitis (LIP), non-specific interstitial pneumonitis (NIP), lymphoma, drug or radiation-related pneumonitis, and pulmonary hypertension can be seen in these patients [2,5].

It is important to highlight that not all lung disease in patients with HIV infection or even AIDS is necessarily related to the HIV infection. Furthermore, the relative frequency of HIV-associated complications is continuously changing as new antiretrovirals and preventive therapies continue to alter the natural history of the disease. Figure 13.1 illustrates the changes in the incidence of selected AIDS index diseases brought about by the development of successful therapeutic strategies [6]. Despite this, PCP still remains the single most frequent AIDS index disease today [7,8].

AIDS in the ICU

Although relatively infrequent, respiratory disease in the context of HIV infection can lead to acute respiratory failure. This is in fact, the leading cause for intensive care unit (ICU) admission among HIV-infected individuals. Of the causes of ICU admission related to HIV infection, acute respiratory failure secondary to PCP is by far the most important, owing to its high frequency and its potentially high mortality. In a recent review of the causes for admission to ICU among HIV-infected individuals, PCP (either alone or in association with other medical problems) was the cause for the admission in 92% of the cases. Cerebral toxoplasmosis and Kaposi's sarcoma were the causes of

ICU admission in 3% of cases each, while bacterial pneumonia, gastrointestinal bleeding, lymphoma, and cardiomyopathy were given as the reasons for ICU admission in 2% of cases, respectively [9].

Recently, a worsening prognosis has been noted among AIDS patients admitted to ICU. This has been attributed to a paradoxical effect of better therapies, and most likely to the use of adjunctive corticosteroids. In brief, early use of corticosteroids has led to a significant decrease in the frequency of acute respiratory failure (ARF) in patients with AIDS-related PCP. Unfortunately, the few cases that fail to respond to this treatment modality have a very poor prognosis. The net effect being a reduction in the number but a worsening prognosis among AIDS cases admitted to the ICU [10].

Differential diagnosis

When dealing with HIV-infected individuals who present with respiratory symptoms, the differential diagnosis will be greatly influenced by the knowledge of the degree of immunosuppression present. In the absence of other signs or symptoms (i.e. oral candida, hairy leukoplakia), this can be readily assessed using the CD4 count. In general, AIDS-defining illnesses are uncommon if the CD4 count is above $300/mm^3$. In particular, most episodes of PCP occur in patients with absolute CD4 counts below $200/mm^3$. On the other hand, bacterial pneumonias or tuberculosis tend to occur at any time during the natural history of HIV disease [8].

Historical data or behavioral factors will also influence the differential diagnosis. As such, the frequency of bacterial pneumonias is particularly high among HIV-infected individuals who use intravenous drugs for recreational purposes [11,12]. Also, the prior knowledge of the PPD status is important, as the chances of reactivation of tuberculous infection among HIV-infected individuals with a positive tuberculin reaction (induration ≥5 mm following a 5TU-PPD) is extremely high [13–15].

Contrary to that which occurs in most other areas of medicine, it must be noted that, when dealing with AIDS, the search for a single diagnosis may be fruitless, since multiple pathological processes often occur simultaneously in this disease [17].

Clinical assessment

As in any other setting, pulmonary involvement in patients with HIV infection generally produces non-specific signs and symptoms. Fever, malaise, and weight loss for several weeks to months before the onset of pulmonary symptoms are not infrequent. In a group of patients with AIDS and pulmonary involvement, Stover et al. reported that cough was the most frequent symptom, being present in 89% of patients. Dyspnea was present in 64%, productive cough in 39%, pleuritic pain in 20%, and hemoptysis in 3% of patients [18]. Acute symptoms were characteristic among patients with bacterial pneumonias who were also more likely to present with shaking chills. In general, symptoms were more indolent among patients with opportunistic infections; however, occasionally they were also rapidly progressive [18]. The physical examination, although often useful in establishing a diagnosis of AIDS or AIDS-related complex, is usually unhelpful in establishing the etiology of the pulmonary involvement.

Laboratory evaluation

A number of laboratory tests are often useful in the assessment of HIV-infected individuals presenting with respiratory complaints. Obviously, this will vary greatly depending on the specific nature of their complaints. In general, the serum level of lactic dehydrogenase (LDH) has proven extremely useful in the clinical setting to rule out PCP. Even mild PCP will usually be accompanied by a significant elevation of the LDH to 1.5–2 times the upper limit of normal. In fact, the degree of the LDH elevation generally correlates with the severity of the PCP episode. Furthermore, changes in the LDH will parallel the clinical course of the underlying disease. This is a useful aid in discriminating worsening PCP following the initiation of therapy from worsening respiratory symptoms, owing to a superimposed process.

It must be emphasized, however, that the LDH, although a very sensitive (95%) marker of PCP, is also non-specific. Hemolysis, lymphoma, pulmonary embolism, and liver disease are among the numerous other causes of an elevated LDH often seen in this patient population. Of particular note, in this context, is the fact that dapsone therapy can lead to the development of methemoglobinemia, which in turn leads to hemolytic anemia and LDH elevation [20–24].

Pulmonary function tests before and after bronchodilators, methacholine challenge, DLCO, oxygen saturation while breathing air at rest and during exercise, and blood gases have also been used in this setting. In some centers if pulmonary function tests are normal, a gallium lung scan is often performed, as increased lung uptake of gallium-67 would suggest direct pulmonary involvement and it would warrant further evaluation in an aim to establish the definitive diagnosis [2]. All of these tests, while very sensitive indicators of lung dysfunction, have relatively low specificity. As such, etiological confirmation of pulmonary disease involves obtaining pulmonary secretions as dictated by signs and symptoms. This is most often done with the use of sputum, sputum induction, or bronchoalveolar lavage. In all instances, respiratory secretions should be examined thoroughly considering the wide variety of organisms that can lead to respiratory involvement in these patients [2,19].

Pneumocystis carinii pneumonia (PCP)

Pneumocystis carinii, recently reclassified as a fungus on the basis of its genomic make-up, is an ubiquitous organism which produces disease in humans throughout the world, usually in the setting of severe immunosuppression. PCP was rarely diagnosed until the early 1980s when it became the index disease that facilitated the clinical recognition of AIDS. Since then, PCP has become the most frequent serious opportunistic infection among individuals infected with

HIV. In North America, PCP represents the AIDS-defining illness in 65% of cases and will eventually affect over 85% of HIV patients during their lifetime. PCP is generally a late event in the evolution of HIV infection as demonstrated by a CD4 count usually below 250/mm^3 [8].

Clinical and radiological features

Dyspnea, non-productive cough, and fever are the classical features of PCP [2,3]. Acute hypoxemic respiratory failure (ARF) requiring mechanical ventilation may occur in as many as 20% of hospitalized patients. Most often this occurs within the first few days of starting antimicrobial therapy. Less frequently, acute hypoxemic respiratory failure develops as a complication of diagnostic bronchoscopy and rarely as the initial presentation at the emergency room [25,26].

Clinically overt PCP usually develops over a period of several days to weeks and, during this time, the radiological picture tends to progress from a normal chest X-ray to a diffuse bilateral interstitial pattern. Varying degrees of alveolar involvement can be seen, including frank consolidation [27]. A number of atypical radiological presentations have been described, including cystic changes, pneumothoraces, nodular or mass-like opacities, and even cavities. Upper lung field involvement, pneumothoraces, and extrapulmonary pneumocystosis have also been increasingly recognized, particularly (but not exclusively) in the context of aerosol pentamidine prophylaxis [27,28].

Diagnosis

Given the non-specific nature of the clinical, laboratory, and radiological picture of PCP, diagnostic confirmation is highly recommended. Sputum induction has been successfully adopted in a number of centers where diagnosis of PCP is frequently made. Bronchoalveolar lavage (BAL) is a rapid, safe, and effective means of obtaining tracheobronchial secretions to provide an adequate diagnostic specimen.

The usual histopathologic picture of PCP consists of a mild to moderate interstitial inflammatory response with predominance of lymphocytes and alveolar macrophages. Additionally, a classic foamy alveolar exudate can be seen when hematoxylin-eosin (H&E) stain is used. The foamy appearance of the alveolar exudate is due to the presence of the organism which is not stained with H&E but can be easily recognized using readily available special stains, such as silver stains and toluidine blue. BAL allows clear identification of the organism provided the specimen is appropriately concentrated and stained [25]. Although *P. carinii* infection is usually confined to the lungs, systemic pneumocystosis involving multiple organs, such as liver, spleen, lymph nodes, adrenals, and eyes, has been recently reported occasionally [28].

The appropriate assessment of the severity of each PCP episode is of utmost importance, since this will dictate the therapeutic approach. Clinical parameters are generally used for this purpose. However, it must be emphasized that these can seriously underestimate the severity of the episode. Arterial blood gases or pulse oxymetry (at rest and/or during exercise) have been used successfully for this purpose. It is generally agreed that an A-a O$_2$ gradient $\geqslant$30 mmHg is indicative of a moderately severe episode which carries a significantly worse prognosis in terms of survival. As discussed above, the LDH is also useful in the assessment and monitoring of these patients [20–24].

Management

Trimethoprim-sulfamethoxazole (TMP-SMX) is effective against *P. carinii* as well as several bacterial pulmonary pathogens. TMP-SMX is administered intravenously or orally at a dose of 20 and 100 mg/kg/day respectively in three or four divided doses for 14–21 days. Tolerance of TMP-SMX creates a significant problem, with adverse drug reactions occurring in over 50% of HIV-infected individuals [29–32].

Pentamidine isoethionate is also effective against *P. carinii*. It is usually given intravenously once daily in 250–500 ml of D5W at a dose of 4 mg/kg for the first 5 days followed by 3 mg/kg to complete a total of 14–21 days. Adverse reactions are common, occurring in over 50% of patients [29].

Dapsone (DPS) at a dose of 100 mg by mouth OD combined with TMP 200 mg by mouth four times a day has similar efficacy and better tolerability than TMP-SMX [31] for the treatment of AIDS-related PCP. Accordingly, DPS-TMP is currently the preferred choice for the treatment of mild to moderate PCP in the ambulatory setting.

A new naphtoquinolone, atovaquone (also known as 566C80 or Mepron®) is well tolerated and, although somewhat less effective than standard treatment, it provides a useful alternative [35]. Clindamycin-primaquine and trimetrexate-leucovorin-DPS are promising therapeutic alternatives currently undergoing clinical testing [36–38].

Recently, attention has focused on the role of corticosteroids as an adjuvant therapy for PCP [26]. Adjunctive corticosteroids prevent the early deterioration in gas exchange often seen shortly after initiating anti-PCP therapy, and are associated with faster defervescence, as well as improvements in respiratory rate, temperature, heart rate, P_aO_2 and LDH [32]. Also, corticosteroids decrease mortality among patients with PCP-related ARF [39–41].

In summary, patients with mild to moderate PCP are usually started on DPS-TMP orally. If there is a concern regarding superimposed bacterial infection, TMP-SMX is a better choice, owing to its broader antimicrobial spectrum. Pentamidine should be generally reserved for hospitalized patients with microbiologically proven PCP and documented sulfa–drug intolerance. Atovaquone is preferred to pentamidine for the oral treatment of mild to moderate PCP among patients who fail or cannot tolerate TMP-SMX. Corticosteroids should be started at once in any patient whose P_aO_2 is ≥70 mmHg while breathing room air. Response to antimicrobials is generally slow and significant improvement usually does not occur until after 5–7 days. With the use of adjunctive corticosteroids, however, significant improvement is usually observed within the first 3 days of treatment. Patients who fail to improve within the first 5 days of therapy should be thoroughly reviewed to rule out potential intercurrent infections or other complications. Even though *P. carinii* resistance to the antimicrobials has not been documented, lack of improvement within 7 days of therapy is generally interpreted as a failure of treatment and, therefore, an indication for a trial of the alternative agent.

Prognosis

Untreated, PCP is universally fatal. With the use of appropriate antimicrobials, mortality is below 10%. However, this clearly increases with the severity of the episode. The expected mortality of a mild first episode of PCP, therefore, is usually negligible. In addition, young age and early diagnosis have been correlated with better outcome. PCP-related ARF was initially reported to have a mortality greater than 80% in most series, but, with the use of adjunctive corticosteroids, this has been reduced to less than 50%. As discussed above, however, if PCP-related acute respiratory failure develops despite early intervention with corticosteroids and appropriate antimicrobial agents, the prognosis remains dismal [10].

Prophylaxis

The relapse rate of PCP among AIDS patients is high, exceeding 65% at 18 months. PCP prophylaxis should, therefore, be initiated in any patient with documented HIV infection once he or she has a CD4 cell count below 200/mm³ regardless of symptoms or anytime after an episode of PCP [8]. The presence of recurrent oral candida, constitutional symptoms, or a CD4 fraction below 15% also suggests the need of PCP prophylaxis regardless of the CD4 count [8].

PCP can be best prevented using TMP-SMX, as one double-strength (DS) tablet daily. Unfortunately, the development of adverse effects or cumulative toxicity with antiretrovirals often preclude its use. Intolerance to this regimen can affect as many as 50% of HIV-infected individuals. It must be emphasized, however, that, if tolerated, TMP-SMX is preferred as it offers the highest success rate [8]. Dapsone 100 mg three times per week [8] should be offered to those with intolerance to TMP-SMX. Alternatively, intermittent aerosol pentamidine at a dose of 300 mg once a month via a RESPIGARD II® (flow-driven nebulizer) is recommended [6,8,42].

Mycobacterium tuberculosis (M TB)

Tuberculosis (TB) occurs with varying degrees of frequency among HIV-infected individuals, reaching 20% in some series. Because the risk of developing TB is proportional to the risk of developing it prior to the acquisition of HIV, its incidence in North America is greatest among intravenous drug users, Blacks, and Latin Americans. TB usually develops within the year prior to the diagnosis of other AIDS-defining conditions. However, it must be noted that, since 1993, TB in an HIV-infected individual is diagnostic of AIDS according to the Centers for Disease Control (CDC) classification of HIV disease [19,43].

The symptoms of TB in the context of HIV are generally non-specific. This is particularly the case because 'classic' TB symptoms, such as fatigue, malaise, weight loss, fever, and night sweats, are common, even in moderately advanced stages of HIV disease. Unlike the immunocompetent host, in the context of HIV disease, TB usually has radiological features similar to those of primary TB, including hilar and/or mediastinal adenopathy, mid and lower lung infiltrates, pleural effusions, or a miliary pattern. Apical infiltrates or cavities are only seen in a minority of patients. As many as 10% of cases have a normal chest X-ray with a positive sputum culture for MTb. Furthermore, PCP is simultaneously diagnosed in as many as 25% of the cases of TB. Prospective tuberculin skin testing (PPD) is useful among HIV-infected individuals, as TB develops more frequently in patients known to have a previously positive test, but at the time of diagnosis of AIDS at least 30% of patients are anergic. MTb can usually be easily diagnosed with smear and culture of sputum or BAL. Of particular note is the fact that blood cultures and stool cultures can often be positive [13–16].

According to the American Thoracic Society (ATS) and CDC, TB in HIV-infected adults should be treated with isoniazid (INH) 300 mg/day and rifampin 600 mg/day (or 450 mg for patients weighing less than 50 kg). Pyrazinamide 20–30 mg/kg/day should be added for the initial 2 months of therapy. Ethambutol 25 mg/kg/day should also be added if INH resistance is suspected or if central nervous system disease or dissemination are present. Treatment should be continued for a minimum of 9 months and not less than 6 months after documented culture conversion [44].

Mycobacterium avium complex

The number of cases of *Mycobacterium avium* complex (MAC)-related disease continues to increase among HIV-infected individuals, particularly since AIDS patients live longer and other opportunistic diseases are more effectively treated. Disease caused by MAC is usually clinically non-specific. Fever, anorexia, wasting, malaise, and night sweats are frequently present. Unlike TB, disease due to MAC occurs late in the course of HIV infection, usually following other opportunistic infections. Specific respiratory signs and symptoms are usually absent. The same can be said with regard to the radiological involvement of the lung [45].

The diagnosis is generally made by recovery of the organism from blood or biopsy material from lymph

node, liver, bone marrow, or bowel. Positive sputum or stool cultures may represent colonization rather than disease. Recently, clarithromycin has been shown to be efficacious among non-HIV-infected individuals [46]. Preliminary data suggest that clarithromycin-based regimens will improve the previously modest response rates to often poorly tolerated combination therapy regimens [47].

Recently, two controlled trials of rifabutin prophylaxis against MAC infection in AIDS indicate that MAC bacteremia developed in 17% and 8% of those treated with placebo and rifabutin, respectively. Since then, consideration of rifabutin (300 mg/day) prophylaxis has been recommended for all HIV-infected individuals whose CD4 count is $\geqslant 100/mm^3$ [48].

Other causes of pulmonary disease

The pathogenic importance of CMV in the lungs in the context of AIDS remains controversial. CMV isolation from pulmonary secretions in AIDS patients appears to have little prognostic value. In fact, despite the addition of corticosteroids to the treatment of PCP, the once much-feared rise in the frequency of CMV pneumonitis has not been documented. On the other hand, the prominent role of CMV as a gastrointestinal or ocular pathogen among these patients is clearly recognized. Admittedly, establishing an unequivocal diagnosis of CMV disease at other sites is more difficult and involves tissue biopsy.

CMV pneumonitis in the context of AIDS should be diagnosed only if hypoxemia and diffuse pulmonary infiltrates coexist with evidence of CMV cytopathic effect (i.e. intranuclear and intracytoplasmic inclusions) in lung tissue and with histologic absence of other likely cause to explain the pulmonary disorder. CMV disease is treated with gancyclovir or foscarnet. Anti-CMV immunoglobulin provides useful adjunctive therapy to gancyclovir in bone marrow transplant-associated CMV pneumonitis, although its role in AIDS-related CMV pneumonitis is unclear. Long-term maintenance therapy is required for CMV retinitis, although its role in other sites of CMV disease is unclear.

Bacterial pneumonias tend to occur with increased frequency among HIV-infected individuals. Community-acquired pneumonias are usually due to

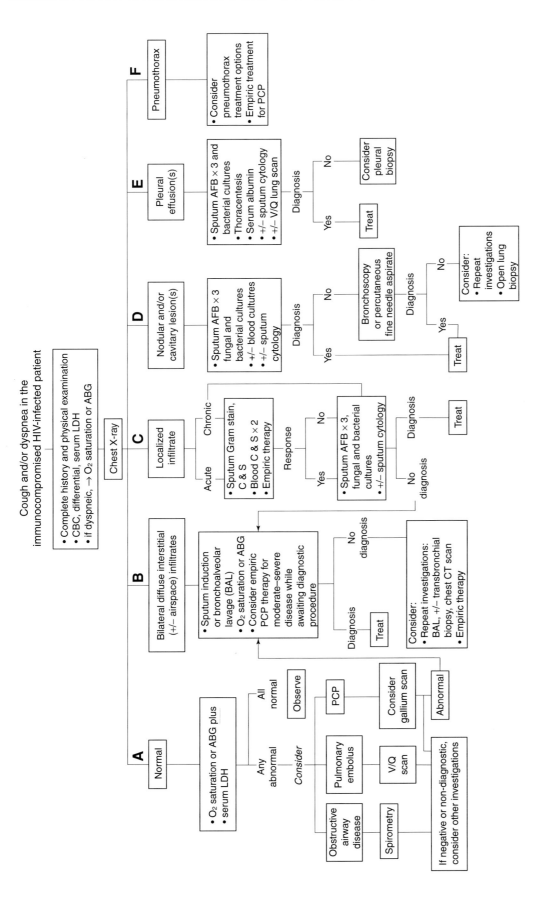

Figure 13.2. Cough and/or dyspnea in the immunocompromised HIV-infected patient

S. pneumoniae, *H. influenzae*, and *S. aureus*. *Legionella* pneumonitis, contrary to early reports, occurs rarely among HIV-infected individuals. Clinical features of community-acquired bacterial pneumonia are indistinguishable from those described in the immunocompetent host. Chest X-rays usually demonstrate segmental or lobar consolidation. Sputum and blood culture are often diagnostically helpful. If this is not the case, bronchoscopic studies will often identify the etiologic agent [9,11,12,50].

Nosocomial pneumonias among HIV-infected individuals are indistinguishable from those occurring in other hospitalized patients. These are usually caused by Gram-negative organisms and tend to have a high mortality despite appropriate antimicrobial therapy [50].

Fungal pneumonias (other than PCP) are an uncommon cause of respiratory disease among HIV-infected individuals. During the first decade of the HIV epidemic, *Aspergillus* pneumonia was a rare complication. However, in the past few years it has been increasingly reported and has become the most frequent pulmonary mycosis in many centers. Others include *Cryptococcus neoformans*, *Histoplasma capsulatum*, and *Coccidioides immitis*, often representing the pulmonary epiphenomenon of disseminated infection. Candidiasis of the trachea, bronchi or lungs, despite being recognized by the CDC as an AIDS-defining condition, is very uncommon among these patients. In addition to acute therapy with appropriate antifungal agents, long-term maintenance therapy is also required [50].

Kaposi's sarcoma involves the lungs in up to 30% of patients with mucocutaneous KS. Clinically significant pulmonary KS without obvious mucocutaneous involvement is exceptionally rare. Pulmonary KS is often indistinguishable from other HIV-related pulmonary diseases. Cough and dyspnea are commonly the presenting features. Fever, wheezing, hoarseness, and even upper airway obstruction can occur. Sputum production is usually absent. Hemoptysis, on the other hand, is relatively frequent. Chest X-ray usually shows nodular opacities of varying sizes coexisting with varying degrees of interstitial disease. Pleural and nodal involvement are also frequent. Bronchoscopic evaluation usually helps to rule out a superimposed treatable HIV-related disease in patients with pulmonary KS. It also may allow visualization of the characteristic red-violaceous lesions in the endobronchial tree. Although biopsy of these lesions at times can provide diagnostic confirmation, this is rarely required. None of the currently available therapies are particularly effective for systemic KS. Interferon has been used with some limited success for the treatment of early disease. Radiation therapy or chemotherapy have had some benefit in providing short-term palliation [51].

Prevention of respiratory disease among HIV-infected individuals

Given the very high frequency of respiratory involvement in this patient population, it is generally recommended that an aggressive preventive strategy be initiated immediately upon the diagnosis of HIV infection. All HIV-infected individuals should receive a one-time pneumococcal vaccine. It has now been demonstrated that this is a cost-effective intervention that should be implemented as soon as possible following the diagnosis of HIV to maximize the chances of an adequate humoral response. Yearly 'flu vaccination during the appropriate time of the year is also recommended for all HIV-infected individuals. The cost effectiveness of this maneuver is less well documented.

A PPD skin test will identify individuals at high risk for the development of tuberculosis. A 5 mm induration following a 5TU-PPD will require one year of INH prophylaxis. PPD skin testing should be repeated on a yearly basis. It should be noted that the predictive value of this test is likely to be compromised as the immunodeficiency progresses [13–16].

As discussed above, PCP prophylaxis should be initiated in all susceptible HIV-infected individuals who have any of the following: a CD4 count below $200/mm^3$; a fraction CD4 count below 15%; unexplained fever; recurrent candidiasis; or a prior episode of PCP. The preferred prophylactic regimen is TMP-SMX, 1 DS tablet once daily, for life. Adverse reactions to TMP-SMX are frequent and at times severe among HIV-infected individuals. Patients should be warned that the drug must be discontinued if generalized rash or fever develops. Alternative prophylactic regimens include DPS at a dose of 100 mg by mouth 3 times weekly or aerosol pentamidine intermittently [8].

Rifabutin at doses of 300 mg daily can significantly decrease the frequency of MAC in patients with advanced immunodeficiency. This intervention is currently recommended for patients who have CD4 counts below 100/mm³ [48].

Despite the availability of preventive or suppressive therapies, we must recognize that these are only partially effective. Furthermore, issues of acceptability, tolerability, compliance, cost, and accessibility of these preventive measures will continue to limit the ability of physicians to reduce the frequency of these respiratory complications of HIV/AIDS [52].

Finally, given the nature of HIV disease, itself, it is quite clear that successful prevention of certain pathologies, in the absence of a cure for the under-lying disease, will invariably give way to the development of newer opportunistic diseases. It is for this reason that the clinician must always maintain a high index of suspicion regarding the possibility of new emerging conditions.

Acknowledgment

Dr Montaner is a National Health Research Scholar of the National Health Research Program (NHRDP), Health and Welfare, Ottawa, Canada.

References

1   Schechter MT, Craib KJP, Gelmon KA, Montaner JSG, Le TN, O'Shaughnessy MV. HIV-1 and the aetiology of AIDS: results of a controlled study. *Lancet* 1993; **341**: 658–659.

2   White DA, Zaman MK. Pulmonary disease. *Med Clini of North Am* 1992; **76**: 19–44.

3   Quieffin J, Hunter J, Schechter MT et al. Aerosol pentamidine-induced bronchoconstriction. *Chest* 1991; **100**: 24–627.

4   Montaner JSG, Guillemi SA, Januszewska M et al. Unexpected lung lesions among patients with advanced HIV disease prior to PCP prophylaxis when using high resolution computed tomography. *American Thoracic Society*, San Francisco, May 1993; **147**: A1003.

5   Mani S, Smith GJ. HIV and pulmonary hypertension: a review. *South Med J* 1994; **87**: 357–362.

6   Montaner JSG, Lawson LM, Gervais A et al. A placebo controlled Canadian study of aerosol pentamidine for the secondary prophylaxis of AIDS-related PCP. *Ann Intern Med* 1991; **114**: 948–953.

7   Montaner JSG, Le T, Hogg R et al. Changing spectrum of AIDS index diseases in Canada. *AIDS* 1994 (in press).

8   US Public Task Force on Antipneumocystis Prophylaxis in Patients with Human Immunodeficiency Virus. Recommendations for prophylaxis against *Pneumocystis carinii* pneumonia for persons infected with human immunodeficiency virus. *J Acquir Immune Defic Synov* 1993; **6**: 46–55.

9   Montaner JSG, Phillips P, Russell JA. In : Hall JB, Schmidt GA,. Wood LDH (eds) *AIDS in the Intensive Care Unit. Principles of Critical Care.* McGraw-Hill, Inc. 1992: 1208–1231.

10 Hawley PH, Ronco JJ, Guillemi SA et al. Decreasing frequency but worsening mortality of acute respiratory failure (ARF) secondary to AIDS-related Pneumocystis carinii pneumonia. Chest (in press).

11 Magnenat JL, Nicod LP, Auckenthaler R, Junod AF. Mode of presentation and diagnosis of bacterial pneumonia in human immunodeficiency virus-infected patients. *Am Rev Respir Dis* 1991; **144**: 917–922.

12 Pesola GR, Charles A. Pneumococcal bacteremia with pneumonia. Mortality in acquired immunodeficiency syndrome. *Chest* 1992; **101**: 150–155.

13 Blatt SP, Hendrix CW, Butzin CA, et al. Delayed-type hypersensitivity skin testing predicts progression to AIDS in HIV-infected patients. *Ann Intern Med* 1993; **119**: 177–184.

14 Markowitz N, Hansen NI, Wilcosky TC et al. Tuberculin and anergy testing in HIV-seropositive and HIV-seronegative persons. *Ann Intern Med* 1993; **119**: 185–193.

15 Moreno S, Baraia-Etxaburu J, Bouza E, et al. Risk for developing tuberculosis among anergic patients infected with HIV. *Ann Intern Med* 1993; **119**: 194–198.

16 Kornbluth RS, McCutchan JA. Skin test responses as predictors of tuberculous infection and of progression in HIV-infected persons. *Ann Intern Med* 1993; **119**: 241–243.

17 Brusch JL. Case records of the Massachusetts General Hospital-Case 34–1993. *N Engl J Med* 1993; **329**: 645–653.

18 Stover DE, White DA, Romano PA et al. Spectrum of pulmonary diseases associated with the acquired immunodeficiency syndrome. *Am J Med* 1985; **78**: 429–437.

19 Haas DW, Des Prez R. Tuberculosis and acquired immunodeficiency syndrome: a historial perspective on recent developments. *Am J Med* 1994; **96**: 439–450.

20 Zaman MK, White DA. Serum lactate dehydrogenase levels and Pneumocystis carinii pneumonia. *Am Rev Respir Dis* 1988; **137**: 796–800.

21 Lipman ML, Goldstein E. Serum lactic dehydrogenase predicts mortality in patients with AIDS and pneumocystic pneumonia. *West J Med* 1988; **149**: 486–87.

22 Kagawa MT, Kirsch CM, Yenokia GG, Levine ML. Serum lactate dehydrogenase activity in patients with AIDS and Pneumocystis carinii pneumonia – an adjunct to diagnosis. *Chest* 1988; **94**: 1031–33.

23 Garay SM, Greene J. Prognostic indicators in the initial presentation of Pneumocystis carinii pneumonia. *Chest* 1989; **95**: 769–72.

24   Meeker DP, Matysik GA, Stelmach K, Rehm S. Diagnostic utility of lactate dehydrogenase levels in patients receiving aerosolized pentamidine. *Chest* 1993; **104**: 386–88.

25   Levine SJ, White DA. *Pneumocystis carinii*. *Clinics Chest Med* 1988; **9**: 395–423.

26   Montaner JSG, Russell JR, Lawson LM, Ruedy J. Acute respiratory failure secondary to *Pneumocystis carinii* pneumonia in the acquired immunodeficiency syndrome: a potential role for systemic corticosteroids. *Chest* 1989; **95**: 881–884.

27   Golden JA, Sollitto RA. The radiology of pulmonary disease. *Clinics Chest Med* 1988; **9**: 481–495.

28   Telzak EE, Cote RJ, Gold JWM, Campbell SW, Armstrong D. Extrapulmonary *Pneumocystis carinii* infections. *Rev Infect Dis* 1990; **12**: 380–385.

29   Wharton, BM, Coleman DL, Wofsy CB et al. Prospective randomized trial of trimethoprim-sulfamethoxazole versus pentamidine for *Pneumocystis carinii* pneumonia in the acquired immunodeficiency syndrome. *Ann Intern Med* 1986; **105**: 37–44.

30   Gordin FM, Simon GL, Wofsy CB, Mills J. Adverse reactions to trimethoprim-sulfamethoxazole in patients with acquired immunodeficiency syndrome. *Ann Intern Med* 1984; **100**: 495–499.

31   Medina I, Mills J, Leoung G et al. Oral Therapy for *Pneumocystis carinii* pneumonia in the acquired immunodeficiency syndrome: a controlled trial of trimethoprim-sulfamethoxazole versus trimethoprim-dapsone. *N Engl J Med* 1990; **323**: 776–82.

32   Montaner JSG, Lawson LM, Levitt N, Belzberg A, Schechter MT, Ruedy J. Corticosteroids prevent early deterioration in patients with moderately severe AIDS-related *Pneumocystis carinii* pneumonia and the acquired immunodeficiency syndrome (AIDS). *Ann Intern Med* 1990; **113**: 15–20.

33   Hughes WT, Gray V, Gutteridge WC, Latter VS, Podney M. A hydroxynapthoquinone, 566C80 is effective in experimental *Pneumocystis carinii* pneumonitis. *Antimicrob Agents Chemother* 1990; **34**: 225–228.

34   Hughes W, Leoung G, Kramer F et al. Comparison of atovaquone (566C80) with trimethoprim-sulfamethoxazole to treat Pneumocystis carinii pneumonia in patients with AIDS. N Engl J Med 1993; **328**: 1521–1527.

35   Masur H. Prevention and treatment of *Pneumocystis* pneumonia. *N Engl J Med* 1992; **327**: 1853–1860.

36   Toma E, Fournier S, Poisson N et al. Clyndamycin with primaquine for *Pneumocystis carinii* pneumonia. *Lancet* 1989; **I**: 1046–1048.

37   Allegra CJ, Chabner BA, Tuazon CU et al. Trimetrexate for the treatment of *Pneumocystis carinii* pneumonia in patients with acquired immunodeficiency syndrome. *N Engl J Med* 1987; **317**: 978–985.

38   Sattler FR, Allegra CJ, Verdegem TD, Akil B, Tuazon CU, Hughlett C. Trimetrexate-leucovorin dosage evaluation study for the treatment of Pneumocystis carinii Pneumonia. *J Infect Dis* 1990; **161**: 91–96.

39   Gagnon S, Boota AM, Fischl MA, Baier H, Kirksey OW, La Voie L. Corticosteroids as adjunctive therapy for severe *Pneumocystis carinii* pneumonia in the acquired immunodeficiency syndrome: a double-blind, placebo-controlled study. *N Engl J Med* 1990; **323**: 1444–1450.

40   Bozette SA, Sattler FR, Chiu J et al. A controlled trial of early adjunctive treatment with corticosteroids for *Pneumocystis carinii* pneumonia in the acquired immunodeficiency syndrome. *N Engl J Med* 1990; **323**: 1451–1457.

41   Consensus statement on the use of corticosteroids as adjunctive therapy for *Pneumocystis carinii* pneumonia in the acquired immunodeficiency syndrome. *N Engl J Med* 1990; **323**: 1500–1504.

42   Leoung GS, Feigal DW, Montgomery AB et al. Aerosolized pentamidine for prophylaxis against *Pneumocystis carinii* pneumonia: the San Francisco Community Prophylaxis Trial. *N Engl J Med* 1990; **323**: 769–775.

43   Centers for Disease Control and Prevention. 1993 revised classification system for HIV infection and expanded surveillance case definition for AIDS among adolescents and adults. *MMWR* 1992; **41**: 1–19.

44   Bass JB, Farer LS, Hopewell PC et al. Treatment of tuberculosis and tuberculosis infection in adults and children. American Thoracic Society. *Am J Respir Crit Care Med* 1994; **149**: 1359–1374.

45   Horsburg CR. *Mycobacterium avium* complex infection in the acquired immunodeficiency syndrome. *N Engl J Med* 1991; **324**: 1332–1338.

46   Wallace RJ Jr, Brown BA, Griffith DE et al. Initial clarithromycin monotherapy for *Mycobacterium avium-intracellulare* complex lung disease. *Am J Respir Crit Care Med* 1994; **149**: 1335–1341.

47   Chiu J, Nussbaum J, Bozette S, et al. Treatment of disseminated *Mycobacterium avium* complex infection in AIDS with amikacin, ethambutol, rifampin and ciprofloxacin. *Ann Intern Med* 1990; **133**: 358.

48   Nightingale SD, Cameron DW, Gordin FM, Sullam PM et al. Two controlled trials of rifabutin prophylaxis against *Mycobacterium avium* complex infection in AIDS patients. *New Engl J Med* 1993; **329**: 828–33.

49   Jacobson MA, Mills J. Cytomegalovirus infection. *Clin Chest Med* 1988; **9**: 443.

50   Fels AOS. Bacterial and fungal pneumonias. *Clin Chest Med* 1988; **9**: 449.

51   Ognibene FP, Shelhamer JH. Kaposi's sarcoma. *Clin Chest Med* 1988; **9**: 459.

52   Montaner JSG, Craib KJP, Le TNet al. Prevention of respiratory disease among HIV infected individuals: compliance with current guidelines within a cohort of homosexual men. *Am Rev Resp Dis* 1993, **147**: A1001.

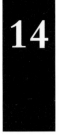

14 THORACIC IMAGING

Catherine A. Staples
Nestor L. Müller

Introduction

Pulmonary complications are frequently identified in patients affected with the human immune deficiency virus (HIV). A wide range of diseases, both infectious and non-infectious, are seen. However, opportunistic infections, particularly *Pneumocystis carinii* pneumonia (PCP), remain most common. In this chapter, the radiographic and computed tomography (CT) features of the pulmonary complications in acquired immune deficiency syndrome (AIDS) will be reviewed, and a guide to the utilization of CT in AIDS will be provided.

Infectious diseases

Protozoan infections

Pneumocystis carinii pneumonia

Pneumocystis carinii pneumonia remains the most common opportunistic infection in AIDS. Although *P. carinii* is genotypically a fungus, it behaves more like a protozoan [1].

PCP usually has an insidious onset presenting over days to weeks. In 10% of patients, the initial chest radiograph may be normal despite documentation of infection [2]. The typical chest radiographic findings include a bilateral perihilar or diffuse symmetric fine to medium reticular or reticulonodular pattern and ground-glass opacification (Figure 14.1). With progression over several days, more homogeneous consolidation is seen, but a reticular pattern is still usually identified in the periphery [3]. Although the radiographic abnormalities are typically diffuse, there may be an upper or lower zone predominance. An upper zone predominance is also increased with the use of prophylactic aerosolized pentamidine

[4–6]. A miliary or coarse interstitial pattern is less commonly seen (Figure 14.2). Atypical patterns of presentation include focal air space disease (which may mimic pyogenic pneumonia), cavitary nodules, hilar and/or mediastinal lymphadenopathy, and effusions.

Thin-walled cystic lesions have been noted on 10% of chest radiographs and on up to 40% of CT scans (Figure 14.3) [7,8]. These thin-walled cysts are often multiple, but may be confluent and have bizarre shapes (Figure 14.4). Thick-walled cavities can occur, but usually signify a secondary infection, particularly by *Aspergillus* species [9]. The majority of cysts are probably due to parenchymal destruction [10]. Many cysts resolve, suggesting partial obstruction and a check valve mechanism [7]. Cysts have been noted with increased frequency in patients receiving prophylactic aerosolized pentamidine [4]. The predominant subpleural location of cysts results in an increased incidence of pneumothorax (Figure 14.5). A pneumothorax presenting in an HIV-infected patient is virtually diagnostic of PCP.

CT is not usually required for diagnosis of classic cases of PCP, but can be helpful in the assessment of symptomatic patients with normal or questionable radiographic findings. The most characteristic finding of PCP on CT consists of extensive areas of ground-glass attenuation often in a patchy or geographic distribution (Figure 14.6). The ground-glass attenuation is frequently non-lobular in distribution and associated with reticulation (Figure 14.7). Confluent consolidation is seen in more severe cases. Although these findings may occasionally be seen with viral and bacterial pneumonia, the presence of ground-glass attenuation is most suggestive of PCP [11,12].

Intense diffuse heterogeneous uptake of gallium-67 in the lungs is strongly suggestive of PCP [13]. Although non-invasive, gallium scanning is expensive and requires 48–72 hours to be completed. Gallium

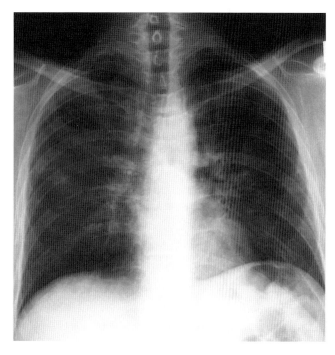

Figure 14.1.   A 48-year-old hemophiliac with PCP. A chest radiograph demonstrates diffuse fine, reticular, and ground-glass opacification with perihilar predominance.

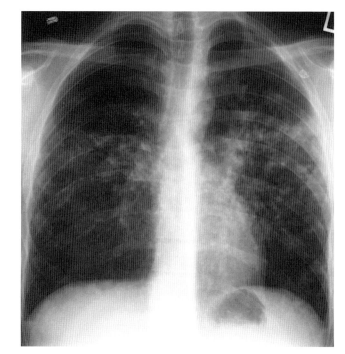

Figure 14.2.   A 31-year-old man with PCP. A chest radiograph shows coarse reticulonodular interstitial opacification, a less common presentation of PCP

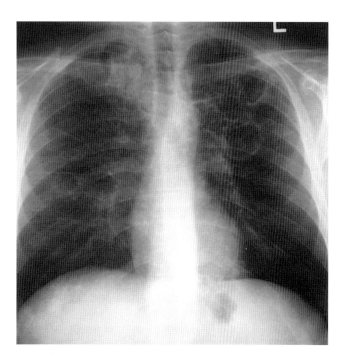

Figure 14.3.   A 37-year-old man with PCP. Diffuse fine reticulation, ground-glass opacification and multiple thin-walled cysts are seen with an upper-zone predominance on this chest radiograph.

scans are most useful in patients with symptoms suggestive of PCP but a normal chest radiograph [13]. In the majority of patients the diagnosis of PCP is confirmed at bronchoscopy. Although *Pneumocystis* organisms can be identified in induced sputum, few centers use this technique.

Pulmonary toxoplasmosis

Toxoplasma gondii is a protozoan that is a well-recognized cause of central nervous system disease in AIDS. Pulmonary involvement, however, is uncommon. Pulmonary toxoplasmosis is usually manifested radiographically by a bilateral, predominantly coarse, nodular pattern distinct from the fine interstitial pattern of PCP [14]. Although rare, toxoplasmosis should be considered in the differential diagnosis of other conditions in AIDS, which may show a similar coarse nodular pattern such as tuberculosis, cryptococcosis, and other disseminated fungal infections.

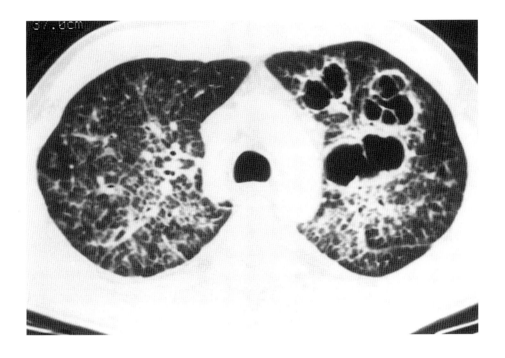

Figure 14.4. A 37-year-old man with PCP. A high-resolution CT scan at the level of the carina shows confluent cysts in the left upper lobe. Interlobular and intralobular lines are seen superimposed on a background of ground-glass attenuation.

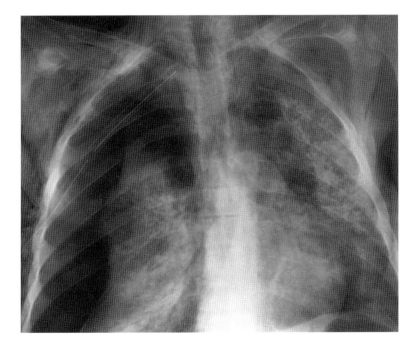

Figure 14.5. A 31-year-old man with PCP. A chest radiograph shows diffuse consolidation. Subpleural cysts are seen in the right upper lobe with a large right pneumothorax, pneumomediastinum and subcutaneous emphysema.

Viral infections

Cytomegalovirus

Although cytomegalovirus (CMV) is the most frequent infectious organism found at autopsy in AIDS, the clinical significance, even when there is cytopathologic evidence of CMV pneumonitis, is uncertain [15].

Some authors postulate that CMV is not a pathogen in the lung of AIDS patients, since they cannot mount the destructive immune response to CMV in the lungs [15]. Recent reports, however, suggest that CMV pneumonia may occur in some patients with AIDS and result in clinically significant complications [16].

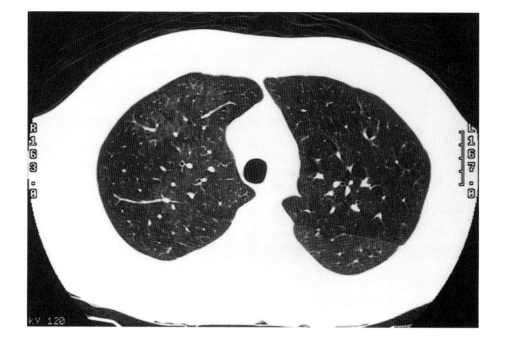

Figure 14.6. A 32-year-old man with bronchoscopically confirmed PCP. A high-resolution CT scan at the level of the aortic arch shows subtle and patchy non-lobular areas of ground-glass attenuation. Chest radiograph was normal.

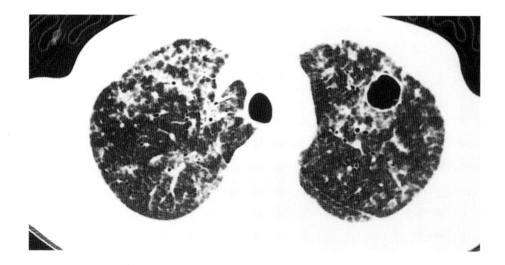

Figure 14.7. A 30-year-old man with PCP. A high-resolution CT scan obtained through upper lung zones shows reticulation with patchy ground-glass attenuation. One of multiple cysts is seen in the left upper lobe.

CMV is reported to produce bilateral interstitial infiltrates indistinguishable from PCP or fibrosis [17,18]. Pulmonary nodules or masses have also recently been described by McGuinness et al. [16]. Diagnosis requires histology either obtained by fine needle aspiration, transbronchial biopsy or open lung biopsy.

Pyogenic infections

Patients with AIDS have an increased incidence of pyogenic infections because they have impairment of both cell-mediated and humoral immunity. Bacterial infections are most common in HIV-infected intravenous drug abusers [19].

The radiographic findings of the most common bacterial infections (*Hemophilus influenzae* and *Streptococcus pneumoniae*) are similar to the presentation in non-HIV-infected patients. Diffuse, patchy or lobar consolidation are the most frequent abnormalities and effusions are common [20]. Sider et al. noted that bacterial infection was the most common cause of segmental unilateral alveolar infiltrates on CT, especially when cavitation or effusions were also present [12].

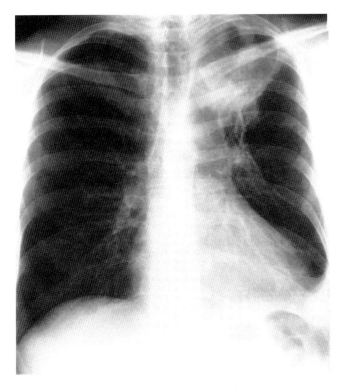

Figure 14.8. A 31-year-old man with nocardia pneumonia. Chest radiograph demonstrates rounded left upper lobe consolidation and a small left pleural effusion.

Septic emboli characteristically produce peripheral nodules or nodular infiltrates with a basal predominance and a high frequency of cavitation (Figure 14.8). CT classically shows feeding vessels leading to the nodules. Effusions or empyema are also commonly seen [18].

Less common bacterial infections in AIDS include *Nocardia* and *Legionella* species (Figure 14.9). Rhodococcus pneumonia (*Corynebacterium equi*, *Rhodococcus equi*) has also been described with increased frequency, and typically produces focal consolidation or a mass with cavitation [21a,b].

Mycobacterial diseases

Tuberculosis

The increasing incidence of tuberculosis (TB) worldwide has largely been attributed to AIDS [22]. This increase is most marked in racial and ethnic minorities, and in intravenous drug abusers. Approximately 10% of AIDS patients develop tuberculosis [2]. Although most patients respond well to treatment, the incidence of multiple drug-resistant tuberculosis is increasing.

Similar to the clinical and pathologic findings, the radiographic appearance is correlated with the degree of immunosuppression [22,23]. In early HIV disease, the radiographic presentation mimics reactivation TB in the non-HIV-infected host, and cavitary infiltrates predominate in the posterior segment of the upper

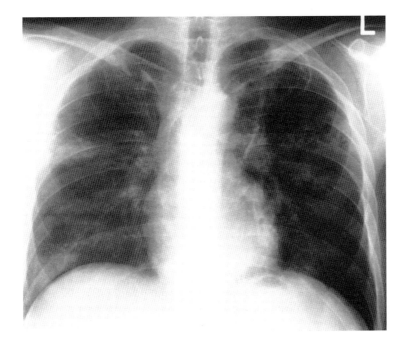

Figure 14.9. A 33-year-old man with septic emboli secondary to an infected indwelling venous catheter. A chest radiograph shows multiple peripheral cavitated nodules and infiltrates.

lobes or the superior segment of the lower lobes [23]. With advanced HIV infection, TB is usually disseminated in the lungs and frequently involves extra-pulmonary sites [22,23]. Diffuse coarse, nodular or reticulonodular infiltrates are common [23] (Figure 14.10). This coarse interstitial pattern should be contrasted with the typically fine interstitial pattern seen with PCP [23]. A miliary pattern is not uncommon (Figure 14.11). Alveolar infiltrates may be focal and are more common in the mid and lower lung zones. Lymphadenopathy occurs in up to 80% of patients and may occur in the absence of infiltrates [23]. Mycobacterial infection is the most common cause of lymphadenopathy in AIDS [12]. Enlarged nodes with central low attenuation owing to necrosis and peripheral rim enhancement after administration of intravenous contrast are characteristic findings at CT [2,24,25] (Figure 14.12). Although most commonly described in tuberculosis, this pattern may also be seen with atypical mycobacterial infection and infrequently with fungal infection or AIDS-related lymphoma [2,24,25] (Figure 14.13).

Mycobacterium avium **complex**

The incidence of *Mycobacterium avium* complex (MAC) in AIDS patients is reported to be 17–28% [23]. It

presents in advanced HIV disease, usually when the CD4 count drops below 50/mm^3. The diagnosis is often difficult to establish. The clinical symptoms and the radiographic findings may be indistinguishable from tuberculosis. However, MAC is usually widely disseminated at the time of diagnosis and lung involvement is relatively unimportant clinically [23].

Approximately 20% of chest radiographs in patients with MAC-related pulmonary disease are normal [26]. Abnormal findings include diffuse bilateral reticulonodular infiltrates, nodules, and focal or diffuse alveolar disease similar to TB, but a miliary pattern is less commonly seen [23]. Cavitation is rare. The incidence of lymphadenopathy and effusions is variable [12,23,26].

Fungal infections

Fungal infections are a frequent complication in AIDS. The most common disseminated fungal infections include cryptococcosis, histoplasmosis, and coccidioidomycosis. Histoplasmosis and coccidioidomycosis are most frequently seen in regions where they are endemic. Aspergillosis is a less common complication,

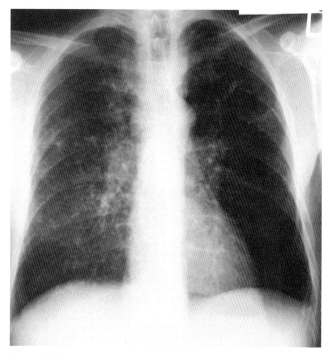

Figure 14.10.   A 43-year-old man with tuberculosis. A chest radiograph demonstrates coarse reticulonodular interstitial infiltrates with mediastinal and hilar adenopathy.

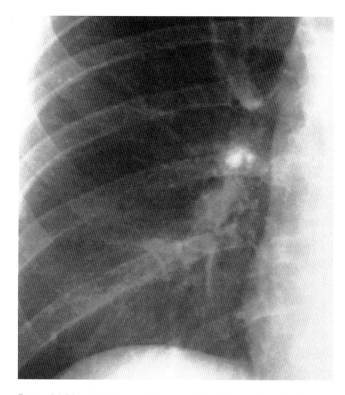

Figure 14.11.   A 39-year-old man with miliary tuberculosis. A chest radiograph, enlarged to show the right lower zone, shows diffuse pin-point nodules.

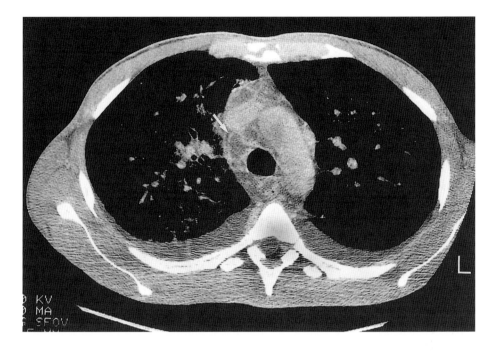

Figure 14.12. A 27-year-old man with tuberculosis. A high-resolution CT scan (mediastinal window) at the level of the aortic arch shows rim-enhancing lymph nodes with central low attenuation (arrow).

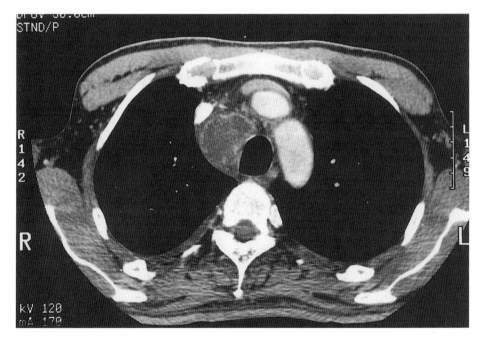

Figure 14.13. A 47-year-old man with *Mycobacterium avium-intracellulare* infection confirmed by CT-guided fine needle aspiration biopsy. An intravenous contrast-enhanced high-resolution CT scan demonstrates a bulky, low-attenuation, right paratracheal node with peripheral rim enhancement.

but the incidence appears to be increasing [27,28]. The disseminated fungal infections are usually treated with amphotericin B or one of the new triazoles, but prognosis is poor [29–31].

Cryptococcosis

Cryptococcosis, caused by the encapsulated yeast *Cryptococcus neoformans*, is the most common deep-seated fungal infection in AIDS and is seen world-wide [29]. It is present in 2–15% of AIDS patients with

pneumonia [32,33]. The lung is the port of entry, but primary pulmonary cryptococcosis is often asymptomatic [29,34]. Most patients with cryptococcosis in AIDS have cryptococcal meningitis and only 27% of these patients will have pulmonary involvement [34].

The most common radiographic findings include diffuse nodular or alveolar infiltrates and/or lymphadenopathy but reports vary significantly [29,32–34] (Figures 14.14 and 14.15). A single nodule or mass, with or without cavitation, or focal consolidation are

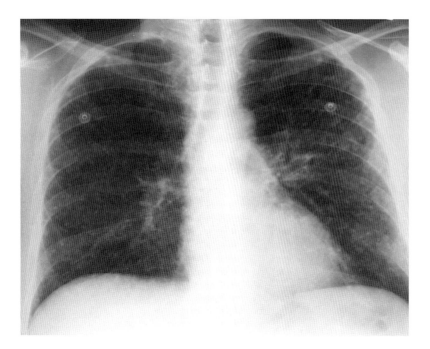

Figure 14.14. A 35-year-old man with disseminated cryptococcosis. A chest radiograph shows diffuse nodules.

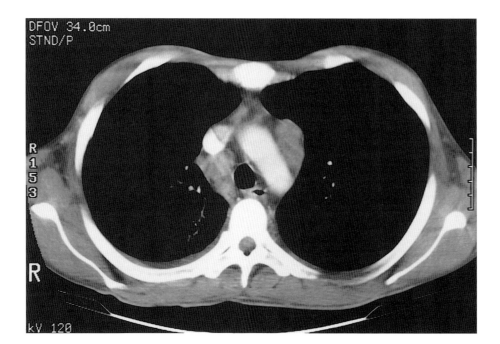

Figure 14.15. A 26-year-old man with disseminated cryptococcosis. A conventional contrast-enhanced CT scan obtained at the level of the aortic arch shows multiple enlarged lymph nodes.

less frequent findings which may mimic malignancy (Figure 14.16).

Histoplasmosis

Histoplasmosis, caused by the fungus *Histoplasma capsulatum*, is seen on all continents [29]. In North America it is endemic in the Ohio, Mississippi, and St Lawrence river valleys. Progressive disseminated histoplasmosis has been seen with increasing incidence in patients with AIDS [35]. Fifty-three per cent of patients have respiratory complaints at the time of presentation and 10% of cases present with a sepsis syndrome [36]. Bone marrow culture is the best diagnostic method [35]. Approximately 40% of AIDS patients with pulmonary

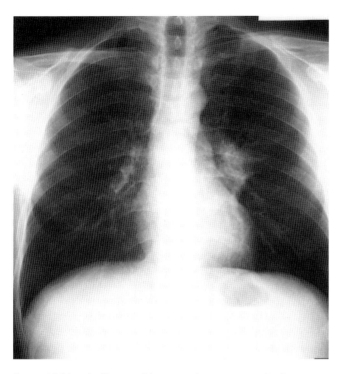

Figure 14.16. A 41-year-old man with cryptococcal infection. A chest radiograph shows a lobulated mass in the lingula. Fine needle aspiration biopsy confirmed the diagnosis.

disseminated histoplasmosis have a normal chest radiograph [35,36]. Diffuse interstitial infiltrates are the most common abnormal radiographic findings [29,35]. A miliary pattern, focal infiltrates, and hilar and mediastinal lymphadenopathy are less common [29,36].

Coccidioidomycosis

This mycosis is caused by *Coccidioides immitis* and is endemic in the south-western USA and Mexico. It also occurs in Central and South America. Respiratory symptoms are common in patients with coccidioidomycosis and AIDS, but only 30% of patients have radiographic abnormalities [37]. Diffuse nodular infiltrates are most frequently seen, but focal opacities, cavities, and lymphadenopathy also occur [29]. Diagnosis requires isolation of *Coccidioides immitis*. Bronchoalveolar lavage and transbronchial biopsy usually have a high diagnostic yield in patients with respiratory symptoms [29].

Aspergillosis

Recent studies suggest that aspergillosis is a more frequent pathogen in AIDS patients than previously thought [27,30]. *Aspergillus* infections are seen most commonly in advanced stages of AIDS [27,30,38]. Obstructing bronchial aspergillosis, pseudomembranous necrotizing tracheobronchial aspergillosis and chronic cavitary forms have been described [27,30,31,38,38a]. Classic angioinvasive aspergillosis also occurs.

Upper-lobe thick-walled cavities are the typical radiographic findings in all forms of aspergillosis [27,30,31,38]. A preexisting cystic lesion which progressively enlarges and becomes thick-walled is highly suspicious of aspergillosis. Cavities may be multiple and

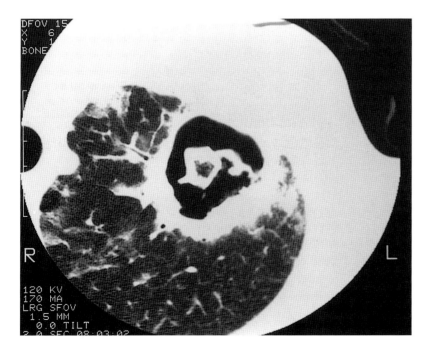

Figure 14.17. A 38-year-old man with invasive aspergillosis confirmed by histologic examination of lobectomy specimen. A targeted high-resolution CT scan of the left upper lobe shows a thick irregular cavity containing a mass. Surrounding interstitial changes were due to granulomatous PCP.

intracavitary masses are not uncommon (Figure 14.17). Associated findings include nodules, which may be pleural-based, consolidation and effusions.

Sputum cultures are of little value in the diagnosis of aspergillosis in HIV-infected patients owing to frequent colonization of airways with *Aspergillus*. Mycologic cultures after bronchoalveolar lavage is the method of choice for diagnosis [27]. Transthoracic needle biopsy is also useful for cavities and nodules [31]. The outcome of *Aspergillus* infections is poor despite treatment.

Malignant diseases

Kaposi's sarcoma

Kaposi's sarcoma (KS), is the most common AIDS-related neoplasm [39]. It occurs almost exclusively in homosexual and bisexual men, suggesting that a second cofactor may be necessary to promote KS [40].

KS usually presents with cutaneous lesions. KS can affect the airways, lungs, and pleura, and is seen in approximately 10% of AIDS patients overall and occurs in 30% of AIDS patients with cutaneous KS [39]. Patients with pulmonary KS usually present with short-ness of breath, cough, fever, and occasionally hemoptysis. Endobronchial lesions are typically raised, red or violet nodules, and when present in association with KS elsewhere, a presumptive diagnosis of lung involvement can often be made [41]. Diagnosis can be difficult, however, because involvement may be patchy and not all patients with lung involvement will have endobronchial lesions [39].

When pulmonary KS is extensive, chest radiographic findings may be characteristic. Diffuse, bilateral, poorly defined nodules, 1–2 cm in size or a reticulonodular interstitial pattern in a perihilar distribution, are common findings [42,43] (Figure 14.18). Coarse and 'wild-looking' chest radiographic features are characteristic of KS [42]. Findings may be less specific and mimic opportunistic infection [43,44]. Lobar or sublobar patchy consolidation and atelectasis may be seen [45]. Effusions are common [42–45]. Adenopathy is less common and usually a late finding [46].

Nodules with irregular margins, or areas of consolidation seen along a predominantly bronchovascular distribution are most characteristic of pulmonary KS at CT [11] (Figure 14.19). Subpleural nodules may

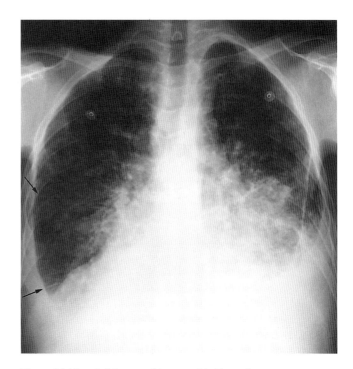

Figure 14.18. A 28-year-old man with Kaposi's sarcoma. A chest radiograph shows perihilar consolidation and extensive reticulonodular infiltrates. Septal lines (arrows) and bilateral effusions are seen.

also be seen [2]. Ground-glass attenuation locally adjacent to nodules or masses suggests areas of hemorrhage [47]. Interlobular septal thickening is seen in 38% of cases and is suggestive of KS [11] (Figure 14.20). In addition to effusions and adenopathy, a high incidence of extrapulmonary KS chest disease is evident on CT, including subcutaneous nodules and lytic lesions in the sternum, ribs, and thoracic spine [48].

The constellation of typical CT findings in a patient with skin KS is frequently sufficient for confident diagnosis of lung involvement [11,48]. CT is also useful in the diagnosis and staging of KS and in monitoring response to chemotherapy [48]. Gallium-67 scans show no lung activity in patients with pulmonary KS, which may be useful when trying to differentiate KS from infection [13].

AIDS-related lymphoma

AIDS-related lymphoma (ARL) occurs less frequently than KS. Lymphoma tends to be highly aggressive, present at an advanced stage and have a poor prognosis in AIDS [49]. Most ARLs are high-grade B-cell lymphomas [50]. It is hypothesized that Epstein-Barr virus infection may contribute to the development of

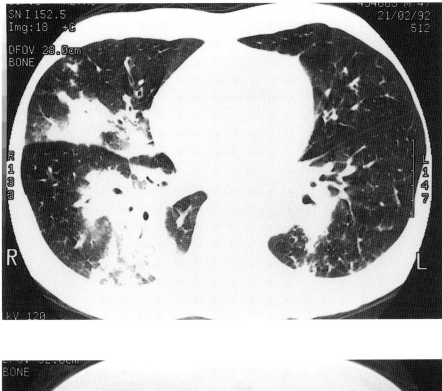

Figure 14.19. A 47-year-old man with Kaposi's sarcoma. A high-resolution CT scan through lower zones shows peribronchovascular interstitial thickening and consolidation. Note the surrounding ground-glass attenuation.

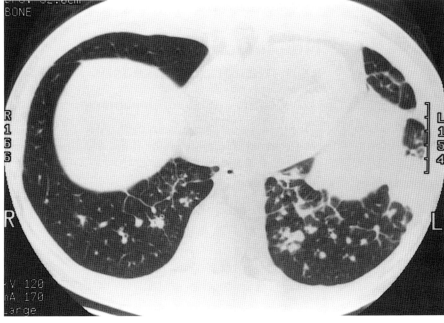

Figure 14.20. A 33-year-old man with Kaposi's sarcoma. A high resolution CT scan through the lung bases shows nodular thickening of the bronchovascular interstitium and smooth thickening of the interlobular septa.

ARL [51]. Although the manifestations of Hodgkin's disease are likely altered with AIDS, the occurrence of Hodgkin's disease in an HIV-infected person is not considered AIDS-related [40].

Extranodal involvement is seen in approximately 90% of patients with ARLs [40,43,49,50]. The most commonly involved sites are the central nervous system, the gastrointestinal tract, and the liver. Intra-

thoracic involvement varies from 0 to 40% [40,49,52,53]. The radiographic features of ARLs are variable. Effusions are reported to be the most common radiographic abnormality and are seen in at least 50% of cases [50,52] (Figure 14.21). They may be unilateral, bilateral or the sole manifestation of thoracic ARL [52]. Solitary or multiple smooth contoured nodules which rapidly enlarge are typical.

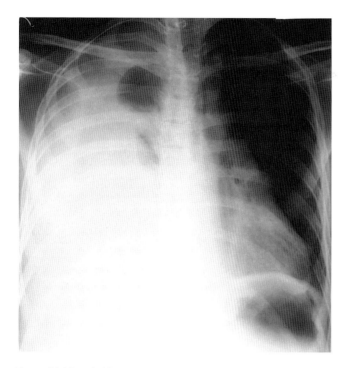

Figure 14.21. A 39-year-old man with non-Hodgkin lymphoma diagnosed by pleural aspiration. A chest radiograph shows a large right pleural effusion.

A doubling time of 4–6 weeks is not unusual [49,50]. Masses may exhibit central cavitation, air bronchograms or chest-wall invasion (Figure 14.22). Unlike lesions of KS, masses in ARL do not usually demon-strate an irregular margin or a bronchovascular distribution. Hilar and mediastinal lymphadenopathy occurs in 25% of cases [50]. Axillary lymphadenopathy occurs more commonly in ARLs than in other AIDS-related complications, but is not specific [12]. Interstitial infiltrates have been reported to be frequent in ARL, but in our experience, this is an uncommon manifestation of lymphoma in AIDS. Alveolar opacities, pericardial effusions or masses and myocardial involvement occur less frequently. Associated lytic bone lesions can also be seen (Figure 14.23).

Solid tumors

Lung cancer has been noted to occur more frequently and at a younger age group in AIDS patients than expected [54]. However, the relationship between AIDS and lung cancer is controversial [2,54]. The radiographic features of lung cancer occurring in an HIV-infected patient (although possibly more aggressive), are not different from lung cancer in an immunocompetent host.

Non-infectious and non-malignant diseases

Lymphocytic interstitial pneumonia

(LIP) is a lymphoproliferative disorder of the lung characterized by diffuse infiltration of the interstitium

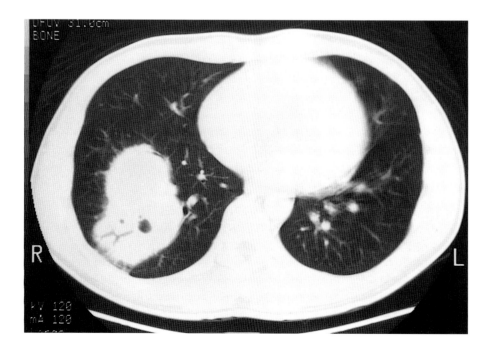

Figure 14.22. A 38-year-old man with non-Hodgkin lymphoma. A conventional CT scan through the lung bases shows a large right lower lobe mass containing an area of necrosis and an air bronchogram.

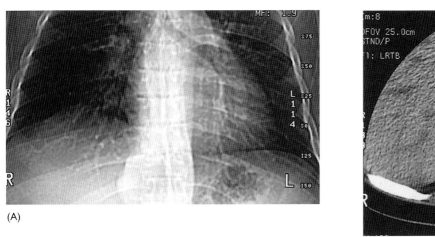

(A)

(B)

Figure 14.23. A 32-year-old man with non-Hodgkin lymphoma. (A) A scanogram obtained at CT shows a right paraspinal mass at T-10 and T-11. (B) A 5 mm collimation CT scan obtained through the mass at the time of fine needle aspiration biopsy shows a retrocrural mass invading the vertebra and an additional lytic lesion involving a posterior left rib.

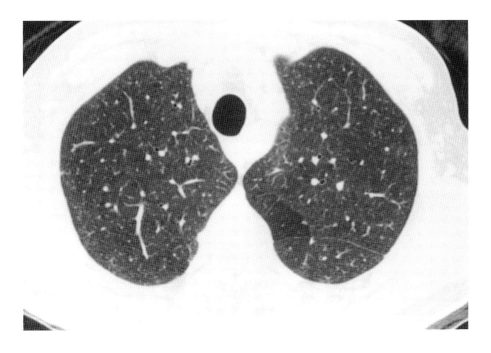

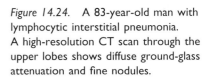

Figure 14.24. A 83-year-old man with lymphocytic interstitial pneumonia. A high-resolution CT scan through the upper lobes shows diffuse ground-glass attenuation and fine nodules.

with a polymorphic mixture of lymphocytes, histiocytes, and plasma cells. It has been associated with various systemic immunologic diseases and the incidence of LIP is also increased in AIDS, particularly in Haitian patients and children [40,55]. It is postulated that LIP represents a direct lung response to the presence of HIV [40,53,55].

The radiographic findings are non-specific and can include a fine to coarse, reticular or reticulonodular pattern as well as patchy alveolar or ground-glass opacities [55] (Figure 14.24). These features can mimic opportunistic infections, but tend to be stable over long periods of time [40]. Open lung biopsy is usually required for diagnosis [40,55]. Fortunately,

Table 14.1. Indications for CT in AIDS.

1. Identification or exclusion of occult disease in a symptomatic patient with a normal chest radiograph (in place of gallium scan).
2. Evaluation of diffuse lung abnormalities when chest radiographic findings confusing or unhelpful.
3. Evaluate suspected lymphadenopathy or mass.
4. Staging malignancies and/or follow-up response to treatment.
5. CT-guided transthoracic needle biopsy or direct mediastinoscopy, bronchoscopy, pleural tap or open lung biopsy.

LIP usually responds to steroid therapy and progression of LIP to lymphoma is rarely seen in AIDS [40,53].

Chest CT and pattern recognition in AIDS

In the majority of AIDS patients with pulmonary complications, a diagnosis can be readily established by a combination of clinical, radiographic and laboratory findings. CT can be helpful and is indicated in the assessment of symptomatic patients with normal or non-specific radiographic, findings and in patients with suspected lymphadenopathy (Table 14.1). CT-based diagnosis may obviate invasive diagnostic procedures in selected cases. CT allows a confident correct diagnosis of up to 94% of patients with PCP and 90% of patients with KS [11a,b].

Several recent studies have shown that specific patterns of disease involvement in AIDS patients, particularly at CT, can help suggest the likely diagnosis and guide further appropriate investigation [11a,12]. The diagnostic possibilities in order of probability for the specific CT and radiographic patterns seen in patients with AIDS are summarized in Quick Reference Table F.

It is important to recognize that multiple pulmonary complications may be present together, especially in late HIV disease. The CT scan may be the first test to suggest the presence of multiple complications when certain findings, which are not usually seen in association, coexist. For example, diffuse ground-glass attenuation, which is highly predictive of PCP, is usually an isolated finding. The association of a mass, lymphadenopathy, or a significant effusion with diffuse ground-glass attenuation indicates the presence of an additional process (Figure 14.25).

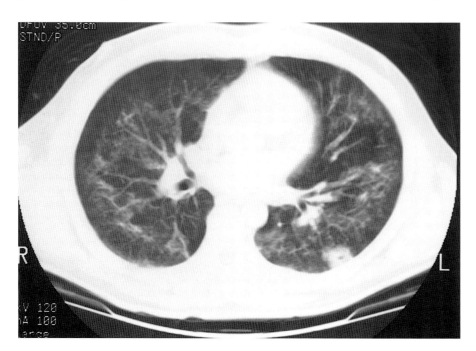

Figure 14.25. A 39-year-old man with PCP and non-Hodgkin lymphoma. A conventional CT scan shows ground-glass and alveolar infiltrates bronchoscopically confirmed due to PCP. Fine needle aspiration biopsy of the left lower lobe mass subsequently confirmed non-Hodgkin lymphoma.

References

1 Edman JC, Kovacs JA, Massur H et al. Ribosomal RNA sequence shows pneumocystis carinii to be a member of the fungi. *Nature* 1988; **334**: 519–522.

2 Naidich DP, McGuinness G. Pulmonary manifestations of AIDS: CT and radiographic correlations. *Radiol Clinics of North Am* 1991; **29**: 999–1017.

3 Goodman PC. Pneumocystis carinii pneumonia. *J Thorac Imag* 1991; **6**: 16–21.

4 Conces DJ Jr, Kraft JL, Vix VA et al. Apical pneumocystis carinii pneumonia after inhaled pentamidine prophylaxis. *AJR* 1989; **152**: 1192–1194.

5 Chaffey MH, Klein JS, Gamsu G, Blanc B, Golden JA. Radiographic distribution of pneumocystis carinii pneumonia in patients with AIDS treated with prophylactic inhaled pentamidine. *Radiology* 1990; **175**: 715–719.

6 Edelstein H, McCabe RE. Atypical presentations of pneumocystis carinii pneumonia in patients receiving inhaled pentamidine prophylaxis. *Chest* 1990; **98**: 1366–1369.

7 Sandhu JS, Goodman PC. Pulmonary cysts associated with pneumocystis carinii pneumonia in patients with AIDS. *Radiology* 1989; **173**: 33–35.

8 Kuhlman JE, Knowles MC, Fishman EK, Siegelman SS. Premature bullous pulmonary damage in AIDS: CT diagnosis. *Radiology* 1989; **173**: 23–26.

9 Kuhlman JE, Kavuru M, Fishman EK, Siegelman SS. *Pneumocystis carinii* pneumonia: spectrum of parenchymal CT findings. *Radiology* 1990; **175**: 711–714.

10 Feuerstein IM, Archer A, Pluda JM et al. Thin-walled cavities, cysts, and pneumothorax in pneumocystis carinii pneumonia: further observations with histopathologic correlation. *Radiology* 1990; **174**: 697–702.

11a Hartman TE, Primack SL, Müller NL, Staples CA. Diagnosis of thoracic complications in AIDS: accuracy of CT. *AJR* 1994; **162**: 547–553.

11b Kang EY, Staples CA, McGuinness G. Detection and differential diagnosis of pulmonary infections and tumors in patients with AIDS: value of chest radiography versus CT. *AJR* 1996; **166**: 15–19.

12 Sider L, Gabriel H, Curry DR, Pham MS. Pattern recognition of the pulmonary manifestations of AIDS on CT scans. *RadioGraphics* 1993; **13**: 771–784.

13 Kramer EL, Sanger JH, Garay SM, Grossman RJ, Tiu S, Banner H. Diagnostic implications of Ga-67 chest-scan patterns in human immunodeficiency virus-seropositive patients. *Radiology* 1989; **170**: 671–676.

14 Goodman PC, Schnapp LM. Pulmonary toxoplasmosis in AIDS. *Radiology* 1992; **184**: 791–793.

15 Millar AB, Patou G, Miller RF et al. Cytomegalovirus in the lungs of patients with AIDS: respiratory pathogen or passenger? *Am Rev Respir Dis* 1990; **141**: 1474–1477.

16 McGuinness G, Scholes JV, Garay SM, Leitman BS, McCauley DI, Naidich DP. Cytomegalovirus pneumonitis: spectrum of parenchymal CT findings with pathologic correlation in 21 AIDS patients. *Radiology* 1994; **192**: 451–459.

17 Naidich DP, Garay SM, Goodman PC, Rybak BJ, Kramer EL. Pulmonary manifestations of AIDS. In: Federle M,

Megibow A, Naidich DP (eds) *Radiology of Acquired Immune Deficiency Syndrome*. New York: Raven Press, 1988: 47–76.

18 Kuhlman JE, Fishman EK, Hruban RH, Knowles M, Zerhouni EA, Siegelman SS. Diseases of the chest in AIDS: CT diagnosis. *RadioGraphics* 1989; **9**: 827–857.

19 Witt DJ, Craven DE, McCabe WR. Bacterial infections in adult patients with the acquired immunodeficiency syndrome (AIDS) and AIDS-related complex. *Am J Med* 1987; **82**: 900–906.

20 Daley CL. Pyogenic bacterial pneumonia in the acquired immunodeficiency syndrome. *J Thorac Imaging* 1991; **6**: 36–42.

21a MacGregor JH, Samuelson WM, Sane DC, Godwin JD. Opportunistic lung infection caused by *Rhodococcus (Corynebacterium) equii*. *Radiology* 1986; **160**: 83–4.

21b Wicky S, Cartei F, Mayor B, Frija J, Gevenois PA, Giron J, Laurent F, Derri G, Schnyder P. Radiological findings in nine AIDS patients with *Rhodococcus equi pneumonia*. *Eur Radiol* 1996; **6**, 826–830.

22 Davis SD, Yankelevitz DF, Williams T, Henschke CI. Pulmonary tuberculosis in immunocompromised hosts: epidemiological, clinical, and radiological assessment. *Semin Roentgenol* 1993; **XXVIII**: 119–130.

23 Goodman PC. Mycobacterial disease in AIDS. *J Thorac Imaging* 1991; **6**: 22–27.

24 Im JG, Song KS, Kang HS et al. Mediastinal tuberculous lymphadenitis: CT manifestations. *Radiology* 1987; **164**: 115–119.

25 Pastores SM, Naidich DP, Aranda CP, McGuinness G, Rom WN. Intrathoracic adenopathy associated with pulmonary tuberculosis in patients with human immunodeficiency virus infection. *J Computer Assisted Tomography* 1993; **103**: 1433–1437.

26 Marinelli DL, Albelda SM, Williams TM, Kern JA, Iozzo RV, Miller WT. Nontuberculous mycobacterial infection in AIDS: clinical, pathologic, and radiographic features. *Radiology* 1986; **160**: 77–82.

27 Lortholary O, Meyohas MC, Dupont B et al. Invasive aspergillosis in patients with acquired immunodeficiency syndrome: report of 33 cases. *Am J Med* 1993; **95**: 177–187.

28 Minamoto GY, Barlam TF, Vander Els NJ. Invasive aspergillosis in patients with AIDS. *Clin Infect Dis* 1992; **14**: 66–74.

29 Stansell JD. Fungal disease in HIV-infected persons: cryptococcosis, histoplasmosis, and coccidioidomycosis. *J Thorac Imaging* 1991; **6**: 28–35.

30 Miller WT Jr, Sais GJ, Frank I, Gefter WB, Aronchick JM, Miller WT. Pulmonary aspergillosis in patients with AIDS: clinical and radiographic correlations. *Chest* 1994; **105**: 37–44.

31 Denning DW, Follansbee SE, Scolaro M, Norris S, Edelstein H, Stevens DA. Pulmonary aspergillosis in the acquired immunodeficiency syndrome. *N Engl J Med* 1991; **324**: 654–62.

32 Cameron ML, Bartlett JA, Gallis HA, Waskin HA. Manifestations of pulmonary cryptococcosis in patients with acquired immunodeficiency syndrome. *Rev Infect Dis* 1991; **13**: 64–67.

33 Sider L, Westcott MA. Pulmonary manifestations of cyrptococcosis in patients with AIDS: CT features. *J Thorac Imaging* 1994; **9**: 78–84.

34 Miller WT Jr, Edelman JM. Cryptococcal pulmonary infection in patients with AIDS: radiographic appearance. *Radiology* 1990; **175**: 725–728.

35 Johnson PC, Sarosi GA, Septimus EJ, Satterwhite TK. Progressive disseminated histoplasmosis in patients with the acquired immune deficiency syndrome: a report of 12 cases and a literature review. *Semin Respir Infect* 1986; **1**: 1–8.

36 Wheat LJ, Slamma TG, Zeckel ML. Histoplasmosis in the acquired immune deficiency syndrome. *Am J Med* 1985; **78**: 203–210.

37 Fish DG, Ampel NM, Galgiani JN et al. Coccidioidomycosis during human immunodeficiency virus infection. A review of 77 patients. *Medicine* 1990; **69**: 384–391.

38 Wright JL, Lawson L, Chan N, Filipenko D. An unusual form of pulmonary aspergillosis in two patients with the acquired immunodeficiency syndrome. *Am J Clin Pathol* 1993; **100**: 57–59.

38a Staples CA, Kang EY, Wright JL et al. Invasive pulmonary aspergillosis in AIDS: radiographic, CT, and pathologic findings. *Radiology* 1995; **196**: 409–414.

39 Mitchell DM, McCarty M, Fleming J, Moss FM. Bronchopulmonary Kaposi's sarcoma in patients with AIDS. *Thorax* 1992; **47**: 726–729.

40 White DA, Matthay RA. State of the art: noninfectious pulmonary complications of infection with the human immunodeficiency virus. *Am Rev Respir Dis* 1989; **140**: 1763–1787.

41 Zibrak JD, Silvestri RC, Costello P et al. Bronchoscopic and radiologic features of Kaposi's sarcoma involving the respiratory system. *Chest* 1986; **90**: 476–479.

42 Goodman PC. Kaposi's sarcoma. *J Thorac Imaging* 1991; **6**: 43–48.

43 Nyberg DA, Federle MP. AIDS-related Kaposi's sarcoma and lymphomas. *Semin Roentgenol* 1987; **XXII**: 54–65.

44 Garay SM, Belenko M, Fazzini E, Schinella R. Pulmonary manifestations of Kaposi's sarcoma. *Chest* 1987; **91**: 39–43.

45 Sivit CJ, Schwartz AM, Rockoff SD. Kaposi's sarcoma of the lungs in AIDs: radiologic-pathologic analysis. *AJR* 1987; **148**: 25–28.

46 Naidich DP, Tarras M, Garay SM et al. Kaposi's sarcoma: CT-radiographic correlation. *Chest* 1989; **96**: 723–728.

47 Leung AN, Miller RR, Müller NL. Parenchymal opacification in chronic infiltrative lung diseases: CT-Pathologic correlation. *Radiology* 1993; **188**: 209–214.

48 Wolff SD, Kuhlman JE, Fishman EK. Thoracic Kaposi sarcoma in AIDS: CT findings. *J Computer Assisted Tomography.* 1993; **17**: 60–62.

49 Haskal ZJ, Lindan CE, Goodman PC. Lymphoma in the immunocompromised patient. *Radiol Clinics North Am* 1990; **28**: 885–899.

50 Goodman PC. Non-Hodgkin's lymphoma in the acquired immunodeficiency syndrome. *J Thorac Imaging* 1991; **6**: 49–52.

51 Purtilo DT, Kipscomb H, Volsky DJ et al. Role of Epstein-Barr virus in acquired immunodeficiency syndrome. *Adv Exp Med Biol* 1985; **187**: 93–96.

52 Sider L, Weiss AJ, Smith MD, Von Roenn JH, Glassroth J. Varied appearance of AIDS-related lymphoma in the chest. *Radiology* 1989; **171**: 629–632.

53 Heitzman ER. Pulmonary neoplastic and lymphoproliferative disease in AIDS: a review. *Radiology* 1990; **177**: 347–351.

54 Braun MA, Killam DA, Remick SC et al. Lung cancer in patients seropositive for human immunodeficiency virus. *Radiology* 1990; **175**: 341–343.

55 Oldham SAA, Castillo M, Jacobson FL, Mones JM, Saldana MJ. HIV-associated lymphocytic interstitial pneumonia: radiologic manifestations and pathologic correlation. *Radiology* 1989; **170**: 83–87.

15 DIAGNOSIS AND TREATMENT OF GASTROINTESTINAL DISEASE IN PATIENTS WITH HIV INFECTION

Joep F.W.M. Bartelsman

HIV seroconversion

The commonest syndrome associated with human immune deficiency virus (HIV)-seroconversion is an acute mononucleosis-like illness. In patients for whom the date of exposure could be established, the incubation period was 11–28 days and the mean duration of acute illness was 12.7 days [1].

The clinical picture is characterized by a sudden onset of fever, sore throat, lymphadenopathy, rash, lethargy, dry cough, headache, myalgia, conjunctivitis, vomiting, nausea, and diarrhea. Some patients experience severe esophageal symptoms, caused by multiple discrete esophageal ulcers [2].

Acute primary HIV esophagitis has been described in a young man who presented with fever and odynophagia [3]. HIV-1–p24 antigen could only be shown in the blood on the first day of hospital admission, 7 days after the onset of the disease. Sero-conversion for HIV-1 antibodies took place 28 days after the onset. Esophageal candidiasis occurring during primary HIV infection has also been reported [4].

AIDS

Mucosal involvement of the gut by viral, bacterial, fungal, and protozoal pathogens as well as by malignant tumors is common in acquired immune deficiency syndrome (AIDS). The gastrointestinal tract can be involved in three different ways [5,6]:

1. Opportunistic tumors: Kaposi's sarcoma, B-cell lymphoma, and squamous carcinoma of the tongue and the anus.

2. Opportunistic infections.
3. Direct HIV effects on the gut.

Over a 10–year period (1982–1992), 550 adult AIDS patients were seen in our hospital. Of these, 527 were male and 23 were female. Seventy per cent of these patients were found to have gastrointestinal disease by radiologic studies, endoscopy, laboratory tests, or autopsy. The most frequent gastrointestinal symptoms and abnormalities were: diarrhea (50%), dysphagia or odynophagia (34%), anorectal disease (16%) and Kaposi's sarcoma (20%).

Esophagus (Figures 15.1–15.9)

Candida infection is the most common cause of esophageal symptoms in AIDS patients. Endoscopy typically shows white pseudomembranes or raised plaques in the esophagus which consist of pseudo-hyphae with fibrin and cellular debris. Pseudohyphae do not extend beyond the muscular layer and perforation associated with *Candida* ulceration is rare [7]. Culture biopsy specimens will allow for specification of the *Candida* organisms and for determination of sensitivities of the pathogen to antifungal agents.

Cytologic brushings are superior to endoscopic biopsies in diagnosing fungal esophagitis. Fluconazole is highly effective in treating esophageal candidiasis and superior to ketoconazole, although isolated cases of fluconazole-resistant *Candida albicans* have been reported [8].

Herpes simplex virus (HSV) can cause severe dysphagia and odynophagia. The earliest lesion at endoscopy are multiple vesicles, which slough to form

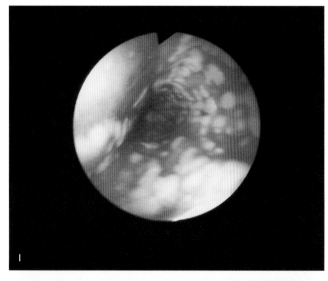

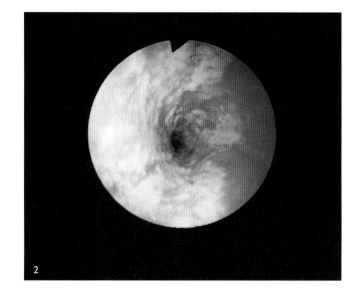

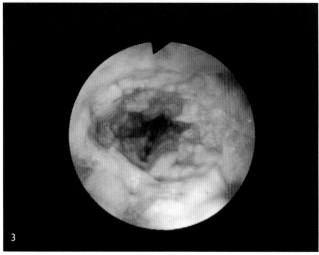

Figures 15.1–15.3.   Esophagus: *Candida* esophagitis.

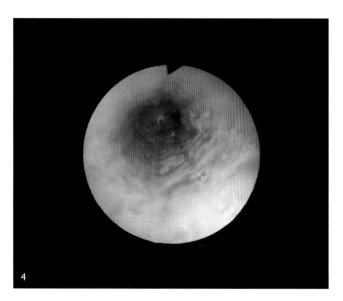

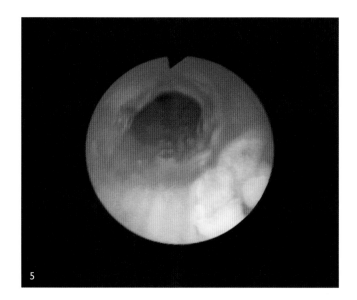

Figures 15.4 and 15.5.   HSV esophagitis.

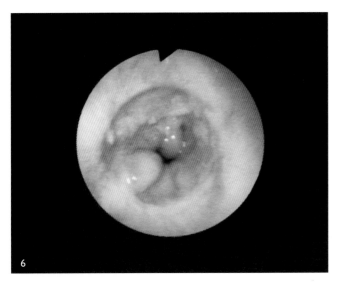

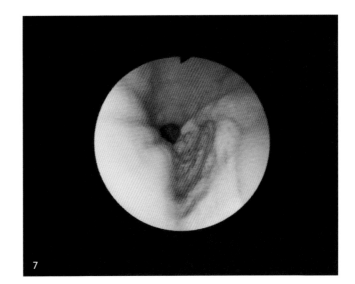

Figures 15.6 and 15.7. CMV esophagitis.

circumscribed ulcers with slightly raised erythematous edges. These ulcers can coalesce to form large ulcers. HSV can be isolated from a swab culture or by biopsies, which may show the typical viral inclusions in the epithelial cells. Culture is slightly more sensitive than microscopic examination for diagnosis [9].

Cytomegalovirus (CMV) can also cause esophageal ulceration with severe complaints. Endoscopy often shows large, solitary, shallow, distal ulcers with relatively normal surrounding mucosa. Infection occurs within submucosal fibroblasts and endothelial cells, not in the epithelium, and is usually part of a widespread visceral infection. However, the demonstration of CMV does not necessarily signify disease. The standard diagnosis of CMV disease has been the finding of cytomegalic cells with typical intranuclear inclusions at histology. Additional methods include viral cultures, immunohistochemical detection of CMV antigens, *in situ* hybridization, and the polymerase chain reaction (PCR) [10].

CMV infection can be treated with ganciclovir, or foscarnet in patients in whom ganciclovir has failed [11]. We diagnosed giant esophageal ulceration in 42 patients with AIDS: 21 of them were probably caused by CMV, 3 by HSV, and 1 by non-Hodgkin lymphoma (NHL). In 17 patients with a large esophageal ulceration, no specific cause could be diagnosed. These patients with idiopathic ulcerations can be successfully treated with corticosteriods. Kaposi's sarcoma (KS) is frequently found in the gut of patients with cutaneous involvement [12]. Lesions in the gastrointestinal tract may occur in the absence of any skin lesions. KS can be in any part of the gastrointestinal tract and is mostly asymptomatic. The endoscopic picture of KS in the gut is:

1. Small, flat, red or violet lesions.
2. Sessile red or violet polyps, sometimes with a central ulceration.
3. Large tumors, sometimes causing obstruction.

Small endoscopic biopsies frequently fail to make the diagnosis of KS, owing to the submucosal nature of most of the KS lesions.

We diagnosed KS endoscopically in the esophagus in 17 out of 65 patients with KS of the gastrointestinal tract. In general, visceral KS lesions require treatment only if symptomatic, since enteric lesions along rarely alter the progression of AIDS or directly lead to death. In case of symptoms, therapeutic alternatives are: excision of localized lesions, radiotherapy, chemotherapy, or immunomodulation with interferon or thymic hormones. Also antiviral therapy for HIV may have an effect of KS [19].

AIDS-related high-grade B-cell lymphoma can involve the esophagus, which is the least common site of involvement in the gastrointestinal tract. NHL can present as a solitary or multiple masses, small polypoid lesions, or large ulcerations, which can be complicated by bleeding or perforation. The overall prognosis of patients with AIDS and NHL is usually poor. Aggressive treatment of lymphomas with combination chemotherapy has resulted in remission rates exceeding 50%, but iatrogenic immunosuppression can hasten the acquisition of infections and shorten survival.

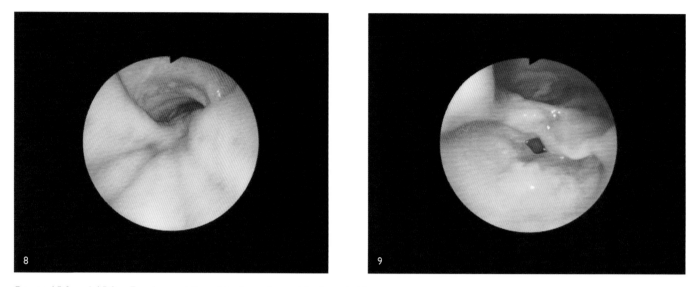

Figures 15.8 and 15.9. Esophagus: idiopathic giant ulcer with tissue bridge.

Stomach (Figures 15.10–15.15)

CMV infection of the stomach causes a diffuse gastritis, multiple erosions, or large demarcated ulcers.

In our hospital, we have diagnosed endoscopic abnormalities in the stomachs of 95 patients (Table 15.1). CMV caused ulcers in four patients, two more ulcers were caused by NHL, and six ulcers had a non-specific cause (including *Helicobacter pylori*). From 13 patients with gastric erosions, CMV could be demonstrated in only 2, and in patients with diffuse gastritis, in only 8 out of 73 patients. In contrast to HIV-seronegative patients, the prevalence of *H. pylori* in HIV-infected patients seems to be low [15,16]. This low prevalence of *H. pylori* can be caused by the immunodeficiency itself or by previous administration of antibiotics for other infectious diseases.

Table 15.1.   Gastric abnormalities in 98 patients with AIDS.

Stomach biopsy	Endoscopic findings		
	Ulcer (n=12)	Erosions (n=13)	Diffuse gastritis (n=73)
CMV	4	2	8
NHL	2	–	–
Cryptosporidiosis	–	–	4
MAI	–	–	2
Non-specific	6	11	59

Small intestine (Figures 15.16–15.18)

Diarrhea, sometimes accompanied by abdominal pain, nausea, and vomiting, is the commonest symptom of small bowel infection. It may be cholera-like and potentially life-threatening. Two hundred and seventy five of our 550 patients with AIDS had diarrhea (50%).

Diarrhea was seen in 54% of homosexual patients and 40% of non-homosexual patients with AIDS in our hospital. A total of 119 patients had 1 or 2 episodes of diarrhea, and 156 patients had 3 or more episodes of chronic diarrhea. In 46% of patients, the cause of the diarrhea could be found by examination of the feces. The infections diagnosed most frequently by feces examination were: *Campylobacter jejuni* (19%), *Cryptosporidium* (16%), *Mycobacterium avium-intracellulare* (MAI) (12%), and *Microsporidium* (10%).

We performed a combined duodenoscopy and sigmoidoscopy with multiple biopsies in 157 patients with diarrhea, with negative findings after repeated feces examination. An additional diagnosis could be obtained in 31 patients (20%): CMV colitis in 20, microsporidiosis in 5, and cryptosporidiosis in 6 patients.

Bacterial enteritis

Diarrhea in AIDS may not only be due to opportunistic infectious diseases. It may also be the result

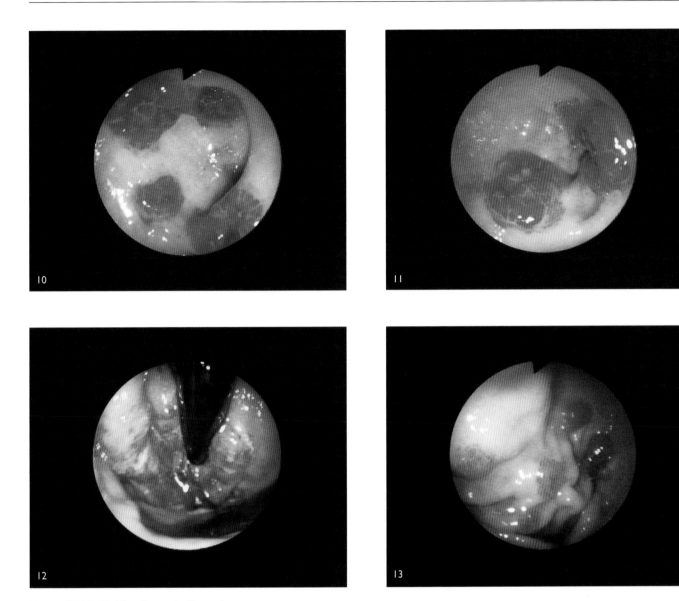

Figures 15.10–15.13.   Stomach: Kaposi's sarcoma.

of a variety of non-opportunistic pathogens [17]. Salmonellosis has been particularly problematic in the HIV population with bacteremia occurring in nearly 50% in one study [18,19]. Bacteremias and relapse rate are increased in patients with low CD4 counts. Also the course of infections with *Campylobacter* and *Shigella* can be more complicated in patients with advanced immunodeficiency. Quinolone antibiotics are mostly chosen for therapy, but cases of resistance and clinical relapse of *Campylobacter* during therapy are reported. MAI may invade the intestine and lodge in macrophages in the lamina propria. It can cause abdominal pain, chronic diarrhea and malabsorption. Accumula-

tion of macrophages with MAI can cause thickening of the villi, which can resemble Whipple's disease during duodenoscopy. A regimen with four drugs (rifampin, ethambutol, clofazimine, ciprofloxacine) has been associated with symptomatic improvement but not with elimination of mycobacteria [20].

Parasitic infections

In AIDS, a variable clinical response to infection with *Giardia lamblia* is observed. Prior exposure may lead to less severe illness in AIDS patients [21].

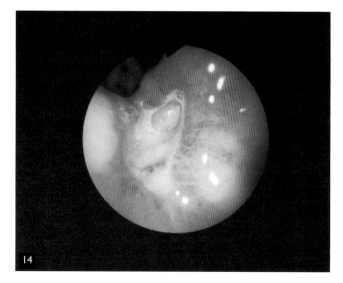

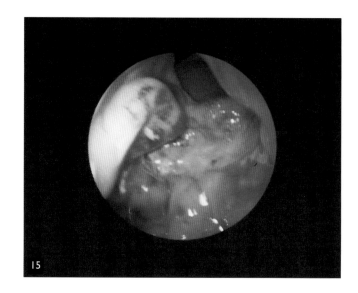

Figures 15.14 and 15.15.   Stomach: B-cell lymphoma.

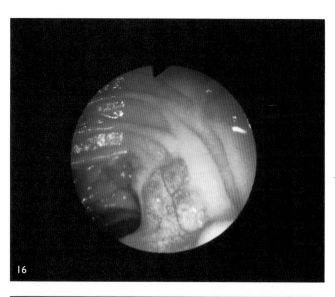

◀ *Figure 15.16.*   Duodenum: Kaposi's sarcoma.

▼ *Figures 15.17 and 15.18.*   Duodenum: pseudo Whipple's disease (*Mycobacterium avium intracellulare*).

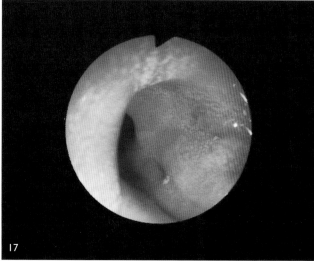

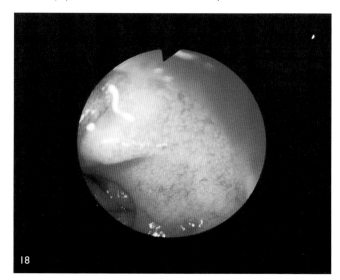

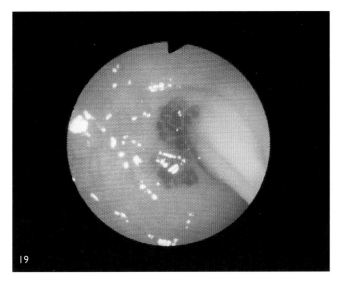

Figure 15.19.   Colon: Kaposi's sarcoma.

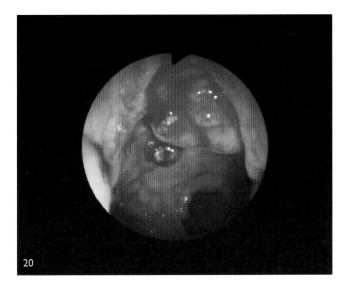

Figure 15.20.   Colon: B-cell lymphoma.

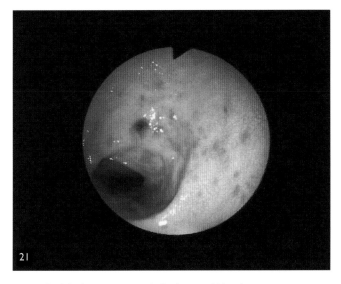

Figure 15.21. Colon: mucosal thickening (*Mycobacterium avium intracellulare*).

Cryptosporidium parvum has long been recognized as a pathogen in HIV-positive patients. It causes profuse watery diarrhea with cramps and weight loss. There is no clear association between the number of oocysts in the stool or those seen on duodenal biopsy and the severity of diarrhea. The duration of the diarrhea in HIV patients is correlated inversely with the total lymphocyte count. Patients with cryptosporidiosis are frequently coinfected with additional pathogens. Successful treatment of those other enteric infections can result in the disappearance of the cryptosporidia and resolution of diarrhea [23,24]. No antimicrobial

agent has proved to be consistently effective against *Cryptosporidium* [15].

Cyclospora cayetanensis, a coccidian organism, has been identified in stools of HIV-positive patients with chronic diarrhea [26]. *Cyclospora* is identified in stool by the modified acid-fast stain and may resemble *Cryptosporidium* oocysts, but *Cyclospora* oocysts are larger.

Microsporidiosis is a well-recognized cause of chronic diarrhea in AIDS-patients. *Enterocytozoon bieneusi* is frequently diagnosed nowadays since new light-microscopical identification techniques for stool and gastrointestinal biopsies have been introduced [27]. Albendazole may be a useful therapy in this infection [28].

Encephalitozoon-like microsporidia are also detected in the duodenum biopsies in patients with HIV infections. This organism is unlike *E. bieneusi*, not confined to enterocytes, but has also been found in lamina propria macrophages [30].

Viral infections

An ulcerating enteritis associated with CMV infection can affect long segments of the small intestine [6]. CMV can cause terminal ileitis and mimic Crohn's disease [31]. CMV ulcers can be complicated by severe bleeding or perforation, requiring exploratory laparotomy. Perforation of duodenal and jejunal CMV ulcers can occur, but ileal perforation is more frequently reported [32].

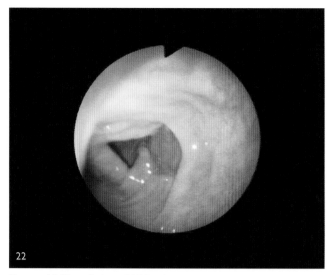

Figures 15.22.   Colon: CMV colitis.

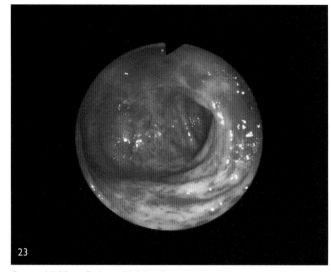

Figure 15.23.   Colon: CMV colitis.

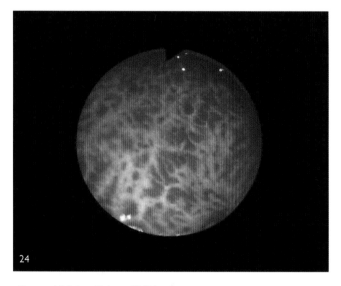

Figures 15.24.   Colon: CMV colitis.

Colon (Figures 15.19–15.24)

Clostridium difficile-associated diarrhea and pseudomembranous colitis have been documented in patients with AIDS, who received antibiotics before the onset of the diarrhea [33]. *C. difficile* may present as a severe infection with prolonged diarrhea, which usually resolves with metronidazole or vancomycine, but compared with HIV-seronegative patients, the strains of *C. difficile* in AIDS patients are from serogroup C, which is often quite resistant to antibiotic agents [34].

CMV is the most frequent cause of colitis in patients with AIDS. The most common presenting symptoms are diarrhea an abdominal pain [32]. Usually the

diarrhea contains blood and mucus, and is accompanied by abdominal cramps. endoscopy shows focal or diffuse mucosal erythema, edema, ulceration, and hemorrhage. Biopsy specimens may reveal the typical cytoplasmic and intranuclear inclusions. CMV colitis can be complicated by toxic megacolon and perforation [35].

Ganciclovir is the treatment of choice for CMV colitis. In one double-blind placebo-controlled study there was a significantly better histopathologic involvement in the ganciclovir group, compared with the placebo group, after 2 weeks of treatment, but diarrhea, abdominal pain, and fever did not significantly improve [36]. After failure of ganciclovir treatment, patients can benefit from the use of foscarnet [11].

Adenoviruses have been found in the stool and in the colonic epithelium in many HIV-infected patients, who have diarrhea of unknown etiology, but the significance of adenovirus as a cause of diarrhea remains unclear [37]. KS and lymphoma can occur throughout the large bowel, but lymphomas most frequently arise in the ileocecal region and the rectum.

Anorectal disease (Figures 15.25–15.28)

Anorectal lesions are common, especially in homosexual AIDS patients. Anorectal ulcers can be caused by HSV, CMV, *Chlamydia*, *Treponema pallidum*, or malignancies such as lymphoma, Kaposi's sarcoma or

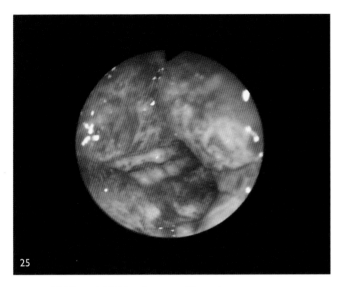

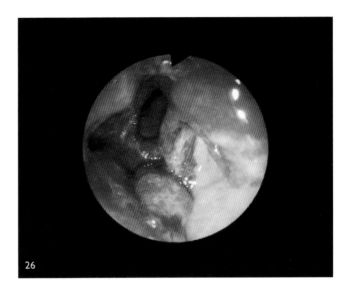

Figures 15.25 and 15.26.   Rectum: Kaposi's sarcoma.

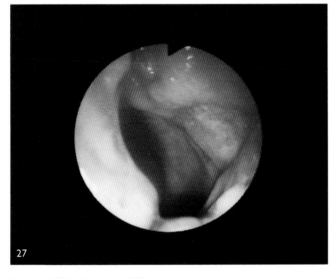

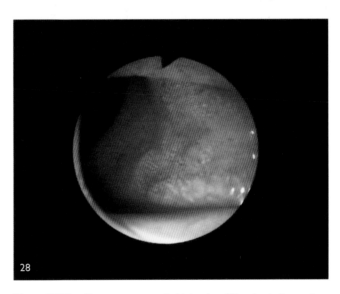

Figure 15.27.   Rectum: HSV proctitis.

Figure 15.28.   Rectum: mucosal thickening (*Mycobacterium avium intracellulare*).

squamous cell carcinoma. Other causes include atypical mycobacteria, *Histoplasma* and *Cryptococus neoformans* [6]. HIV-positive patients can develop anorectal sepsis, including abscesses and fistulas, in which no specific agents can be found [38].

Some patients develop very large and deep anorectal ulcerations, which cause severe pain, tenesmus, blood loss, and sometimes require surgical intervention [39]. The etiology of many of those ulcers remains unclear.

References

1   Gaines H, van Sydow M, Pehrson PO et al. Clinical picture of primary HIV-infection presenting as a glandular fever-like illness. *Br Med J* 1988; **297**: 1363–1368.

2   Rabeneck L, Popovic M, Gartner S et al. Acute HIV-infection presenting with painful swallowing and esophageal ulcers. *JAMA* 1990; **236**: 2318–2322.

3   Bartelsman JFWM, Lange JMA, Van Leeuwen R. Acute primary HIV-esophagitis. *Endoscopy* 1990; **22**: 184–185.

4   Tindall B, Hing M, Edwards P et al. Severe clinical manifestations of primary HIV infection. *AIDS* 1989; **3**: 747–749.

5   Dancygier H. AIDS and gastrointestinal endoscopy. *Endoscopy* 1994: **26**: 175–184.

6   Claydon EJ, Tanner A. Gastrointestinal emergencies in HIV-infection. *Baillière's Clin Gastroenterol* 1991; **5**: 887–911.

7   René E, Verdon R. Upper gastrointestinal tract infections in AIDS. *Baillière's Clin Gastroenterol* 1990; **4**: 339–359.

8   Laine L, Dretler RH, Conteas CN et al. Fluconazole compared with ketonazole for the treatment of candida esophagitis in AIDS. A randomized trial. *Ann Intern Med* 1992; **117**: 665–660.

9   McBane RD, Gross JB. Herpes esophagitis: clinical syndrome, endoscopic appearance and diagnosis in 23 patients. *Gastrointest Endoscopy* 1991; **37**: 600–603.

10 Theise ND, Rotterdam H, Dieterich D. Cytomegalovirus esophagitis in AIDS: diagnosis by endoscopic biopsy. *Am J Gastroenterol* 1991; **86**: 1123–1126.

11 Dieterich DT, Poles MA, Dicker M et al. Foscarnet treatment of cytomegalovirus gastrointestinal infections in acquired immunodeficiency syndrome patients who have fained Ganciclovir induction. *Am J Gastroenterol* 1991; **88**: 542–548.

12 Saltz RK, Kurtz RC, Lightdale CJ et al. Kaposi's sarcoma. Gastrointestinal involvement. Correlation with skin findings and immunological function. *Dig Dis Sci* 1984; **29**: 817–823.

13 Friedman SL. Kaposi's sarcoma and lymphoma of the gut in AIDS. *Baillière's Clin Gastroenterol* 1990; **4**: 455–475.

14 Dieterich DT. Cytomegalovirus: a new gastrointestinal pathogen in immunocompromised patients. *Am J Gastroenterol* 1987; **82**: 7643–7765.

15 Marano BJ, Smith F, Bonanno CA. Helicobacter pylori prevalence in acquired immunodeficiency syndrome. *Am J Gastroenterol* 1993; **88**: 687–690.

16 Edwards PD, Carrick J, Turner J et al. Helicobacter pylori-associated gastritis is rare in AIDS: antibiotic effect or a consequence of immunodeficiency? *Am J Gastroenterol* 1991; **86**: 1761–1764.

17 Riecken EO, Zeitz M, Ullrich R. Non-opportunistic causes of diarrhea in HIV infection. *Baillière's Clin Gastroenterol* 1990; **4**: 385–403.

18 Wanke CA. Small intestinal infections. *Curr Opin Gastroenterol* 1994; **10**: 59–65.

19 Nelson MR, Shanson DC, Hawkins DA et al. Salmonella, Campylobacter and Shigella in HIV-seropositive patients. *AIDS* 1992; **6**: 1495–1498.

20 Kemper CA, Meng TC, Nussbaum J et al. Mycobacterium avium complex bacteremia in AIDS with a four-drug oral regimen: rifampin, ethambutol, clofazimin and ciprofloxacin. *Ann Intern Med* 1992; **116**: 466–472.

21 Janoff EN, Smith PD. Perspectives on gastrointestinal infections in AIDS. *Gastroenterol Clin North Am* 1988; **17**: 451–463.

22 Goodgame RW, Genta RM, White AC et al. Intensity of infection in AIDS-associated Cryptosporidiosis. *J Clin Infect Dis* 1993; **167**: 704–709.

23 McGowan I, Hawkins AS, Weller IVD. The natural history of Cryptosporidial diarrhea in HIV-infected patients. *AIDS* 1993; **7**: 349–354.

24 Blanshard C, Jackson AM, Shanson DC et al. Cryptosporidiosis in HIV-seropositive patients. *Q J Med* 1992; **85**: 813–823.

25 Cevallos AM, Farthing MJG. Parasitic infections of the gastrointestinal tract. *Curr Opin Gastroenterol* 1994; **10**: 80–87.

26 Wurtz RM, Kocka FE, Peters CS et al. Clinical characteristics of seven cases of diarrhea associated with a novel acid-fast organism in the stool. *Clin Infect Dis* 1993; **16**: 136–138.

27 Weber R, Bryan RT, Owen RL et al. Improved light-microscopical detection of microsporidia spores in stool and duodenal aspirates. *N Engl J Med* 1992; **326**: 161–166.

28 Blanshard C, Ellis DS, Tovey DG et al. Treatment of intestinal microsporidiosis with albendazole in patients with AIDS. *AIDS* 1992; **6**: 311–313.

29 Field AS, Hing MC, Milliken ST et al. Microsporidia in the small intestine of HIV-infected patients. A new diagnostic technique and a new species. *Med J Aust* 1993; **158**: 390–394.

30 Ornstein JM, Dieterich DT, Kotler DP. Systemic dissemination by a newly recognized intestinal microsporidia species in AIDS. *AIDS* 1992; **6**: 1143–1150.

31 Wajsman R, Cappell MS, Biempica L et al. Terminal ileitis associated with cytomegalovirus and the acquired immune deficiency syndrome. *Am J Gastroenterol* 1989; **84**: 790–793.

32 Jacobson MA, Mills J. Serious cytomegalovirus disease in the acquired immunodeficiency syndrome (AIDS). *Ann Intern Med* 1988; **108**: 585–594.

33 Cappell MS, Philogene C. Clostridium difficile infection is a treatable cause of diarrhea in patients with advanced immunodeficiency virus infection: a study of seven consecutive patients admitted from 1986 to 1992 to a university teaching hospital. *Am J Gastroenterol* 1993; **88**: 891–897.

34 Barbut F, Depitre C, Delmée M et al. Comparison of enterotoxin production, cytotoxin production, serogrouping and antimicrobial susceptibilities of clostridium difficile strains isolated from AIDS and human immunodeficiency virus-negative patients. *J Clin Microbiol* 1993; **31**: 740–741.

35 Wolkomir AF, Barone JE, Hardy HW et al. Abdominal and anorectal surgery and the acquired immunodeficiency syndrome in heterosexual intravenous drug users. *Dis Col Rectum* 1990; **33**: 267–270.

36 Dieterich DT, Kotler DP, Busch DF et al. Ganciclovir treatment of cytomegalovirus colitis in AIDS: a randomized, double-blind, placebo controlled multicenter study. *J Infect Dis* 1993; **167**: 278–282.

37 Durepaire N, RangerRogez S, Gandji et al. Enteric prevalence of adenovirus in human immunodeficiency virus seropositive patients. *J Med Virol* 1995; **45**: 56–60.

38 Carr ND, Mercey D, Slack WW. Non-condylomatous perianal disease in homosexual men. *Br J Surg* 1989; **76**: 1064–1066.

39 Consten ECJ, Slors JFM, Danner SA et al. Local excision and mucosal advancement for anorectal ulceration in patients infected with human immunodeficiency virus. *Br J Surg* 1995; **82**: 891–894.

16 IMAGING OF THE LUMENAL GASTROINTESTINAL TRACT IN AIDS

Susan D. Wall
Judy Yee
Jacques W.A.J. Reeders

Introduction

Most patients with acquired immune deficiency syndrome (AIDS) will exhibit gastrointestinal symptoms at some time during the course of their illness. In fact, clinical AIDS often is determined by identifying an opportunistic pathogen of neoplasm of the gastrointestinal (GI) tract. AIDS patients will often have multifocal abnormalities of the GI tract [1]. GI symptoms in patients with AIDS often are non-specific and so present diagnostic and management challenges. Radiology plays a key role in helping to make the diagnosis as well as in directing the management.

A seroconversion illness may occur soon after the initial infection by human immune deficiency virus (HIV). In addition to neurological signs and symptoms of acute HIV infection, a mononucleosis-like illness can occur. This may include symptoms related to the GI tract, such as nausea and diarrhea. Usually this is self-limited and resolves spontaneously. Some patients complaint of pain on swallowing or, less commonly, dysphagia. Both endoscopy and double-contrast esophagrams may demonstrate giant (>2 cm), well-defined shallow ulceration of the esophagus with surrounding normal mucosa. Multiple lesions may occur, but solitary lesions are more frequent. Because biopsies, brushings, cultures, and histopathologic examination have failed to identify another causative organism, these lesions have been termed idiopathic esophageal ulcerations associated with HIV infection [2]. Electron microscopy of biopsy specimens taken at ulcer margins have demonstrated retrovirus-like particles supporting the diagnosis of HIV infection as the etiology [3]. Corticosteroid treatment of the esophageal ulceration is effective with 92% of patients having complete symptomatic response with prednisone, usually within a week [4]. HIV-related esophageal ulcers also can occur later in the course of the disease, after recovery from the seroconversion illness [5]. The lower GI tract may also be involved directly by HIV. This seroconversion illness often includes a sore throat, malaise, and myalagias. A maculopapular rash involves the upper trunk, arms, and face in 80% of patients [3]. HIV has been isolated within the gut tissue in up to 50% of patients with AIDS [6].

Idiopathic AIDS enteropathy is a chronic diarrheal illness without other identified infectious etiology. It is thought to be due to enteric HIV infection. Infection of the gut by HIV is associated with a decrease in the total number of intestinal T-lymphocytes as well as a significant reversal of the normal mucosal helper/suppressor T-cell ratio [7]. HIV-infected mucosal cells demonstrate hypoproliferative changes with mucosal atrophy [8]. Consequently, the structure and function of the gut is thought to be directly affected by the virus itself.

The course of HIV disease involves a latent period following initial infection. The likelihood of developing clinical AIDS is directly related to the duration of HIV infection. An estimated cumulative incidence of AIDS of 54% has been reported 11 years following seroconversion [9]. During the period of time between seroconversion and the development of clinical AIDS, HIV-positive patients often demonstrate non-specific findings on cross sectional imaging. For instance, hepatosplenomegaly often is present without associated focal lesions. Fatty infiltration of the liver may also be seen. Multiple small lymph nodes (<0.5 cm) may be present in the retroperitoneum and mesentery. Circumferential rectal wall thickening and infiltration

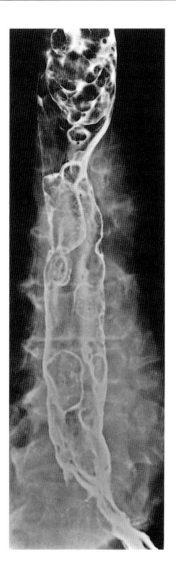

Figure 16.1. Kaposi's sarcoma of the esophagus: multiple small and larger polypoid smooth delineated lesions, diffusely spread throughout the esophagus.

of the perirectal fat may occur in homosexual or bi-sexual individuals owing to repeated episodes of proc-titis. None of these findings are necessarily indicative of opportunistic infection or HIV-related malignancy.

AIDS malignancies

Kaposi's sarcoma

Kaposi's sarcoma (KS) is a neoplasm believed to orig-inate in the lymphoreticular system. Until the AIDS epidemic, KS was a relatively uncommon and indo-lent neoplasm found primarily in elderly men. Today,

it is common among AIDS patients. Some reports have indicated that as many as one-third of AIDS patients have KS [10,11]. The incidence of KS is highest among homosexual or bisexual AIDS patients as com-pared with other risk groups.

Up to 50% of homosexual/bisexual men with AIDS develop KS during their lifetime [12] and are approx-imately 20 times more likely to develop this neoplasm than hemophiliac men at AIDS diagnoses [13]. The dramatic difference in KS rates between different HIV-transmission groups, as well as studies suggesting that KS is associated with specific sexual risk factors [14] and geographic clustering [14,15] implies that an exogenous infection may be the primary cause of this disease [16]. Unique herpesvirus-like DNA sequences belonging to a new human gamma herpesvirus, desig-nated KS-associated herpesvirus (KSHV), have been found in >90% of KS lesions from North America, Africa, Asia, and Europe [17], indicating that KSHV is found in all forms of KS in a variety of settings.

HIV-associated KS is much more aggressive than that found in elderly men prior to the epidemic. It generally is multifocal with visceral, cutaneous and lymph node involvement being common. An associ-ated increased incidence of second primary neoplasms, particularly HIV-related lymphoma, has also been found in these patients [18]. Common sites of involve-ment by KS listed in order of frequency include the following: skin, lymph nodes, GI tract, lung, liver, and spleen. Cutaneous KS usually precedes the develop-ment of GI disease but not always. Visceral involvement has been found in more than 50% of homosexual patients [10,11].

One of the most common sites of AIDS-related KS is the luminal gastrointestinal tract. Any or all portions may be affected from the oropharynx to the rectum. However, the most frequent site of involvement within the GI tract is the duodenum [10,11]. Patients are often asymptomatic if lesions are small, unless the oropharynx is involved when even early lesions may cause odynophagia or dysphagia. Barium pharyngog-raphy is useful for diagnosis. Double contrast images, especially with a lateral view, can detect even small lesions [19].

Other enteric KS lesions are often found inciden-tally unless there is extensive involvement which can cause symptoms that lead to imaging studies. Early disease consists of flat lesions that are not demonstrated on barium studies even when a double-contrast tech-nique is used. However, the appearance of these

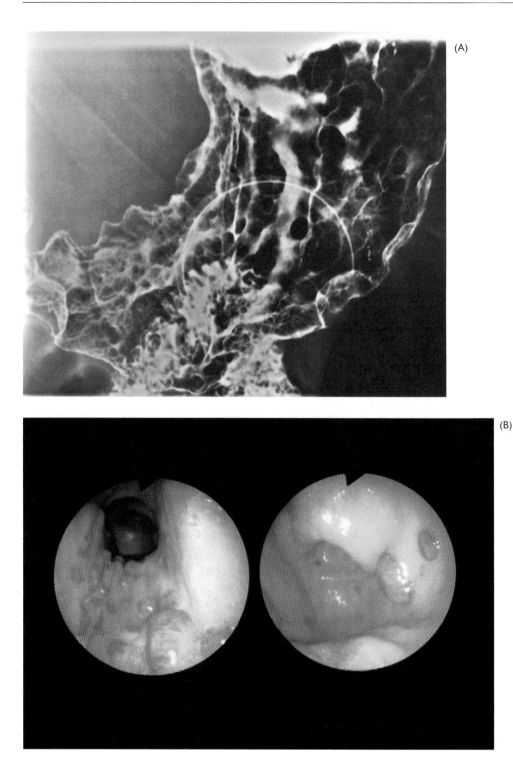

Figure 16.2. Kaposi's sarcoma of the stomach: multiple submucosal nodules visible after barium meal (A) and during gastroscopy (B).

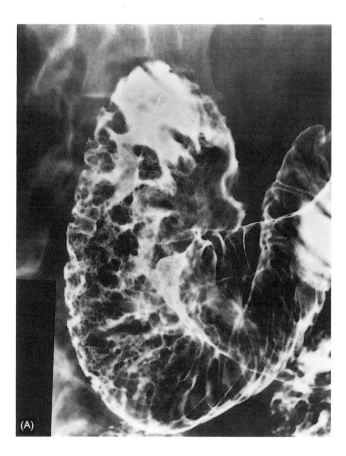

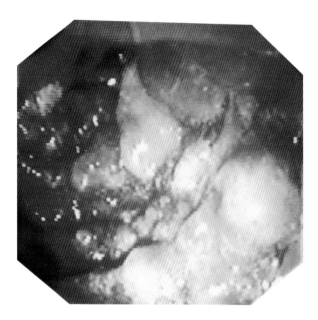

(B)

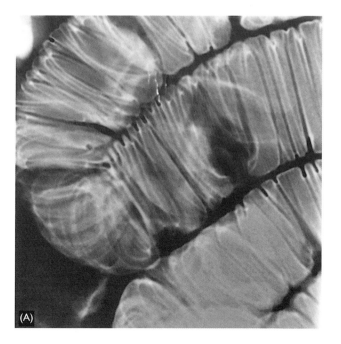

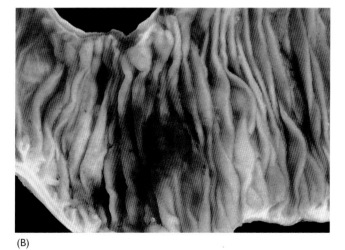

(B)

Figure 16.3. Kaposi's sarcoma of the duodenum: thickening of mucosal folds with submucosal nodules scattered throughout the duodenum. (A) Duodenography, (B) gastroscopy.

Figure 16.4. Kaposi's sarcoma of the small bowel (enteroclysis): multiple submucosal nodules (arrows) on normal intervening nucosa of the jejunum. (A) Enteroclysis, (B) gross specimen.

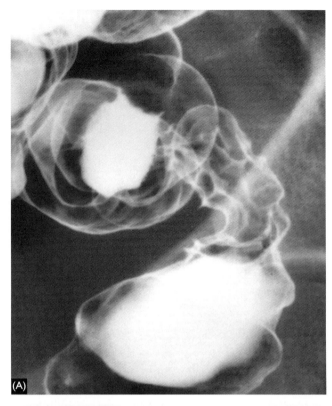

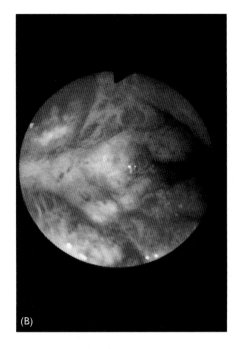

Figure 16.5. Kaposi's sarcoma of the rectum: nodular filling defects in the proximal part of the rectum. (A) Rectography, (B) colonoscopy.

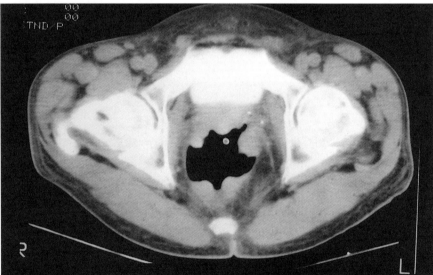

Figure 16.6. Kaposi's sarcoma of the rectum: asymmetric, irregular nodular thickening of the anterior rectal wall due to Kaposi's sarcoma, demonstrated on CT. Stranding of the perirectal fat is also present in this homosexual patient who also has proctitis.

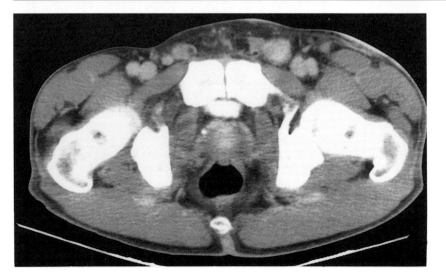

Figure 16.7. Disseminated Kaposi's sarcoma: CT scan with intravenous contrast demonstrating high-density inguinal adenopathy due to disseminated Kaposi's sarcoma. Enhancement of the lymph nodes involved reflects the vascular nature of this tumor.

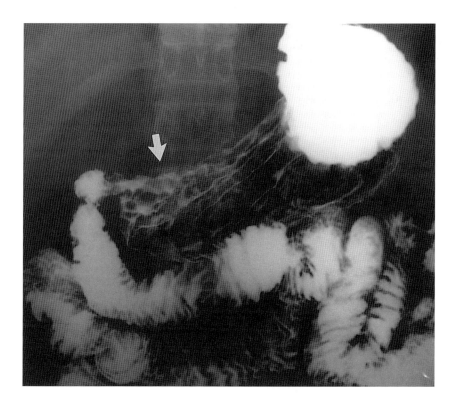

Figure 16.8. Gastric lymphoma: irregularly thickened folds are present in the distal antrum (arrow) which was found to be a non-Hodgkin lymphoma on biopsy.

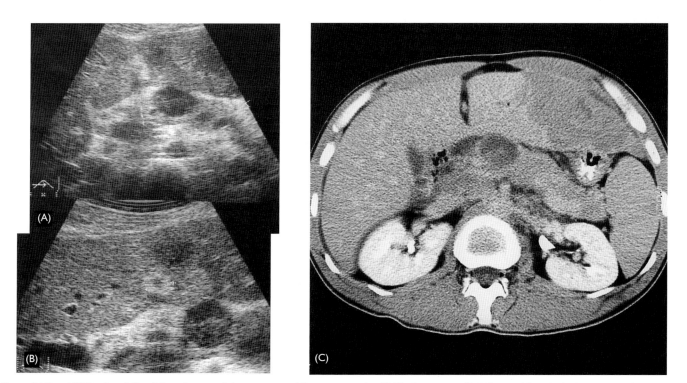

Figure 16.9. AIDS-related B cell lymphoma of the pancreas. Ultrasonography (A,B) shows a well delineated hypoechoic mass at the corpus of the pancreas, which is non-attenuating, hypodense on CT. (C) After i.v. contrast injection.

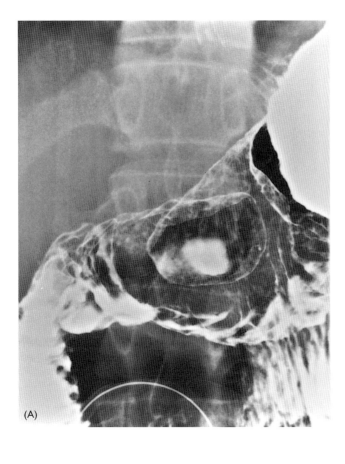

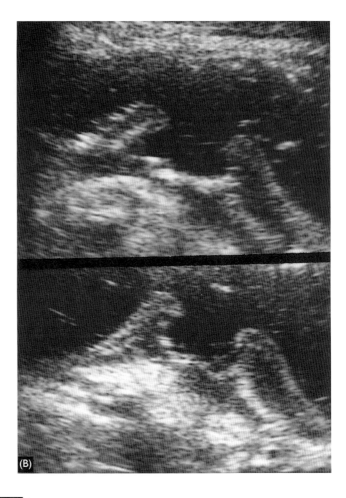

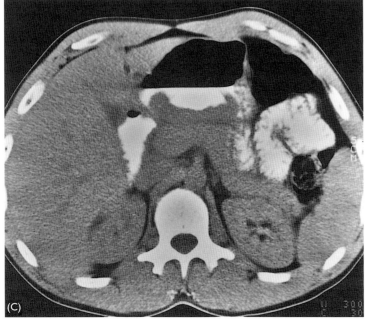

Figure 16.10. AIDS-related B-cell lymphoma of the stomach. (A) Double-contrast barium study, (B) ultrasonography, (C) CT of the stomach. Smoothly delineated ulcer crater surrounded by localized wall thickening/edema.

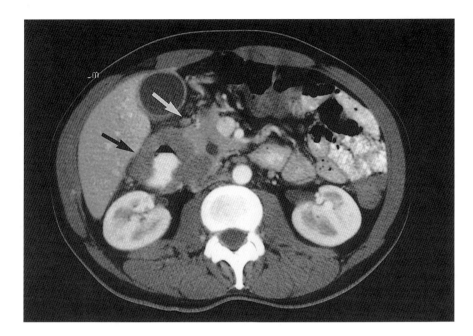

Figure 16.11. Duodenal lymphoma. Large lobulated mass encircling the contrast-filled second portion of the duodenum (black arrow). This mass is causing biliary ductal obstruction. A small node is present near the pancreatic head (white arrow).

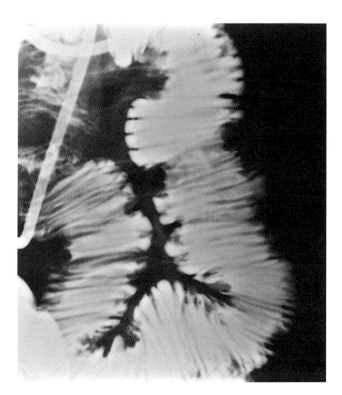

Figure 16.12. AIDS-related lymphoma of the small bowel. Enteroclysis: irregular nodular narrowing and fold thickening of the proximal jejunal loops.

lesions on endoscopy is characteristic and diagnosis can be made by visual inspection. KS lesions typically appear as violaceous macules or nodules measuring 5–15 mm. Positive biopsy specimens contain spindle cells with numerous vascular clefts and hemorrhage [18]. Endoscopic biopsy has a low yield owing to the submucosal location of the tumor, making biopsy specimens too superficial to be diagnostic.

Only 23% of endoscopic biopsies of KS lesions were positive for KS in one series yielding a 77% false-negative rate [18]. As KS lesions coalesce, they enlarge and become more nodular and can then be detected on barium studies. Smooth submucosal nodules with or without central umbilication are typical for KS. The 'bull's-eye' or 'target' appearance often is absent, and is a helpful sign only when present. As the disease progresses, there is extension into the muscularis and mucosa of the bowel wall. Large bulky polypoid masses and irregular fold thickening may be seen (Figures 16.1, 16.2 and 16.3). Differential diagnosis of enteric AIDS-related KS includes lymphoma, multiple polyps, metastases, opportunistic infection and Crohn's disease. Complications include GI bleeding, intussusception, perforation, diarrhea, protein-losing enteropathy and rarely intestinal obstruction [20]. Enteric KS lesions have been found to respond to systemic chemotherapy, with the likelihood of response related to total tumor bulk [21].

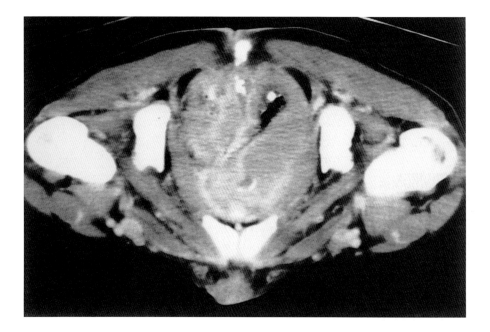

Figure 16.13. AIDS-related lymphoma of the rectum: large intramural/intralumenal inhomogeneous soft tissue mass at the rectal wall. (Courtesy: A.J. Megibow, M.D., New York Medical Center, New York, USA.)

Kaposi's sarcoma of the small bowel (Figure 16.4) is demonstrated by nodules or nodular wall thickening which is typically segmental (Figure 16.5) and often evident on computed tomography (CT) (Figure 16.6). Diffuse wall thickening is more suggestive of lymphoma or infectious enteritis. High-attenuation adenopathy on dynamic bolus CT scan in AIDS patients is suggestive of disseminated KS [22] (Figure 16.7). Contrast-enhancing adenopathy is believed to reflect the vascular nature of this tumor. Kaposi's sarcoma is present in 10–15% of liver biopsies and tends to involve the periportal regions of the liver [23]. Hepatic and splenic involvement in KS has characteristic but nonspecific ultrasound (US) and CT scan findings. These include hepatosplenomegaly and on ultrasound small (5–12 mm) hyperechoic nodules in the liver and spleen. Small, low-attenuation lesions are seen on CT scan where delayed imaging may demonstrate enhancement [24]. The differential diagnosis includes fungal microabscesses, metastatic disease, and multiple hemangiomas. Lymphoma and mycobacterial infections tend to produce hypoechoic lesions on ultrasound.

HIV-related lymphoma

HIV-related lymphoma occurs frequently among AIDS patients, although it is less common than KS.

Less than 10% of AIDS patients will develop lymphoma [24]. Non-Hodgkin lymphoma is more common than Hodgkin's disease or Burkitt's lymphoma. HIV-related lymphomas are poorly differentiated high-grade subtypes with a poor prognosis. They tend to be highly aggressive. Advanced disease usually is present at the time of diagnosis. Often they are present in unusual extranodal sites, particularly in the brain, bone marrow, and abdominal viscera [26]. Peripheral adenopathy often is absent. Stomach, enteric and rectal lymphoma will appear as irregular fold thickening on barium studies (Figures 16.8–10,16.12,16.13). CT is helpful in demonstrating the extraluminal extent of enteric lymphomatous masses (Figure 16.11). CT and US may also demonstrate non-specific hepatosplenomegaly.

Lymphomatous involvement of the liver, spleen and pancreas in AIDS patients is suggested by single or multiple, focal, homogeneous low-density masses on CT scan, or focal hypoechoic lesions on ultrasound (Figures 16.9a,b,c). Bulky retroperitoneal or mesenteric adenopathy is a common manifestation of AIDS-related lymphoma. However, the differential diagnosis includes KS and mycobacterial infection. Small (<15 mm) retroperitoneal nodes are often due to reactive hyperplasia in AIDS patients and should be interpreted cautiously [27]. AIDS-related lymphomas may also present as isolated pelvic adenopathy or rarely with diffuse peritoneal seeding or lymphomatosis [28].

Opportunistic infections

Candidiasis

Oral thrush is one of the earliest and most common findings in HIV-positive individuals, and *Candida albicans* is the most frequent cause of esophageal infection in AIDS. *Candida* esophagitis in association with HIV seropositivity defines clinical AIDS in that patient. Patients with esophageal candidiasis typically present with sudden onset of odynophagia or dysphagia.

Chest pain can develop and may be intense. Endoscopic findings are characteristic with creamy, white plaques covering a friable, erythematous mucosa. However, therapy is often instituted based on clinical symptoms, especially if typical findings are present on barium swallow [29]. The earliest detectable lesions on double-contrast esophagram are mucosal plaques causing small filling defects, usually oriented along the long axis of the esophagus. Fold thickening and abnormal motility may be present, although they are non-specific findings. A typical 'cobblestone' appearance develops with progression of the infection and represents edema of the submucosa and surrounding tissues (Figure 16.14). Advanced cases will demonstrate the classic 'shaggy' contour of the esophagus, owing to trapping of barium within the interstices of confluent plaques and pseudomembranes. Deep ulcers, in addition to sloughed mucosa contribute to the irregular appearance of advanced disease. AIDS patients tend to present clinically at more advanced stages of infection. Systemic candidiasis is a potentially fatal complication. Hematogenous dissemination of the infection can lead to the development of micro-abscesses in the liver, spleen, and kidneys [30]. Contrast-enhanced CT scan will demonstrate multiple tiny (<5 mm) foci of low-attenuation microabscesses in these organs (Figure 16.15).

Herpes

Odynophagia is the most common symptom associated with *Herpes simplex* virus (HSV) esophagitis.

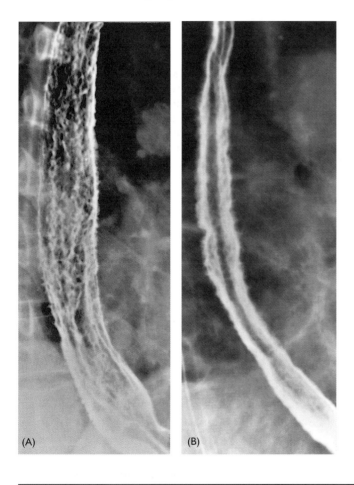

(A)   (B)

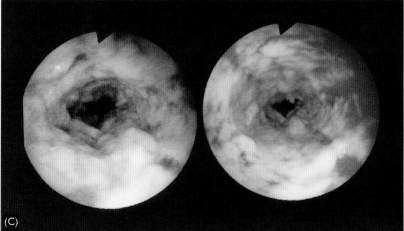

(C)

Figure 16.14. Severe *Candida* esophagitis: 'shaggy esophagus'. (A) Double contrast, (B) mucosal relief esophagogram, (C) endoscopy.

AIDS patients may develop esophagitis owing to either HSV 1 or HSV 2. Herpetic lesions in the mouth may provide a clue to the diagnosis although this does not exclude concomitant candidal infection of the esophagus. In the early stage, endoscopy may reveal small vesicles, although these are not commonly seen. There is progression to shallow ulcerations, which then enlarge and coalesce. In the late stage, diffuse ulcerations and inflammatory exudates may be indistinguishable from *Candida* esophagitis. The features of *Herpes* esophagitis, which are best demonstrated on double-contrast esophagram, consist of multiple

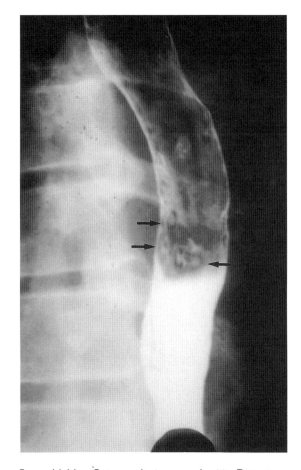

Figure 16.16. Cytomegalovirus esophagitis. Discrete small ulcerations are present in the esophagus (arrows) with normal appearance of intervening mucosa. *Herpes* esophagitis may also have a similar appearance.

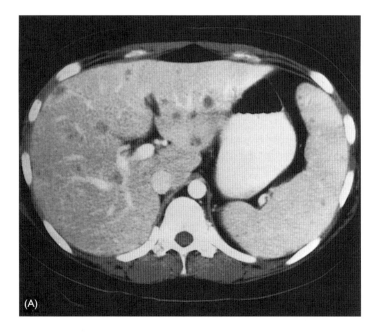

(A)

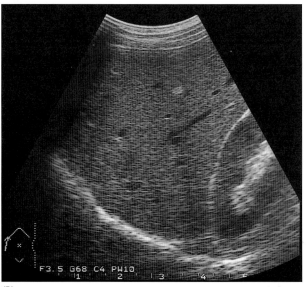

(B)

◄ *Figure 16.15.* Hepatosplenic microabscesses owing to hematogeneous dissemination of *Candida albicans*. Multiple tiny foci of (A) low density (using CT) or (B) hyperechogenicity (using ultrasonography) are seen scattered throughout the liver and spleen.

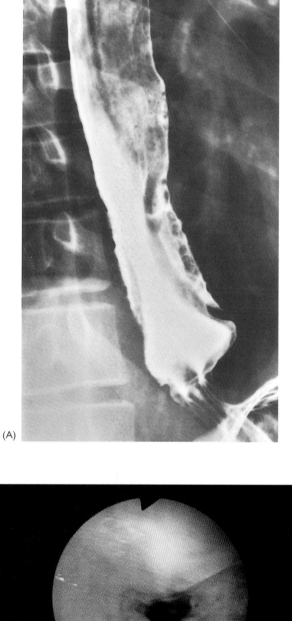

(A)

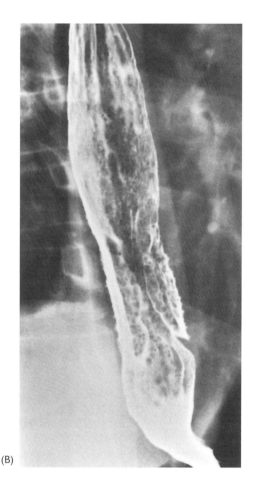

(B)

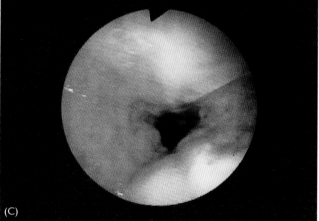

(C)

Figure 16.17. Cytomegalovirus esophagitis: longitudinal, semilunar, deep, penetrating ulcerations at the midesophagus opposite each other. (A) Single-contrast and (B) double-contrast esophagogram. (C) Endoscopy.

scattered shallow ulcers, which are separated by normal appearing mucosa. These ulcers typically have a diamond or stellate configuration and demonstrate a lucent halo of edema. Advanced cases of *Herpes* esophagitis will appear as diffuse nodularity with cobblestoning and a grossly irregular esophageal contour identical to the findings of monilial infection. Consequently, biopsy and histologic analysis are necessary for diagnosis. Characteristic findings on histology include multinucleated giant cells and Cowdry type-A intranuclear inclusion bodies which are found typically along ulcer margins [31].

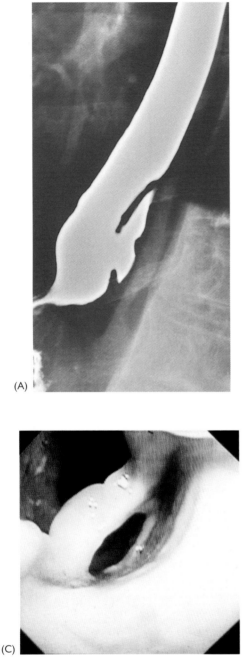

(A)

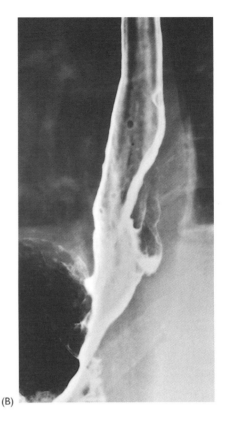

(B)

(C)

Figure 16.18.   Cytomegalovirus esophagitis: localized, deep, penetrating ulceration undermining the normal esophageal mucosa, causing bridging. (A) Single-contrast and (B) double-contrast esophagogram. (C) Endoscopy.

Cytomegalovirus

Cytomegalovirus (CMV) is the most common pathogen identified in AIDS patients. It may involve any segment of the luminal GI tract. The colon and small bowel are infected more commonly than the esophagus or stomach. Biopsy allows histologic diagnosis if the typical cytoplasmic and intranuclear inclusion bodies are found within the ulcer base [32]. Ulcers are caused by ischemia owing to a CMV-induced vasculitis [33]. This is demonstrated by the presence of CMV inclusion bodies in the endothelial cells of the blood vessel wall supplying the ulcers.

The radiographic appearance of CMV esophagitis differs from that of *Candida* esophagitis. CMV esophagitis is demonstrated by the presence of discrete

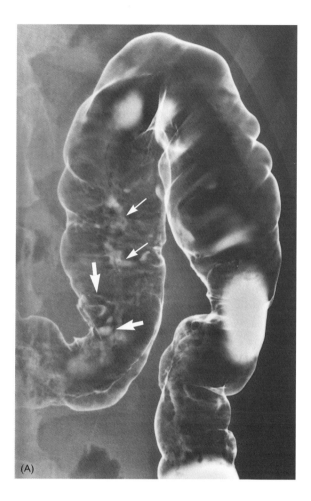

(A)

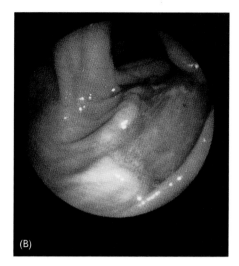

(B)

Figure 16.19. Cytomegalovirus colitis: shallow, poorly defined, oval, serpiginous, and semilunar ulcers with a halo (small arrows) on a background of normal mucosa. Note the diamond-shaped ulcer at the mid-portion of the transverse colon (large arrows). (A) Double-contrast barium enema, (B) colonoscopy.

ulceration of the esophagus with a normal intervening mucosa (Figure 16.16). The most characteristic finding of CMV esophagitis, both on barium esophagram and endoscopy is a giant (>2 cm) superficial ulceration usually located in the distal esophagus (Figures 16.17 and 16.18). A lucent halo of edema may be present. This appearance is similar to the large, flat, idiopathic, esophageal ulceration associated with the seroconversion illness of early HIV infection. Definitive diagnosis is made by endoscopic biopsy and histopathologic examination. In the AIDS population, CMV ulcers of the distal esophagus have been found to extend into the esophagogastric junction and may cause rugal fold thickening of the proximal stomach. CMV gastritis frequently involves the antrum and appears on barium radiography as nodular wall thickening, as well as circumferential antral narrowing with decreased distensibility [33].

CMV colitis presents with mucosal ulcerations that are shallow initially, but deeper later when associated edema and wall thickening are noted. These findings may be observed on both barium study and CT

scan (Figures 16.19–16.22). CMV colitis commonly involves the ascending colon and cecum with extension into the terminal ileum. Sometimes the entire colon is involved [34]. CT scan following intravenous contrast demonstrates low-density edematous bowel wall with marked mucosal and serosal enlargement (Figure 16.23). In advanced cases, hemorrhage into the bowel wall may cause increased density as well as thickening. Pneumatosis, toxic megacolon, and colonic perforation are findings associated with significant mortality [30]. CMV hepatitis has been reported in association with multiple small hyperechoic lesions on US and focal low-density liver lesions seen on CT scan. These foci of infection have been noted histologically to represent focal areas of fatty infiltration [35].

Mycobacterial infections

Mycobacterium tuberculosis

Mycobacterium tuberculosis frequently involves several areas of the GI tract in AIDS patients. Tuberculous

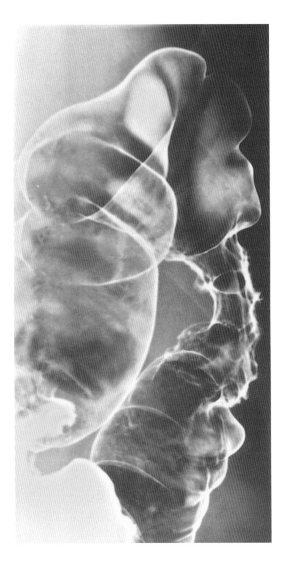

esophagitis is usually due to local extension from the adjacent mediastinum, where infected necrotic mediastinal lymph nodes are present. The findings on esophagram and CT scan include focal extrinsic mass impression, deep ulcerations, sinus tract, and fistula formation. Sinus tracts extend to the mediastinum and bronchial tree, and esophagoesophageal fistulae may occur [36]. Traction diverticula and strictures are seen in chronic tuberculous esophagitis. Other radiographic findings that suggest the diagnosis of esophageal tuberculosis (TB) include widening of the mediastinum, pulmonary nodules, and pleural effusions. Tuberculous colitis may occur in AIDS patients and typically involves the ileocecal region. Circumferential thickening of the wall of the cecum and terminal ileum may be identified both on barium enema and CT scan. In addition, the presence of regional low-attenuation necrotic adenopathy is a helpful diagnostic finding on CT scan. A complication of TB colitis is fistula formation, which is best demonstrated on barium studies.

Atypical *mycobacterium*

Mycobacterium avium-intracellulare (MAI) infection of the GI tract occurs most commonly in the small bowel. Patients present with a clinical enteritis characterized

Figure 16.20. Cytomegalovirus colitis: segmental circumferential ulcerated stricture at the proximal descending colon with a sharp demarcation towards normal mucosa.

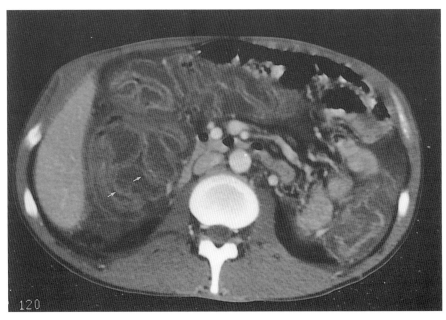

Figure 16.21. Cytomegalovirus colitis: CT scan with intravenous contrast demonstrates a low-density markedly edematous colonic wall with significant mucosal and serosal enhancement (arrows).

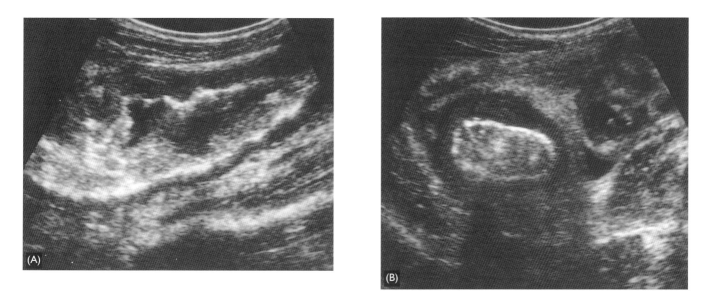

Figure 16.22. Sagittal (A) and transverse (B) ultrasonographic scans in a HIV-positive patient with acute CMV typhlitis, histologically confirmed. (Courtesy: S.R. Wilson, M.D., F.R.C.P.(C), The Toronto Hospital, Toronto, Canada.)

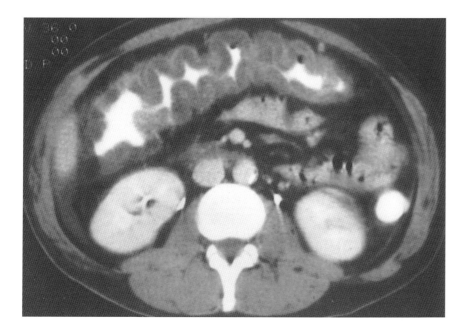

Figure 16.23. Cytomegalovirus colitis. CT: thickening of the wall of the transverse colon. (Courtesy: A.J. Megibow, M.D., New York Medical Center, New York, USA.)

by diarrhea, fever, and weight loss. Because the histologic and radiographic findings of MAI enteritis are similar to Whipple's disease, it is often described as 'pseudo-Whipple disease' (Figure 16.24). Barium study shows mild small bowel dilatation and diffuse, irregular fold thickening. Small bowel loops are separated or displaced owing to adenopathy. CT scan demonstrates similar findings and hepatosplenomegaly as well. Moderate-sized mesenteric and retroperitoneal adenopathy often is present and may appear in low

density owing to necrosis. Some researchers have found this pattern of low-density lymph adenopathy to be more common with *M. tuberculosis* infection than with MAI [37]. Marked hepatosplenomegaly is often present. However, focal low-density MAI microabscesses within the liver and spleen, owing to hematogenous dissemination, are an uncommon finding. Discrete hepatosplenic low-density lesions are more commonly seen with disseminated TB infection [37,38].

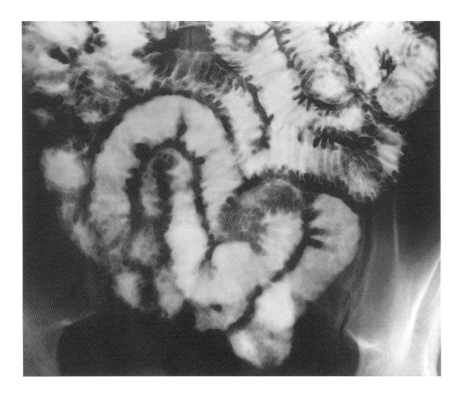

Figure 16.24. MAI infection of the small bowel: enteroclysis shows radiographic findings (irregular fold thickening, dilation), similar to Whipple's disease ('pseudo-Whipple').

Cryptosporidiosis

Cryptosporidium is a small parasitic protozoan that causes severe chronic enteritis in AIDS patients, which is clinically manifested by abdominal pain and voluminous watery diarrhea.

Dehydration and electrolyte abnormalities contribute to the morbidity and sometimes mortality of these patients. Fecal-oral contamination and sexual contact are the most common routes of spread in AIDS patients. Histologically, mucosal damage occurs, owing to partial villous atrophy, crypt hyperplasia, and cellular infiltrates [38]. The diagnosis of intestinal cryptosporidiosis is made by stool examination, although the organism may be identified on intestinal biopsy specimens.

Fold thickening is most prominent in the duodenum and jejunum, although the entire small bowel may be involved. Mild, small bowel dilatation and hypersecretion are seen. This may occasionally produce a sprue-like appearance. Differential diagnosis includes other opportunistic bowel infections such as giardiasis and infection by *Isospora belli*. The latter is another protozoan that often is present in association with *Cryptosporidium*. CT scan may demonstrate small bowel wall thickening and dilatation with increased luminal fluid. Non-specific mesenteric lymphadenopathy (small

sized) may be present but usually is not. At present there is no effective treatment of cryptosporidiosis, although octreotide, spiramycin, and various antibiotics have provided some palliation [21].

Biliary disease

Recent attention has been directed to the involvement of the biliary tract in AIDS patients. Most reported cases described acalculous cholecystitis secondary to CMV or cryptosporidial infection [40,41].

The radiographic findings in AIDS patients with right upper quadrant pain, jaundice, or abnormal liver function tests have been reported [42,43]. Eight of the nine imaging studies disclosed intrahepatic or extrahepatic bile duct changes similar to those seen in sclerosing cholangitis. Isolated papillary stenosis and ductal dilatation were present in one patient. Eight patients had some stricturing of the distal common bile duct. Cholangitis caused by CMV or cryptospridium is the proposed pathologic mechanism [42,43]. In the series by Teixidor et al. [44], one patient was shown to have CMV infection of the biliary tree. The findings in this case was that of a stenosing papillitis. CMV and reovirus II have a tropism for bile duct epithelium in the neonate [41]. Reflux of the organisms through the ampulla of Vater in case of superinfection in the duodenum or small bowel may cause this disorder.

In any AIDS patient with abnormal liver function tests, imaging generally will be performed to evaluate the presence of heptomegaly or space-occupying lesions within the liver. Careful attention should be paid to the bile ducts. If segmental dilatation of any portion of the biliary tree is seen, direct cholangiography may be useful to document the presence of AIDS-related cholangitis. Ultrasonic visualization of gallbladder wall thickening, bile duct dilatation, and altered echogenicity in the periportal regions have been shown to be suggestive of AIDS-related cholangitis [45–49].

Between 1982 and 1992, 608 patients with AIDS were referred to the Academic Medical Center, Amsterdam, the Netherlands. Data for evaluation were available in 550 patients: 487 male homosexuals; 23 female and 40 male heterosexuals. Endoscopic biopsies from ulcers in esophagus, stomach, or duodenum showed CMV in only about half of the cases (52%). Cryptosporidium was found in 3.2%. Biopsies from

erosions or diffuse abnormalities (gastritis, duodenitis) showed CMV, cryptospridium, MAI, and microsporidium in 12.5%, 5.8%, 4.1% and 0.8%, respectively. Only in two patients we have seen CMV or cryptosporidium of the bile duct. However, clinically we were not focused on the bile duct system in most of our patients, due to a lack of clinical symptomology (e.g., cholangitis). We do not yet know what the exact etiopathologic mechanisms are causing abnormalities of the bile duct system. It could well be the case that many AIDS patients in a terminal stage may have already similar biliary tract changes [47,48].

Farman et al. [49] evaluated the ERCP appearances of AIDS-associated cholangitis in 26 patients, as a reflection of seven major US hospitals. The radiographic finding ranged from intrahepatic ductal abnormalities with or without involvement of the extrahepatic biliary tree to irregularities and strictures involving the ampulla of Vater or the intrapancreatic

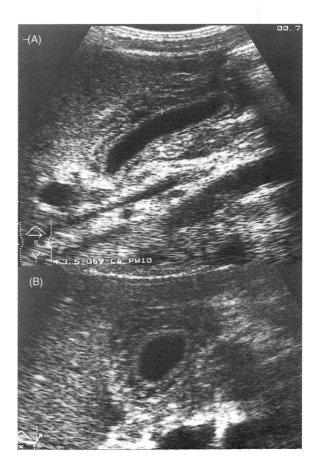

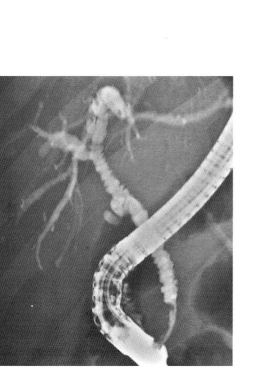

Figure 16.25. AIDS cholangiopathy: cryptosporidiosis. Multifocal extra- and intrabiliary ductal strictures with intervening areas of relative dilation. More marked dilatation of the left ductal system is noted.

Figure 16.26. Acalculous cholecystitis: longitudinal (A) and transverse (B) ultrasonography: CMV infection of the gallbladder; severe thickening of the gallbladder wall, due to the inflammation and edema.

portion of the common bile duct with proximal dilatation and acalculous cholecystitis (Figs 16.25, 16.26). Twenty one of the 26 patients had associated infections including cryptosporidium, MAI, CMV, microsporidium and isospora.

References

1   Wall SD, Ominsky S, Altman DF et al. Multifocal abnormalities of the gastrointestinal tract in AIDS. *AJR* 1986; **146**: 1–5.

2   Frager D, Kotler DP, Baer J. Idiopathic esophageal ulceration in the acquired immunodeficiency syndrome: radiologie reappraisal in 10 patients. *Abdom Imaging* 1994; **19**: 2–5.

3   Rabeneck L, Popovic M, Gartner S et al. Acute HIV infection presenting with painful swallowing and esophageal ulcers. *JAMA* 1990; **263**: 2318–2322.

4   Wilcox CM, Schwartz DA. A pilot study of corticosteroid therapy for idiopathic esophageal ulcerations associated with human immunodeficiency virus infection. *Am J Med* 1992; **93**: 131–134.

5   Levine MS, Loercher G, Katzka DA et al. Giant, human immunodeficiency virus-related ulcers in the esophagus. *Radiology* 1991; **180**: 323–326.

6   Nelson JA, Reynolds-Kohler C, Margaretten W et al. HIV detected in bowel epithelium from patients with gastrointestinal symptoms. *Lancet* 1988; **1**: 259—262.

7   Rodgers VD, Fassett R, Kagnoff MF. Abnormalities in intestinal mucosal T cells in homosexual populations including those with lymphadenopathy syndrome and AIDS. *Gastroenterology* 1986; **90**: 552–558.

8   Ullrich R, Zeitz M, Heise W et al. Small intestinal structure and function in patients infected with HIV: evidence for HIV-induced enteropathy. *Ann Intern Med* 1989; **111**: 15–21.

9   Rutherford GW, Lifson AR, Hessol NA et al. Course of HIV-1 infection in a cohort of homosexual and bisexual men: an 11 year follow up study. *Br Med J* 1990; **301**: 1183–1188.

10 Wall SD, Friedman SL, Margulis AR: gastrointestinal Kaposi's sarcoma in AIDS: radiographic manifestations. *J Clin Gastroenterol* 1984; **6**: 165–171.

11 Reeders JWAJ, Bartelsman JF, Antonides HR, et al. The spectrum of gastrointestinal radiology in AIDS. *Eur Radiol* 1991; **1**: 33–45.

12 Katz MH, Hessol NA, Buchbinder SP, Hirozawa A, O'Malley P, Holmbereg SD. Temporal trends of opportunistic infections and malignancies in homosexual men with AIDS. *J Infect Dis* 1994; **170**: 198–202.

13 Beral V, Peterman TA, Berkelman RL, Jaffe HW. Kaposi's sarcoma among persons with AIDS: a sexually transmitted infection? *Lancet* 1990; **335**: 123–128.

14 Archibald CP, Schechter MT, Le TN, Craib KJP, Montaner JSG, P'Shaughnessy MV. Evidence for a sexually transmitted cofactor for AIDS-related Kaposi's sarcoma in a cohort of homosexual men. *Epidemiology* 1992; **3**: 203–209.

15 Beral N, Bull D, Jaffe J et al. Is risk of Kaposi's sarcoma in AIDS patients in Britain increased if sexual partners came from United States or Africa? *Br Med J* 1991; **302**: 624–625.

16 Beral V. epidemiology of Kaposi's sarcoma. In: Beral V. (ed.) *Cancer, HIV and AIDS*. London: Imperial Cancer Research Fund, 1991: 5–22.

17 Chang Y, Cesarman E, Pessin MS et al. Indentification of herpesvirus-like DNA sequences in AIDS-associated Kaposi's sarcoma. *Science* 1994; **265**: 1865–1869.

18 Friedman SL, Wright TL, Altman DF. Gastrointestinal Kaposi's sarcoma in patients with acquired immunodeficiency syndrome: endoscopic and autopsy findings. *Gastroenterology* 1985; **89**: 102–108.

19 Emery CD, Wall SD, Federle MP et al. Pharyngeal Kaposi's sarcoma in patients with AIDS. *AJR* 1986; **147**: 919–922.

20 Rose HS, Balthazar EJ, Megibow AJ. Alimentary tract involvement in Kaposi's sarcoma: radiographic and endoscopic findings in 25 homosexual men. *AJR* 1982; **139**: 661–666.

21 Friedman SL. Gastrointestinal manifestations of the acquired immunodeficiency syndrome. In: Sleisenger MH, Fordtran JS (eds) *Gastrointestinal Disease*, 5th edn. Philadelphia: W.B. Saunders, 1993: 239–267.

22 Herts BR, Megibow AJ, Birnbaum BA et al. High-attenuation lymphadenopathy in AIDS patients: significance of findings at CT. *Radiology* 1992; **185**: 777–781.

23 Cappell MS. Hepatobiliary manifestations of the acquired immune deficiency syndrome. *Am J Gastroenterol* 1991; **86**: 1–15.

24 Luburich P, Bru C, Ayuso MC et al. Hepatic Kaposi sarcoma in AIDS: US and CT findings. *Radiology* 1990; **175**: 172–174.

25 Bessen LJ, Hymes KB, Greene JB. HIV: epidemiology, biology and spectrum of clinical syndromes. In: Federle MP, Megibow AJ, Naidich DP (eds) *Radiology of AIDS*. New York: Raven Press, 1988: 3–5.

26 Townsend RR, Laing FC, Jeffrey RB et al. Abdominal lymphoma in AIDS: evaluation with US. *Radiology* 1989; **171**: 719–724.

27 Townsend RR. CT of AIDS-related lymphoma. *AJR* 1991; **156**: 969–974.

28 Nyberg DA, Jeffrey RB, Federle MP et al. AIDS-related lymphomas: evaluation by abdominal CT. *Radiology* 1986; **159**: 59–63.

29 Mathieson R, Dutta S. Candida esophagitis. *Dig Dis Sci* 1983; **28**: 365–370.

30 Wall SD, Jones B. Gastrointestinal tract in the immunocompromised host: opportunistic infections and other complications. *Radiology* 1992; **185**: 327–335.

31 Solammandevi S, Patwardhan R. Herpes esophagitis. *Am J Gastroenterol* 1982; **77**: 48–50.

32 Balthazar EJ, Megibow AJ, Hulnick D et al. Cytomegalovirus

esophagitis in AIDS: radiographic features in 16 patients. *AJR*; 1987; **149**: 919–923.

33 Balthazar EJ, Megibow AJ, Hulnick D. Cytomegalovirus esophagitis and gastritis in AIDS. *AJR* 1985; **144**: 1201–1204.

34 Balthazar EJ, Megibow AJ, Fazzini E et al. Cytomegalovirus colitis in AIDS: radiographic findings in 11 patients. *Radiology* 1985; **155**: 585–589.

35 Vieco PT, Rochon L, Lisbona A. Multifocal cytomegalovirus associated hepatic lesions simulating metastases in AIDS. *Radiology* 1990; **176**: 123–124.

36 Goodman P, Pinero SS, Rance RM et al. Mycobacterial esophagitis in AIDS. *Gastrointest Radiol* 1989; **14**: 103–105.

37 Radin DR. Intra-abdominal mycobacterium tuberculosis vs. *Mycobacterium avium-intra cellulare* infections in patients with AIDS: distinction based on CT findings. *AJR* 199 **156**: 487–491.

38 Radin R. HIV Infection: Analysis in 259 consecutive patients with abnormal abdominal CT findings. *Radiology* 1995, **197**: 712–722.

39 Berk RN, Wall SD, McArdle CB et al. Cryptosporidiosis of the stomach and small intestine in patients with AIDS. *AJR* 1984; **143**: 549–554.

40 Kavin H, Jonas RB, Choudhury L, et al. Acalculous cholecystitis and cytomegalovirus infection in acquired immune deficiency syndrome. *Ann Intern Med* 1986; **104**: 53–54.

41 Blumberg RS, Kelsey P, Perrone T et al. Cytomegalovirus and cryptosporidia associated with acalculous cholecystitis. *Ann J Med* 1986; **76**: 118–123.

42 Galloway PG. Widespread cytomegalovirus infection involving the gastrointestinal tract, biliary tree and gallbladder in immuno-compromised patients. *Gastroenterology* 1984; **87**: 1407.

43 Dolmatch BL, Laing FC, Federle MP et al. AIDS-related cholangitis: radiographic findings in nine patients. *Radiology* 1987; **163**: 313.

44 Teixidor HS, Honig CL, Norsoph E, Alberts S, Mouradian JA, Whalen JP. Cytomegalovirus infection of the alimentary canal: radiographic findings with pathologic correlation. *Radiology* 1987; **164**: 317–325.

45 Romano AL, van Sonnenberg E, Casola G et al. Gallbladder and bile duct abnormalities in AIDS: sonographic findings in eight patients. *AJR* 1988: **15**: 123.

46 Defalque D, Menu Y, Girard P, Couland L. Sonographic diagnosis of cholangitis in AIDS patients. *Gastrointest radiol* **14**: 143.

47 Reeders JWAJ, ed. *Diagnostic Imaging of AIDS*. New York: Thieme, 1992: 92–123.

48 Reeders JWAJ, Bartelsman JFWM, Huibregtse K. AIDS-Related Manifestations of the Bile Duct System: A Common Finding? (Editorial Commentary) *Abdom Imaging* 1994; **19**: 423–424.

49 Farman J, Brunetti J, Baer JW, Freiman H, Comer GM, Scholz FJ, Koehler RE, Laffey K, Green P, Clemett AR. AIDS-Related Cholangiopancreatographic changes. *Abdom Imaging* 1994; **19**: 417–422.

17 HEPATOBILIARY AND PANCREATIC ULTRASOUND IN AIDS

John R. Mathieson
Frederick J. Smith

Ultrasound: advantages and technique

Ultrasound is the most commonly used imaging modality in acquired immune deficiency syndrome (AIDS) patients with suspected hepatobiliary or pancreatic disease [1]. Ultrasound is widely available and relatively inexpensive. AIDS patients are often excellent subjects for ultrasound examination, as the paucity of body fat in these patients allows for exquisite visualization of small structures. Often, very fine detail can be appreciated, and with the high quality of modern equipment one can often visualize very small structures that are not usually seen. For example, in the past, if one could visualize intrahepatic bile ducts, this was termed the 'parallel channel' or 'too many tubes' sign, indicating that the bile ducts were abnormally dilated. However, in thin cachectic AIDS patients, particularly using 5 and 7 MHz transducers, one can frequently visualize non-dilated bile ducts and hepatic arteries (Figure 17.1). In these cases, it is important to correlate the findings with liver function tests, such as alkaline phosphatase. Additionally, one can differentiate between hepatic arteries and small bile ducts with the use of color Doppler ultrasound (Figure 17.2).

Hepatic abnormalities in AIDS patients are often quite subtle, and require optimal sonographic technique to be visualized [2]. Rather than attempting to visualize large portions of the liver at once, we have found it useful to investigate only a small portion of the liver using high-frequency (5–10 MHz), small parts transducers in high-resolution mode. One can then frequently visualize subtle nodularity within the liver parenchyma, which may indicate the need for liver biopsy.

Pathological conditions

Diffuse liver disease

Clinical hepatomegaly and abnormal liver function tests are extremely common in AIDS patients, being found in up to 70% of cases [3]. This can be due to the direct consequences of human immune deficiency virus (HIV) infection, or to other conditions which occur with increased frequency in AIDS patients, owing to their particular lifestyle. Homosexual men and intravenous drug abusers are at increased risk of transmission of hepatitis viruses, and may be more frequently exposed to hepatotoxic drugs, notably including alcohol.

The majority of patients presenting with clinical hepatomegaly or abnormal liver function tests have no focal abnormalities on ultrasound.

The commonest sonographic finding in AIDS patients is hepatomegaly, found in approximately 20% of AIDS patients on routine sonography [1]. Causes of hepatomegaly include benign conditions such as steatosis, granulomatous hepatitis, hepatotoxic drugs and a non-specific response to hepatic inflammation [3–6], and malignant causes are most commonly due to diffuse infiltration with Kaposi's sarcoma or lymphoma [3,5]. In practical terms, the underlying cause is eventually determined in only a small minority of cases.

Another frequent abnormality consists of diffuse or patchy areas of increased echogenicity and attenuation. This is usually presumed to be due to fatty infiltration and has been found in 10–50% of patients [1,7]. In some cases, the pattern of fatty infiltration can be extremely inhomogeneous and give rise to quite bizarre appearing liver ultrasound images (Figure 17.3).

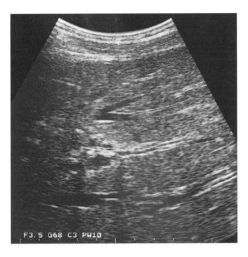

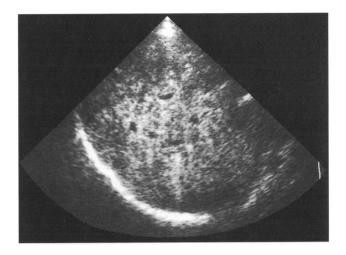

Figure 17.1. Transverse sonogram through the left lobe of the liver shows that normal structures not usually well seen on ultrasound, such as bile ducts and hepatic arteries, are clearly visible.

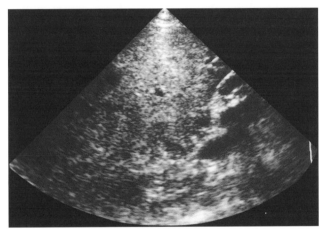

Figure 17.3. Sagittal sonograms through the liver of two AIDS patients show heterogeneous patterns of increased echogenicity due to patchy fatty infiltration.

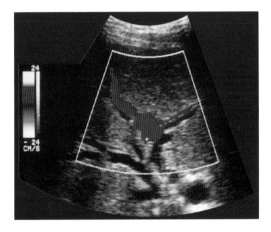

Figure 17.2. Colour Doppler ultrasound shows flow within hepatic vessels, allowing differentiation from dilated bile ducts.

In such cases, non-contrast computed tomography (CT) scans may be helpful in demonstrating focal areas of decreased hepatic attenuation, reflecting the increased amount of fat within the liver.

Pathologically, steatosis can be due to a number of factors, most commonly malnutrition. The classical form of steatosis in AIDS patients is macrovesicular, usually caused by protein malnutrition [3]. This may also be compounded by treatment with total parenteral nutrition. One may also encounter varying amounts of associated microvesicular steatosis, but if the

microvesicular pattern is dominant, this implies another cause, such as hepatotoxic drugs. Ultrasound-guided core liver biopsy may be useful in making this determination [6,8]. In our institution, this procedure is usually performed under direct ultrasound guidance. We use an automated biopsy gun. When a portal tract-based disease is suspected, an 18-gauge needle is used, but in cases where the only concern is to separate macrovesicular from microvesicular steatosis, the sample size obtained by a 20-gauge core needle is sufficient.

Since a large number of AIDS patients are also either homosexual men or intravenous drug abusers, viral hepatitis is common [6]. However, viral hepatitis is no more common in AIDS patients than in homosexual men who are HIV-negative. Nevertheless, 80–95% of AIDS patients will also be hepatitis B-positive.

Similarly, the incidence of cirrhosis is not increased in homosexual men with AIDS compared to those without AIDS. This is due not only to the much shorter latency period of the hepatitis viruses compared to HIV, but also to the decreased ability of AIDS patients to mount the inflammatory response which leads to cirrhosis [3]. However, the sonographic stigmata of cirrhosis are seen in many AIDS patients, including a nodular liver surface, ascites, and evidence of portal venous hypertension.

AIDS patients are subjected to a wide variety of the different hepatotoxic drugs, including sulfonamides, rifampin, isoniazid, ketoconazole, and many others [9,10]. In patients with abnormal liver functions and an ultrasound demonstrating liver enlargement, without focal lesions, a simple trial of medication withdrawal may be diagnostic.

Finally, in a large proportion of patients with hepatomegaly, no specific etiology is found. It has been proposed that this may be due to a non-specific response to hepatic infection [11,12]. In fact, there is very little actual pathologic data in the literature. One of the largest series in which pathologic proof was available was reported by Wilkins in 1991 [13]. In their series of 101 liver biopsies in patients who were HIV-positive or who had AIDS, only nine were pathologically normal. They found 50 cases of chronic hepatitis secondary to viral infection, 43 cases of steatosis, 15 cases of hepatic granulomas, and 8 cases of iron overload. Uncommon findings included cirrhosis (3), cytomegalovirus (CMV) (4), fungal infections (4) and non-Hodgkin lymphoma (2), and non-specific hepatitis (1).

Focal lesions

Although a wide variety of infections and neoplastic conditions can give rise to focal sonographic abnormalities in the liver of AIDS patients, focal lesions in the liver are much less common than generalized hepatomegaly. Also, the sonographic features of focal lesions almost never allow a specific diagnosis to be made, but ultrasound can be used to guide a fine-needle aspiration biopsy (FNAB).

Infectious granulomatous hepatitis and mycobacterial infection

Granulomatous hepatitis is a frequent finding at autopsy and at random liver biopsy. Usually the gran-

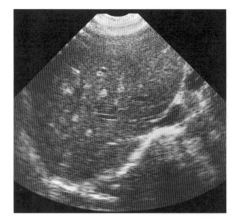

Figure 17.4. Transverse sonogram shows multiple small echogenic nodules throughout the liver in this patient with granulomatous hepatitis. No organism was found.

ulomas are microscopic and not sonographically visible, and simply give rise to hepatomegaly. Occasionally, the granulomas may be macroscopic, and very small hypoechoic or hyperechoic nodules may be seen on ultrasound (Figure 17.4). Granulomatous hepatitis can either due to an identifiable organism, or it can be idiopathic, with cultures and stains for mycobacteria being negative [14].

Both typical and atypical mycobacterial infection can cause focal liver lesions in AIDS patients. Typical *Mycobacterium tuberculosis* (MTb) infection usually present earlier in the course of AIDS than atypical *Mycobacterium avium intracellulare* (MAI) infection, as it is a more virulent infection, requiring a lesser degree of immune system compromise to spread [15]. This information can be used to separate the two conditions, and is particularly helpful as the imaging findings are often similar [16]. Widespread echo-poor lesions are seen throughout the liver, spleen, pancreas, and lymph nodes on ultrasound in both conditions (Figure 17.5). Most patients will have at least some degree on hepatomegaly and splenomegaly in both MAI and MTb, but when liver or spleen enlargement is particularly marked, MAI is more likely. On the other hand, homogeneously enlarged lymph nodes are usually seen with MAI, and large nodes with necrotic, fluid-containing centers are more commonly found with MTb [16,17]. These differences are due to the greater degree of immune dysfunction in MAI patients: they are unable to mount sufficient immune response to cause lymph node necrosis. In practice, there can be a good deal of overlap between the two conditions,

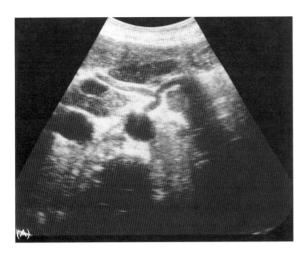

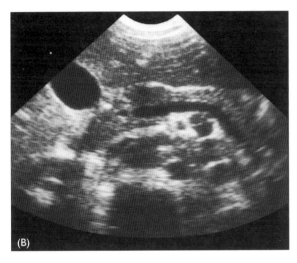

Figure 17.5. Transverse sonograms through the upper abdomen in two AIDS patients show multiple enlarged lymph nodes in the celiac (A) and peripancreatic (B) regions. Both patients had disseminated *Mycobacterium avium intracellulare* infection.

and ultrasound-guided FNAB can give a rapid diagnosis.

Rarely, other forms of mycobacteria such as *M. kansasii* or *M. xenopi* may be a cause of hepatic infection. Other causes of granulomatous hepatitis include systemic talcosis, drug reactions, cryptococcosis, histoplasmosis, and toxoplasmosis [3–5].

Bacterial infections

Hepatic abscesses are not particularly common in AIDS patients, and are not of increased frequency compared to the general population. Nevertheless, they may occur in AIDS patients, particularly in those with a bacterial infection in some other body region. We

have seen liver abscesses in AIDS patients with appendicitis, skin and soft tissue infections, and bacterial endocarditis, as well as in patients without a distant infectious source. As in other patients, hepatic abscesses will begin as small hypoechoic nodules, and gradually increase both in size and in fluid content as a mature abscess forms. If the patient is in a relatively advanced state of immune dysfunction, the process of abscess development can be quite incomplete and interrupted. The centers of the lesions may not actually liquefy, and the wall of the abscess may be poorly formed, giving rise to confusing ultrasound appearances. The center of an abscess may not appear echo-free, and may even mimic a solid lesion. The issue of liver abscesses in AIDS patients is further complicated by the fact that AIDS patients are often on a wide variety of antibiotics for other purposes, and it may be difficult to grow organisms on cultures from blood or FNAB specimens. Therefore, if a large echo-poor liver

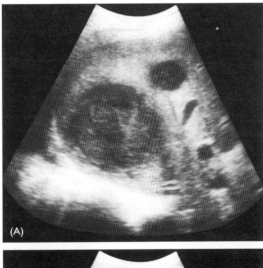

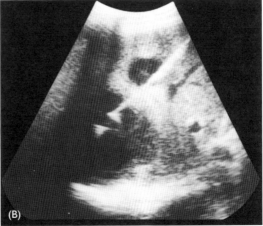

Figure 17.6. Sonogram through the liver (A) shows two large hypoechoic lesions in the right lobe. FNAB produced pus, and percutaneous abscess drainage was performed (B).

lesions is found, the diagnosis of bacterial abscess must still be considered, and if fluid is obtained on FNAB, a percutaneous drainage procedure should be performed (Figure 17.6).

Fungal infections

Fungal infections are quite common in AIDS patients, but, fortunately, disseminated fungal infections involving the liver and spleen are uncommon, and can occur very late in the course of AIDS [18]. These may be difficult to detect with ultrasound, as lesions can be very small, and very little immune reaction may occur. When multiple small (>3 cm) or very small (>1 cm) echo-poor lesions are found throughout the liver and spleen, the diagnosis of fungal infection should be considered.

Although mucocutaneous candidiasis is very common in AIDS patients, disseminated candidiasis is much less common, and is more often seen in patients with other immune disorders who also have profound neutropenia [19]. In patients with AIDS and reactivation of histoplasmosis, focal liver and spleen lesions are rarely seen, as the only imaging findings in most patients consists of hepatomegaly or splenomegaly and lymphadenopathy [20,21]. Cryptococcosis is much more likely to involve the brain or lungs than the abdomen, and, even when disseminated, usually gives rise to non-specific hepatosplenomegaly and lymphadenopathy. We have seen cases of end-stage disseminated cryptococcosis in which a strikingly large number of 1–3 cm lymph nodes were found throughout all regions of the peritoneal cavity.

Peliosis hepatis

Peliosis hepatis is a relatively rare condition in which the liver contains multiple focal nodules, consisting of blood-filled cavities. The nodules are usually small, ranging from microscopic size to 3–4 cm, sometimes have an epithelial lining, and usually communicate with dilated sinusoids. Peliosis hepatis was first described in patients with marasmus, owing to chronic infection or malignancy [22,23], and has since been reported in patients treated with a variety of drugs, particularly steroids [24]. It has been thought to arise from a combination of factors, including destruction of sinusoidal walls, increased hepatic venous pressure, and hepatocellular damage [24,25]. Peliosis was found pathologically in AIDS patients early in the AIDS

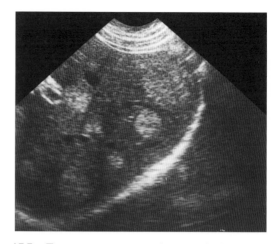

Figure 17.7. Transverse sonogram shows multiple echogenic nodules throughout the liver in an AIDS patient with peliosis hepatis.

epidemic, as described by Devars et al. in 1985 [26]. It was not until 1991 that the CT findings of peliosis hepatis were reported by Radin and Kanel [27].

Peliosis hepatis has now been associated with another unusual vascular lesion, bacillary angiomatosis. This is a proliferative pseudoneoplastic lesion most commonly found on the skin. Both of these are now thought to be caused by *Rochalimaea hensalae*, an unusual bacteria which has only recently been identified [23,26,28]. Although lesions may be confined to the skin, they may also be found in the spleen and in visceral lymph nodes [29].

The ultrasound findings of peliosis are variable, but usually, small echo-poor nodules, 4 cm or less in diameter, are found throughout the liver (Figure 17.7). Similar lesions may also be seen in the spleen and in lymph nodes [30–32]. Sometimes, the nodules may show increased echogenicity, becoming isoechoic or hypoechoic with respect to normal liver. The reason for this is unknown, but may be due to the presence of thrombus. When severe, peliosis may give rise to portal hypertension, and its associated sonographic findings.

When multiple echo-poor liver nodules are found in patients who also have skin lesion, the diagnosis may most easily be diagnosed from the skin lesions. CT can also be extremely useful to make the diagnosis, showing low-density lesions on the non-contrast, which become isodense or hyperdense with intravenous contrast [27,33]. Biopsy may be done, but the bacteria are extremely difficult to isolate, and false-negative results are common. Core biopsy or open liver biopsy are more likely to show the typical morphologic features of the blood-filled spaces in definitive fashion.

Rarely, peliosis may be severe enough to cause anemia [34] and even splenic rupture [35].

Ultrasound is also useful to follow patients once the diagnosis has been made. The liver and spleen lesions will gradually disappear with antibiotic treatment [34,36].

Pneumocystis carinii

In the early days of the AIDS epidemic, *Pneumocystis carinii* became recognized as a common pulmonary pathogen, and a variety of treatments evolved. Regular use of aerosolized Pentamidine became widely used as an effective preventative or suppressive therapy against *Pneumocystis carinii* pneumonia (PCP). However, since the delivery of the drug was primarily to the lung, disseminated *Pneumocystis carinii* disease began to be reported, involving the liver, spleen, kidneys, lymph nodes, gastrointestinal (GI) tract, and a variety of other sites distant from the lungs [37–41].

The commonest sites of extrapulmonary *Pneumocystis carinii* infections are the liver, spleen, and kidneys. The lesions begin as microabscesses, and are often echogenic on ultrasound. The lesions can also be echo-poor, and, in later stages, can become calcified. The lesions are usually very small, measuring 2–5 mm, and can be extremely numerous. It was initially thought that the sonographic finding of innumerable punctate echogenic lesions found in the solid abdominal organs of an AIDS patient was specific for *Pneumocystis carinii* infection [42]. Since then, identical findings have been shown to be caused by disseminated *Candida*, *Aspergillus*, and *Mycobacterium* infections [43–45] (Figure 17.8). In all of these diseases, concurrent involvement of lymph nodes, the pancreas, omentum, and peritoneum can be found. When these findings are encountered, ultrasound or CT-guided biopsy should be done promptly to allow rapid and definitive treatment.

Malignancies

Kaposi's sarcoma

Disseminated Kaposi's sarcoma can involve almost any part of the body, but it is unusual to find liver, spleen, or pancreatic lesions on abdominal ultrasound

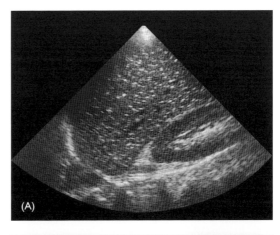

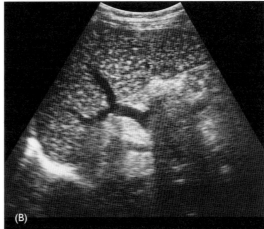

Figure 17.8. Sonograms show innumerable punctate echogenic lesions throughout the liver (A) and spleen (B). Although first described in disseminated *Pneumocystis* infection, biopsy in this case showed *Mycobacterium avium intracellulare*. This can also be seen in disseminated candidiasis and *Aspergillus* infections.

[1,46,47]. This is partly due to the fact that significant involvement of these organs is a relatively late event in the natural history of disseminated Kaposi's sarcoma. It is also due to the fact that Kaposi's sarcoma tends to grow as an infiltrative lesion, along portal tracts, rather than as a large mass [48]. Imaging findings can, therefore, remain quite subtle even in advanced disease [49]. Altered echogenicity of the portal triads, often with a hypoechoic rim, may be the only ultrasound finding. Less commonly, focal echogenic nodules can be found throughout the liver and/or spleen [50] (Figure 17.9). Biopsies may be difficult to interpret, and false-negative results are common. Magnetic resonance imaging may prove helpful in some cases, showing periportal high-signal changes on proton density and T_2-weighted images [47].

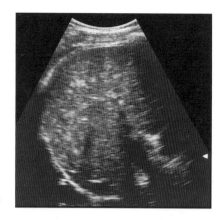

(A)

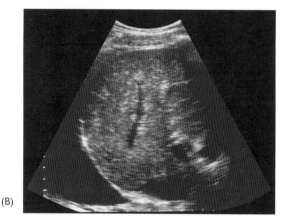

(B)

Figure 17.9. (A,B) Sonograms through the liver show multiple small echogenic nodules. (B) shows that the lesions are distributed preferentially around the portal triads, typical for Kaposi's sarcoma. The patient also had extensive thoracic involvement, with large pleural effusions.

Lymphoma

Non-Hodgkin lymphoma commonly involves the liver and upper abdomen in AIDS patients [3,51–54]. The disease is often extranodal, and the liver is the second most common site of involvement in the abdomen, next to the GI tract [55].

We have observed three main morphological patterns in intraabdominal AIDS-related lymphomas: (1) large masses; (2) multiple, small, focal nodules; and (3) a diffuse infiltrating pattern. The first two are by far the most common, with the diffuse pattern seen only rarely.

When a large mass is found in lymphoma, it will tend to grow around other structures, causing displacement rather than obstruction [52]. Lymphomatous masses can reach extremely large sizes before causing any obstructive symptoms. On ultrasound the masses can be very homogeneous, and are usually hypoechoic relative to liver (Figure 17.10). They can be almost anechoic, and mimic fluid, owing to the bland architecture of lymphoma, which is lacking in acoustic interfaces. However, they can usually be distinguished from fluid by the lack of enhanced through-transmission. When a lymphomatous mass is very large, it can be difficult or impossible to determine the organ of origin, and multiple organs can be displaced or distorted. When a mass such as this is found, there is little else in the differential diagnosis (Figure 17.11).

When AIDS-related lymphoma presents with multiple focal hypoechoic nodules, involvement is

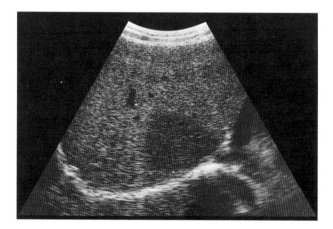

Figure 17.10. Transverse sonogram through the liver shows a large homogeneously hypoechoic mass in the posterior segment of the right lobe. FNAB showed large-cell lymphoma.

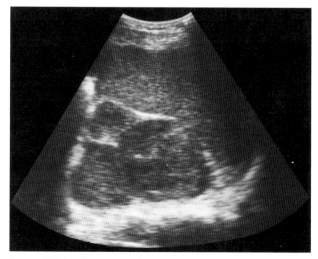

Figure 17.11. Sonogram through the left upper quadrant showing a large mass in the splenic hilum due to AIDS-related lymphoma.

(A)

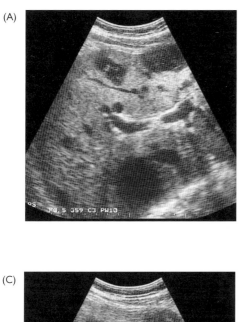

(B)

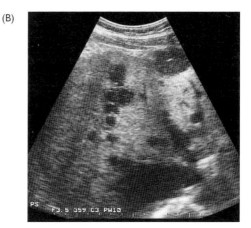

(C)

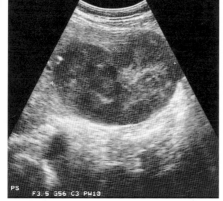

Figure 17.12. Sonograms through the liver showing multiple hypoechoic lesions of widely varying sizes in this AIDS patient with immunoblastic lymphoma.

often not confined to one organ. Nodules may be found throughout the liver, spleen and kidneys, as well as in retroperitoneal lymph nodes, the pancreatic bed and mesentery of the large and small bowel (Figure 17.12). The differential diagnosis includes a wide variety of infectious agent, particularly including mycobacteria.

The least common morphological pattern of intra-abdominal lymphoma in AIDS patients is one of diffuse infiltration. In these patients, the disease can spread throughout the mesentery and peritoneal cavity with an unusual gelatinous or fluid-like character, filling in the spaces between organs and leaves of the mesentery (Figure 17.13). Although the lymphomatous infiltrate is actually solid, it can be almost anechoic on ultrasound, and very low density on CT [56]. Furthermore, the lymphomatous infiltrate can also be associated with ascites. It can, therefore, be difficult or impossible to separate fluid from solid components with imaging. The borders of abdominal organs such as the liver can be very difficult to visualize, and tumor

may infiltrate directly into the liver from the peritoneal cavity. These lymphomas are usually high grade and poorly differentiated. As such, there is often an initially dramatic response to chemotherapy, and ultrasound and CT findings can even return to normal. However, because of the very rapid cell turnover, recurrence and death occur quickly.

The role of ultrasound-guided FNAB in AIDS-related lymphoma is extremely important, and is different than in non–AIDS-related lymphoma patients. First, FNAB is very useful just to establish the diagnosis of lymphoma, particularly in cases where infectious conditions are high on the differential diagnosis. This can usually be done in a matter of minutes, using a variety of quick-stain cytopathology techniques. Second, FNAB specimens may be sufficient to allow staging of the lymphoma sufficiently to allow a treatment regimen to be decided upon. This is particularly true in AIDS patients, whose lymphomas tend to be high grade, and tend to be pathologically diffuse rather than nodular [51]. Successful lymphoma

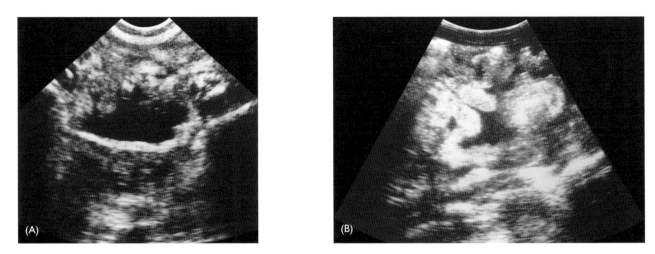

Figure 17.13. Abdominal sonograms show a very hypoechoic infiltrating mass mimicking fluid, enveloped around multiple loops of bowel in this AIDS patient with peritoneal lymphomatosis. FNAB confirmed that the apparent free fluid was in fact solid, with cytopathology showing very poorly differentiated immunoblastic lymphoma. The abdominal sonographic appearance rapidly returned to normal with chemotherapy, but the patient had a relapse and died within 2 months.

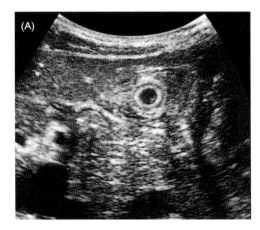
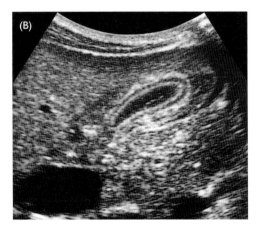

Figure 17.14. Long-axis (A) and short-axis (B) sonograms through the right upper quadrant show marked thickening of the gallbladder wall. Note that the lumen is not distended. This was an asymptomatic incidental finding.

staging requires a close working relationship between the radiologist, the pathologist, and the oncologist [57].

Gallbladder and bile ducts

Gallbladder wall thickening is a very frequent ultrasound finding in AIDS patients (Figure 17.14). However, this finding must be interpreted cautiously, as in the majority of patients it is an incidental finding of no clinical significance. In our survey of abdominal ultrasound in 399 AIDS patients, gallbladder wall thickening was found in 30 patients (7.5%), but was the cause of symptoms in only three of these patients [1]. When gallbladder wall thickening is found in AIDS patients without tenderness over the gallbladder, or a 'sonographic Murphy's sign', and no evidence of bile duct thickening, it can be dismissed as an incidental finding (Figure 17.15). On the other hand, if the gallbladder is tender, thick walled and distended, the diagnosis of acalculous cholecystitis must be entertained [58,59] (Figure 17.16). This condition is usually found only in hospital in-patients who are seriously ill, often suffering from multiple illnesses, who have

(A)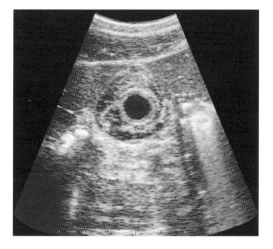

(B)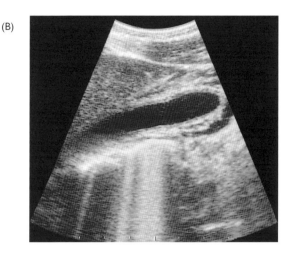

Figure 17.15. Gallbladder wall thickening and edema is shown on long-axis (A) and short-axis (B) sonograms. The gallbladder was not tender, and this was considered an incidental finding.

not been fed orally for a prolonged period of time. In our practice, the only exception to the rule that 'acalculous cholecystitis does not occur in out-patients' has been in AIDS patients. Indeed, we have seen several cases where an episode of acalculous cholecystitis was the first hint that the patient had AIDS, and we began to consider this as an 'AIDS-defining illness'. We have also found that AIDS-associated acalculous cholecystitis can be treated successfully with a temporary ultrasound-guided percutaneous cholecystostomy, and that surgical cholecystectomy is usually not needed.

The drainage catheter should be left in place until a cholangiogram demonstrates that the cystic duct occlusion, presumably due to an opportunistic infection, has resolved. In many cases, bile cultures produce no growth, but a variety of infectious agents including cryptosporidia and CMV have been reported [60–65].

AIDS-related cholangitis has also been described [66–69]. Inflammatory strictures can be quite diffuse, or can be focal and isolated to any part of the biliary tree [70–72] (Figure 17.17). When the common bile or hepatic ducts are involved, patients can present with

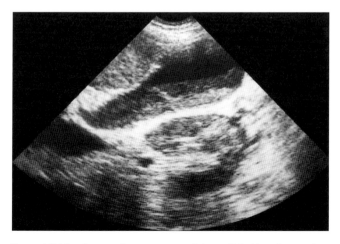

Figure 17.16. Long-axis sonogram of the gallbladder shows that the gallbladder is distended and contains multilayered sludge. This patient's gallbladder was very tender, and his symptoms resolved with percutaneous cholecystostomy. Bile cultures showed cryptosporidia.

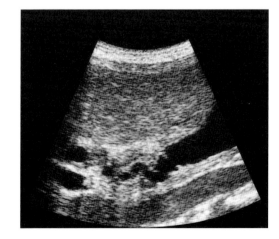

Figure 17.17. Sonogram through the right upper quadrant shows marked thickening of the wall of the cystic duct. Although this was an incidental finding in this patient, this could lead to gallbladder obstruction and acute acalculous cholecystitis.

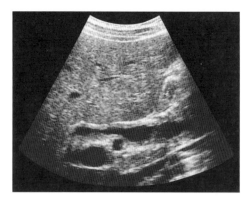

Figure 17.18. Sonogram through the porta hepatis showing thickening of the wall of the common hepatic duct in a patient with AIDS cholangitis.

jaundice, with or without fever. The findings on ultrasound can be quite subtle, and easily overlooked [59,73]. Bile duct walls become slightly thickened, and may appear hypoechoic, isoechoic or even hyperechoic. Even with high-resolution ultrasound equipment, and careful scanning technique, the abnormal bile duct walls can be difficult to demonstrate (Figure 17.18). If the inflammatory change is significant enough to cause obstruction, the dilated ducts above the stricture are usually readily demonstrated with ultrasound. Intrahepatic abscesses, owing to stricture and stasis, can also be found. Sometimes, the inflammation can be confined to the periampullary region, causing papillary stenosis [74]. Endoscopic cholangiography can be very helpful, (Figures 17.19 and 17.20) and endoscopic sphincterotomy can relieve obstruction. When a stricture involves a longer segment of the common duct, either temporary placement of a nasobiliary drain, or longer term use of a biliary endoprosthesis can be considered.

Even though infectious agents cause most gallbladder and bile duct disease in AIDS patients, malignant strictures may also occur. We have seen a few patients with both AIDS and pancreatic cancer, and we have been impressed with the unusually rapid downhill course in these patients, with quite rampant tumor growth leading to death within a very short

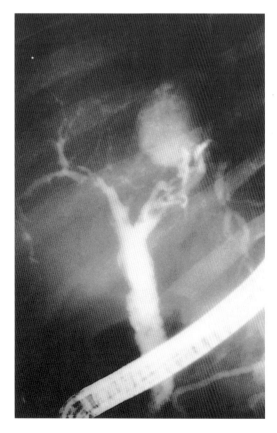

Figure 17.19. Endoscopic retrograde cholangiogram shows irregular strictures of the intrahepatic bile ducts, communicating with a large abscess cavity.

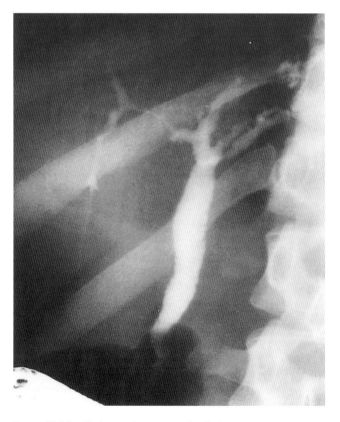

Figure 17.20. Endoscopic retrograde cholangiograms in two patients with AIDS cholangitis show irregular strictures of the intrahepatic bile ducts. No bile duct wall thickening was detected with ultrasound in either case.

period of time. Finally, a lymphomatous mass can occasionally cause biliary obstruction but, as mentioned above, lymphoma tends to cause displacement of the bile duct rather than obstruction.

Pancreas

AIDS-related diseases rarely cause isolated abnormalities of the pancreas, and when pancreatic lesions are found, it is usually in the context of widely disseminated disease. In fact, abnormalities of the pancreas are quite common in end-stage AIDS patients. One autopsy series [75] found that 52 out of 82 (65%) of AIDS patients had abnormal findings in the pancreas, mostly related to subclinical (29%) or clinical pancreatitis (22%). Opportunistic infections or cancers were found in 28%, some of whom also had signs of pancreatitis. It was postulated that AIDS patients may have an increased incidence of pancreatitis, owing to ductal strictures induced by opportunistic infections or malignancies. Pancreatitis in AIDS patients has also been reported to be caused by medications [76]. Pancreatic ductal strictures can be seen with or without associated bile duct abnormalities on endoscopic retrograde cholangiopancreatography [77]. The most common site for pancreatic duct abnormalities to be recognized is in the periampullary region, but pathologically, any portion of the pancreas can be involved. The organisms responsible for pancreatic duct narrowing are similar to those found in AIDS cholangitis [77].

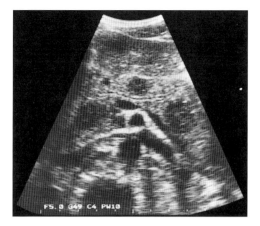

Figure 17.21. Transverse sonograms show multiple echo-poor lesions in the pancreas in this AIDS patient with lymphoma. Similar lesions were also seen in the liver, spleen, and kidneys.

Although a variety of organisms can cause pancreatic infections [78,79] disseminated toxoplasmosis seems to be somewhat unique in causing a particularly virulent necrotizing pancreatitis, often leading to death [80–83]. Concurrent involvement of the brain, heart, lungs and multiple abdominal organs has been found at autopsy. Lymphomatous involvement of the pancreas is also usually associated with multiple organ involvement, most frequently seen in patients with multiple focal nodules (Figure 17.21).

References

1 Smith FJ, Mathieson JR, Cooperberg PL. Abdominal abnormalities in AIDS: detection at US in a large population. *Radiology* 1994; **192**: 691–695.

2 Murray JG, Patel MD, Lee S, Sandhu JS, Feldstein VA. Microabscesses of the liver and spleen in AIDS: detection with 5–MHz sonography. *Radiology* 1995; **197**: 723–727.

3 Schneiderman DJ. Hepatobiliary abnormalities of AIDS. *Gastroenterol Clin North Am* 1988; **17**: 615–630.

4 Glasgow BJ, Anders K, Layfield LJ, Steinsapir KD, Gitnick GL, Lewin KJ. Clinical and pathologic findings of the liver in the acquired immune deficiency syndrome (AIDS). *AJCP* 1985; **83**: 582–588.

5 Cappell MS. Hepatobiliary manifestations of the acquired immune deficiency syndrome [clinical review]. *Am J Gastroenterol* 1991; **86**: 1–15.

6 Dworkin BM, Stahl RE, Giardina MAet al. The liver in aquired immune deficiency syndrome: emphasis on patients with intravenous drug abuse. *Am J Gastroenterol* 1987; **82**: 231–236.

7 Beale TJ, Wetton CW, Crofton ME. A sonographic-pathological correlation of liver biopsies in patients with the acquired immune deficiency syndrome (AIDS). *Clin Radiol* 1995; **50**: 761–764.

8 Cappell MS. Clinical utility of liver biopsy in patients with serum antibodies to the human immunodeficiency virus. *Am J Med* 1990; **88**: 123–130.

9 Shriner K, Goetz MB. Severe hepatotoxicity in a patient receiving both acetaminophen and zidovudine. *Am J Med* 1992; **93**: 94–96.

10 Muñoz P, Moreno S, Berenguer J, de Quirós JCLB, Bouza E. Fluconazole-related hepatotoxicity in patients with acquired immunodeficiency syndrome. *Arch Intern Med* 1991; **151**: 1020–1021.

11 Lebovics E, Thung SN, Schaffner F et al. The liver in the acquired immunodeficiency syndrome: a clinical and histologic study. *Hepatology* 1985; **5**: 293–298.

12 Schneiderman DJ, Arenson DM, Cello JP et al. Hepatic disease in patients with acquired immune deficiency syndrome (AIDS). *Hepatology* 1987; **7**: 925–930.

13 Wilkins MJ, Lindley R, Dourakis SP, Goldin RD. Surgical pathology of the liver in HIV infection. *Histopathology* 1991; **18**: 459–464.

14 Kahn SA, Saltzman BR, Klein RS, Mahadevia PS, Friedland GH, Brandt LJ. Hepatic disorders in the acquired immune deficiency syndrome: a clinical and pathological study. *Am J Gastroenterol* 1986; **81**: 1145–1148.

15 Aubry P, Reynaud JP, Nbonyingingo C, Ndabaneze E, Mucikere E. Ultrasonographic data of the solid organs of the abdomen in stage IV human immunodeficiency virus infection. A prospective study of 101 cases in central Africa [in French]. *Ann Gastroenterol Hepatol* 1994; **30**: 43–52.

16 Radin DR. Intra-abdominal mycobacterium tuberculosis vs. mycobacterium avium-intra cellulare infections in patients with AIDS: distinction based on CT findings. *AJR* 199; **156**: 487–491.

17 Nyberg DA, Federle MP, Jeffrey RB, Bottles K, Wolfsy CB. Abdominal CT findings of disseminated mycobacterium avium-intracellulare in AIDS. *AJR* 1985; **145**: 297–299.

18 Diamond RD. The growing problem of mycoses in patients infected with the human immunodeficiency virus. *Rev Infect Dis* 1991; **13**: 480–486.

19 Shirkhoda A. CT findings in hepatosplenic and renal candidiasis. *J Computer Assisted Tomography* 1987; **11**: 795–798.

20 Radin DR. Disseminated histoplasmosis: abdominal CT findings in 16 patients. *AJR* 1991; **157**: 955–958.

21 Minamoto G, Armstrong D. Fungal infections in AIDS: histoplasmosis and coccidioidomycosis. *Infect Dis Clin North Am* 1988; **2**: 447–456.

22 Simon DM, Krause R, Galambos JT. Peliosis hepatis in a patient with marasmus. *Gastroenterology* 1988; **95**: 805–809.

23 Perkocha LA, Geaghan SM, Yen TSB et al. Clinical and pathological features of bacillary peliosis hepatis in association with human immunodeficiency virus infection. *N Engl J Med* 1990; **323**: 581–586.

24 Leong SS, Cazen RA, Yu GS, LeFevre L, Carson JW. Abdominal visceral peliosis associated with bacillary angiomatosis. Ultrastructural evidence of endothelial destruction by bacilli. *Arch Path Lab Med* 1992; **116**: 866–871.

25 Reed JA, Brigati DJ, Flynn SD et al. Immunocytochemical identification of Rochalimaea henselae in bacillary (epithelioid) angiomatosis, parenchymal bacillary peliosis, and persistent fever with bacteremia. *Am J Surg Path* 1992; **16**: 650–657.

26 Devars du Mayne JF. Hepatic vascular lesions in AIDS. *JAMA* 1985; **254**: 53–54.

27 Radin DR, Kanel GC. Peliosis hepatis in a patient with human immunodeficiency virus infection. *AJR* 1991; **156**: 91–92.

28 Relman DA, Loutit JS, Schmidt TM, Falkow S, Tompkins LS. The agent of bacillary angiomatosis: an approach to the identification of uncultured pathogens. *N Engl J Med* 1990; **323**: 1573–1580.

29 Slater LN, Welch DF, Hensel D, Coody DW. A newly recognized fastidious gram-negative pathogen as a cause of fever and bacteremia. *N Engl J Med* 1990; **323**: 1587–1593.

30 Steeper TA, Rosenstein H, Weiser J, Inampudi S, Snover DC. Bacillary epithelioid angiomatosis involving the liver, spleen, and skin in an AIDS patient with concurrent Kaposi's sarcoma. *Am J Clin Radiol* 1992; **97**: 713–718.

31 Moore EH, Russell LA, Klein JS et al. Bacillary angiomatosis in patients with AIDS: multiorgan imaging findings. *Radiology* 1995; **197**: 67–72. [Published] erratum appears in *Radiology* 1995; **197**: 549.

32 Jamadar DA, D'Souza SP, Thomas EA, Giles TE. Case report: radiological appearances in peliosis hepatis. *Br J Radiol* 1994; **67**: 102–104.

33 Slater LN, Welch DF, Min KW. Rochalimaea henselae causes bacillary angiomatosis and peliosis hepatis. *Arch Intern Med* 1992; **152**: 602–606.

34 Wyatt SH, Fishman EK. Hepatic bacillary angiomatosis in a patient with AIDS. *Abdom Imaging* 1993; **18**: 336–338.

35 Garcia-Tsao G, Panzini L, Yoselevitz M, West AB. Bacillary peliosis hepatis as a cause of acute anemia in a patient with the acquired immunodeficiency syndrome. *Gastroenterology* 1992; **102**: 1065–1070.

36 Kohr RM, Haendiges M, Taube RR. Peliosis of the spleen: a rare cause of spontaneous splenic rupture with surgical implications [review]. *Am Surg* 1993; **59**: 197–199.

37 Radin DR. Spontaneous resolution of peliosis of the liver and spleen in a patient with HIV infection [letter] [see comments]. *AJR* 1992; **158**: 1409.

38 Lubat E, Megibow AJ, Balthazar EJ, Goldenberg AS, Birnbaum BA, Bosniak MA. Extrapulmonary pneumocystis carinii infection in AIDS: CT findings. *Radiology* 1990; **174**: 157–160.

39 Spouge AR, Wilson SR, Gopinath N, Sherman M, Blendis LM. Extrapulmonary pneumocystis carinii in a patient with AIDS: sonographic findings. *AJR* 1990; **155**: 76–78.

40 Sachs JR, Greenfield SM, Sohn M et al. Disseminated pneumocystis carinii infection with hepatic involvement in a patient with the acquired immunodeficiency syndrome. *Am J Gastroenterol* 1991; **86**: 82–85.

41 Radin DR, Baker EL, Klatt EC et al. Visceral and nodal calcification in patients with AIDS-related pneumocystis carinii infection. *AJR* 1990; **154**: 27–31.

42 Abati AD, Opitz L, Brones C, Burstein DE, Gallo L. Cytology of extrapulmonary pneumocystis carinii infection in the acquired immunodeficiency syndrome. *Acta Cytol* 1992; **36**: 440–444.

43 Bray HJ, Lail VJ, Cooperberg PL. Tiny echogenic foci in the liver and kidney in patients with AIDS: not always due to disseminated pneumocystis carinii [see comments]. *AJR* 1992; **158**: 81–82.

44 Towers MJ, Withers CE, Hamilton PA, Kolin A, Walmsley

S. Visceral calcification in patients with AIDS may not always be due to pneumocystis carinii. *AJR* 1991; **156**: 745–747.

45   Keane MA, Finlayson C, Joseph AE. A histological basis for the 'sonographic snowstorm' in opportunistic infection of the liver and spleen. *Clin Rad* 1995; **50**: 220–222.

46   Luburich P, Bru C, Ayuso MC, Azón A, Condom E. Hepatic Kaposi sarcoma in AIDS: US and CT findings. *Radiology* 1990; **175**: 172–174.

47   Valls C, Cañas C, Turell LG, Pruna X. Hepatosplenic AIDS-related Kaposi's sarcoma. *Gastrointest Radiol* 1991; **16**: 342–344.

48   Buetow PC, Buck JL, Ros PR, Goodman ZD. Malignant vascular tumors of the liver: radiologic-pathologic correlation. *Radiographics* 1994; **14**: 153–166.

49   Khalil AM, Carette MF, Cadranel JL, Mayaud CM, Bigot JM. Intrathoracic Kaposi's sarcoma. CT findings. *Chest* 1995; **108**: 1622–1626.

50   Valls C, Cañas C, Turell LG, Pruna X. Hepatosplenic AIDs-related Kaposi's sarcoma. *Gastrointest Radiol* 1991; **16**: 342–344.

51   Ziegler JL, Beckstead JA, Volberding PA et al. Non-Hodgkin's lymphoma in 90 homosexual men. Relation to generalized lymphadenopathy and the acquired immunodeficiency syndrome. *N Engl J Med* 1984; **311**: 565–570.

52   Nyberg DA, Jeffrey, Jr. RB, Federle MP, Bottles K, Abrams DI. AIDS-related lymphomas: evaluation by abdominal CT. *Radiology* 1986; **159**: 59–63.

53   Dodd GD III, Greenler DP, Confer SR. Thoracic and abdominal manifestations of lymphoma occurring in the immunocompromised patient. *Radiol Clin North Am* 1992; **30**: 597–610.

54   Towsend DR. CT of AIDS-related lymphoma. *AJR* 1991; **156**: 969–974.

55   Radin DR, Esplin JA, Levine AM, Ralls PW. AIDS-related non-Hodgkin's lymphoma: abdominal CT findings in 112 patients. *AJR* 1993; **160**: 1133–1139.

56   Lynch MA, Cho KC, Jeffrey RB Jr, Alterman DD, Federle MP. CT of peritoneal lymphomatosis. *AJR* 1988; **151**: 713–715.

57   Sandrasegaran K, Robinson PJ, Selby P. Staging of lymphoma in adults [review]. *Clin Radiol* 1994; **49**: 149–161.

58   Iannuzzi C, Belghiti J, Erlinger S, Menu Y, Fékété F. Cholangitis associated with cholecystitis in patients with acquired immunodeficiency syndrome. *Arch Surg* 1990; **125**: 1211–1213.

59   Romano AJ, vanSonnenberg E, Casola G et al. Gallbladder and bile duct abnormalties in AIDS: sonographic findings in eight patients. *AJR* 1988; **150**: 123–127.

60   Teixidor HS, Godwin TA, Ramirez E. Cryptosporidiosis of the biliary tract in AIDS. *Radiology* 1991; **180**: 51–56.

61   Gross TL, Wheat J, Bartlett M, O'Connor KW. AIDS and multiple system involvement with cryptosporidium. *Am J Gastroenterol* 1986; **81**: 456–458.

62   Kavin H, Jonas RB, Chowdhury L, Kabins S. Acalculous cholecystitis and cytomegalovirus infection in the acquired immunodeficiency syndrome. *Ann Intern Med* 1986; **104**: 53–54.

63   Blumberg RS, Kelsey P, Perrone T, Dickersin R, Laquaglia M, Ferruci J. Cytomegalovirus – and cryptosporidium-associated acalculous gangrenous cholecystitis. *Am J Med* 1984; **76**: 1118–1123.

64   Keshavjee SH, Magee LA, Mullen BJ, Baron DL, Brunton JL, Gallinger S. Acalculous cholecystitis associated with cytomegalovirus and sclerosing cholangitis in a patient with acquired immunodeficiency syndrome. *Can J Surg* 1993; **36**: 321–325.

65   Forbes A, Blanshard C, Gazzard B. Natural history of AIDS related sclerosing cholangitis: a study of 20 cases. *Gut* 1993; **34**: 116–121.

66   Farman J, Brunetti J, Baer JW et al. AIDS-related cholangiopancreatographic changes [see comments]. *Abdom Imaging* 1994; **19**: 417–422.

67   Ducreux M, Buffet C, Lamy P et al. Diagnosis and prognosis of AIDS-related cholangitis. *AIDS* 1995; **9**: 875–880.

68   Bouche H, Housset C, Dumont JL et al. AIDS-related cholangitis: diagnostic features and course in 15 patients. *J Hepatol* 1993; **17**: 34–39.

69   Dolmatch BL, Laing FC, Federle MP, Jeffrey RB, Cello J. AIDS-related cholangitis: radiographic findings in nine patients. *Radiology* 1987; **163**: 313–316.

70   Knollmann FD, Adler A, Maurer J et al. Vergleichende darstellung HIV-assoziierter erkrankungen des hepatobiliaren systems in computertomographie und cholangiographie. *Aktuelle Radiol* 1995; **5**: 216–221.

71   Colins CD, Forbes A, Harcourt-Webster JN, Francis ND, Gleeson JA, Gazzard BG. Radiological and pathological features of AIDS-related polypoid cholangitis. *Clin Radiol* 1993; **48**: 307–310. [Published erratum appears in *Clin Radiol* 1994; **49**: 146.]

72   Benhamou Y, Caumes E, Gerosa Y et al. AIDS-related cholangiography. Critical analysis of a prospective series of 26 patients. *Dig Dis Sci* 1993; **38**: 1113–1118.

73   Defalque D, Menu Y, Girard PM, Coulaud JP. Sonographic diagnosis of cholangitis in AIDS patients. *Gastrointest Radiol* 1989; **14**: 143–147.

74   Da Silva F, Boudghene F, Lecomte I, Delage Y, Grange JD, Bigot JM. Sonography in AIDS-related cholangitis: prevalence and cause of an echogenic nodule in the distal end of the common bile duct. *AJR* 1993; **160**: 1205–1207.

75   Dowell SF, Moore GW, Hutchins GM. The spectrum of pancreatic pathology in patients with AIDS. *Mod Pathol* 1990; **3**: 49–53.

76   Harris AG, Caroli-Bosc FX, Demarquay JF, Hastier P, Delmont J. Acute pancreatitis in an octreotide-treated AIDS patient-suggested alternative mechanisms [letter]. *Pancreas* 1995; **11**: 318–319.

77   Farman J, Brunetti J, Baer JW et al. AIDS-related cholangiopancreatographic changes [see comments]. *Abdom Imaging* 1994; **19**: 417–422.

78   Jaber B, Gleckman R. Tuberculous pancreatic abscess as an initial AIDS-defining disorder in a patient infected with the human immunodeficiency virus: case report and review. *Clin Infect Dis* 1995; **20**: 890–894.

79   Bonacini M, Nussbaum J, Ahluwalia C. Gastrointestinal, hepatic, and pancreatic involvement with Cryptococcus neoformans in AIDS. *J Clin Gastroenterol* 1990; **12**: 295–297.

80   Ahuja SK, Ahuja SS, Thelmo W, Seymour A, Phelps KR. Necrotizing pancreatitis and multisystem organ failure

associated with toxoplasmosis in a patient with AIDS. *Clin Infect Dis* 1993; **16**: 432–434.

81   Liu DC, Lin CS, Seshan V. AIDS complicated with disseminated toxoplasmosis: a pathological study of 9 autopsy cases. *Chung-hua Ping Li Hsueh Tsa Chih* 1994; **23**: 166–169.

82   Hofman P, Michiels JF, Mondain V, Saint-Paul MC, Rampal A, Loubière R. Acute toxoplasmic pancreatitis. An unusual cause of death in AIDS. *Gastroenterol Clin Biol* 1994; **18**: 985–987.

83   Jautzke G, Sell M, Thalmann U et al. Extracerebral toxoplasmosis in AIDS. Histological and immunohistological findings based on 80 autopsy cases. *Pathol Res Pract* 1993; **189**: 428–436.

18 HEPATO-PANCREATO AND BILIARY IMAGING IN AIDS: COMPUTED TOMOGRAPHY

D. Randall Radin

Introduction

Many patients with human immunodeficiency virus (HIV) infection undergo computed tomography (CT) examination of the abdomen for evaluation of unexplained fever, abdominal pain, weight loss, palpable mass, organomegaly, or abnormal liver chemistries. The three most common sites of abnormal abdominal CT findings due to acquired immune deficiency syndrome (AIDS)-related opportunistic infection or neoplasm are the lymph nodes, the liver, and the spleen. Often the radiologist can suggest a specific diagnosis or a short list of possible diagnoses on the basis of careful evaluation of abdominal CT findings. In many cases, diagnosis of the infection or neoplasm is made by analysis of blood, stool, or sputum specimens or by biopsy of an enlarged peripheral lymph node or bone marrow biopsy. However, in a significant percentage of cases, percutaneous fine-needle aspiration or core biopsy of an abdominal nodal or visceral lesion with sonographic or CT guidance may be the best or even the only means, other than open surgical biopsy, to establish the diagnosis.

Mycobacterial infections

Disseminated infections due to *Mycobacterium avium intracellulare* (MAI) and *Mycobacterium tuberculosis* (MTb) are among the most common causes of abnormal abdominal CT findings in patients with AIDS. Ubiquitous in soil and natural water supplies, MAI is rarely pathogenic in immunocompetent patients. However, disseminated MAI infection is common in AIDS patients, diagnosed in as many as 25–50% of cases during life or at autopsy [1]. Infection with MAI tends to occur in the late stage of AIDS, when immune deficiency is severe [2]. A successful treatment regimen has not yet been established.

The AIDS epidemic has caused a secondary epidemic of MTb infection. The outcome for patients infected with both HIV and MTb depends on which infection occurred first [3]. In the more common situation, reactivation of previously controlled primary MTb infection develops in a patient in whom cell-mediated immunity becomes impaired, owing to more recently acquired HIV infection. In these patients, response to standard antituberculosis treatment is good. In the less common situation, a patient with preexisting HIV infection is exposed to MTb and develops primary infection, the severity of which will depend on the degree of immune dysfunction. In contrast to disseminated MAI infection, disseminated MTb infection is often the initial AIDS-related illness in affected patients [4,5].

In patients with AIDS and disseminated mycobacterial infection, evaluation of abdominal CT findings may help to distinguish between MTb infection and MAI infection [5]. In the majority of patient with either infection, the liver and spleen are either normal in size or mildly enlarged. In the minority (<25%) of patients with mycobacterial infection and moderate or marked enlargement of the liver (cephalocaudal span ≥21 cm) or spleen (cephalocaudal span ≥16 cm), the diagnosis is much more likely to be MAI than MTb.

Small hypodense lesions may be seen in the liver, spleen, kidneys, and pancreas in patients with disseminated mycobacterial infection (Figure 18.1). However, these lesions are found three to four times more often in MTb infection than in MAI infection, occurring in about half of patients with MTb compared with only 10–15% of patients with MAI. Most of these lesions are 1 cm or less in diameter. They are most easily identified in the spleen.

Enlargement of abdominal lymph nodes (short-axis diameter ≥10 mm) is the rule in patients with disseminated mycobacterial infection. However, while some or all of these nodes have central or diffuse low density

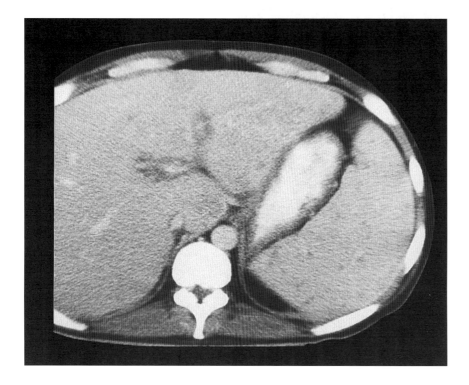

Figure 18.1. Mycobacterium tuberculosis infection. Enhanced CT scan shows multiple tiny hypodense lesions in the spleen and liver.

in at least 90% of patients with MTb infection, only 10–15% of patients with MAI infection have nodes with a low-density center [5,6]. In 85–90% of patients with disseminated MAI infection, all lymph nodes have homogeneous soft-tissue density. It has been suggested that the greater frequency of hypodense visceral lesions and of necrotic lymph nodes in patients with MTb than in patients with MAI may be due to differences in cell-mediated immunity [5]. Compared to patients with MTb infection, patients with MAI infection tend to be at a much later stage of AIDS and thus have a markedly diminished ability to mount an inflammatory response.

In summary, in patients with disseminated mycobacterial infection, the presence of hypodense visceral lesions and necrotic lymph nodes suggests MTb, whereas marked enlargement of the liver and spleen, and enlarged homogeneous soft-tissue-density lymph nodes suggest MAI.

Bacillary peliosis

Peliosis hepatis refers to the presence of multiple blood-filled cavities in the liver [7]. Originally found at autopsy in patients who died of chronic wasting, owing to metastatic disease or tuberculosis, peliosis

has been reported most commonly in the past several decades in patients treated with any of a wide variety of drugs. Most recently, peliosis has been seen in patients with HIV infection or other causes of immunodeficiency. In these immunocompromised patients, peliosis is due to infection by a newly described rickettsial organism, Rochalimaea henselae [8]. This Gram-negative bacillus, which can be shown by means of Warthin–Starry staining, can cause prolonged fever associated with bacteremia, bacillary angiomatosis (a cutaneous vascular lesion), and peliosis of the liver, spleen, and lymph nodes.

Abdominal CT findings in patients with bacillary peliosis include enlargement of the liver and spleen, hypodense hepatic and splenic nodules, and enlarged lymph nodes (Figure 18.2) [7,9]. The hypodense visceral lesions range in size from several millimeters to several centimeters. Hepatic peliotic lesions that communicate with sinusoids may become isodense with intravenous (IV) contrast enhancement.

Although these CT findings are non-specific and are more commonly due to mycobacterial or fungal infection, it is important to include bacillary peliosis in the differential diagnosis. If cutaneous bacillary angiomatosis is present, then appropriate antibiotic treatment, usually with erythromycin or doxycycline, and clinical and radiologic follow-up to confirm

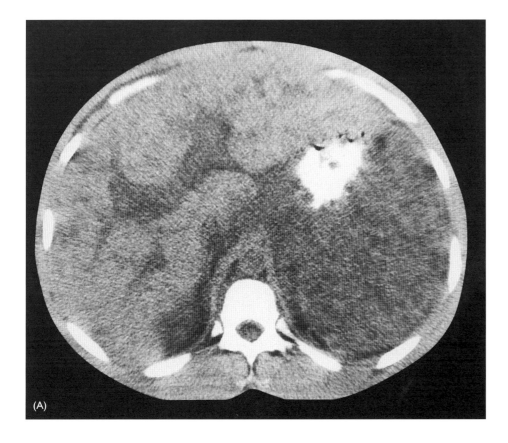

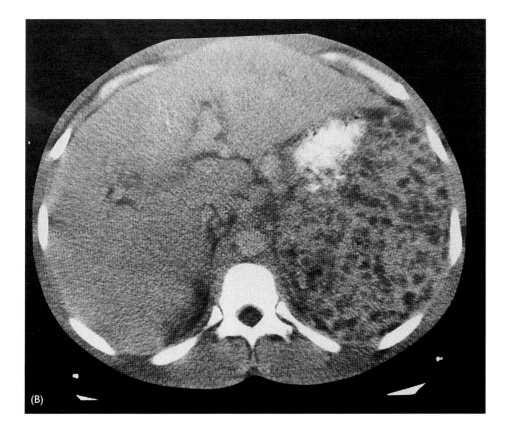

Figure 18.2. Bacillary peliosis. (A) Unenhanced CT scan shows multiple small hypodense lesions in the liver and spleen. (B) After IV contrast enhancement, most hepatic lesions are isodense.

response to therapy, may be sufficient. However, in the absence of cutaneous lesions, the diagnosis of bacillary peliosis may require open biopsy because the organism may be difficult to culture from blood or percutaneous biopsy specimens.

Pneumocystis carinii

Awareness of the AIDS epidemic began about 1980 when two rare diseases, *Pneumocystis carinii* pneumonia and Kaposi's sarcoma, were seen with startling frequency in homosexual men in New York and California, USA. However, reports of radiologic findings of abdominal involvement by *Pneumocystis carinii* infection did not appear until 1990 [10,11]. The reason for the delay in recognition of extrapulmonary dissemination is not known. Possible factors include the increasing number of patients with AIDS, the improved survival of patients, modification of the immune dysfunction by treatment with drugs, such as azidodeoxythymidine (AZT), and the use of aerosolized pentamidine, which may eradicate *Pneumocystis carinii* in the lungs but fail to affect the organism at extrapulmonary sites, owing to inadequate systemic absorption. It is important to note that patients with

extrapulmonary *Pneumocystis* infection may have no clinical or radiologic evidence of previous or concurrent *Pneumocystis carinii* pneumonia nor a history of any medical therapy.

Abdominal CT findings in patients with disseminated *Pneumocystis* infection include visceral and nodal calcifications and, less often, focal hypodense visceral lesions [10,11]. Calcifications are seen most commonly in the spleen, liver, and kidneys, but may also occur in lymph nodes, adrenal glands, peritoneum, and bowel wall (Figure 18.3). When the liver, spleen, and lymph nodes are involved, they may be either normal in size or enlarged. The calcifications are usually multiple and may be fine, punctate, coarse, irregular, or rim like. Involvement of a viscus or lymph node can be focal, multifocal, confluent, or diffuse. Occasionally, hepatic and splenic calcifications seen clearly on unenhanced CT examination may be undetectable after IV contrast administration. In addition, sonographic evidence of hepatic and splenic infection by *Pneumocystis* (multiple tiny echogenic foci without shadowing) may precede the appearance of abnormal CT findings by weeks or months.

Multiple focal hypodense visceral lesions are seen most commonly in the spleen (Figure 18.4). These lesions range in size from several millimeters to 8 cm

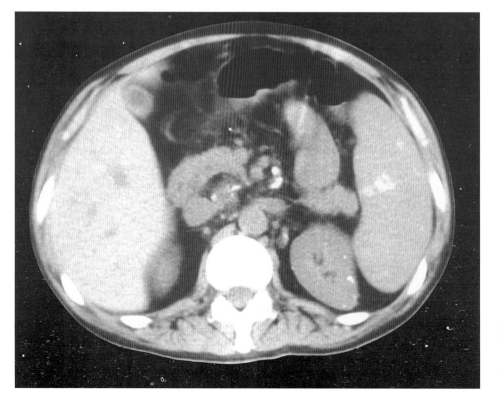

Figure 18.3.   *Pneumocystis carinii* infection. Unenhanced CT scan shows calcifications in the spleen, left kidney, and lymph nodes. Hepatic calcifications are subtle.

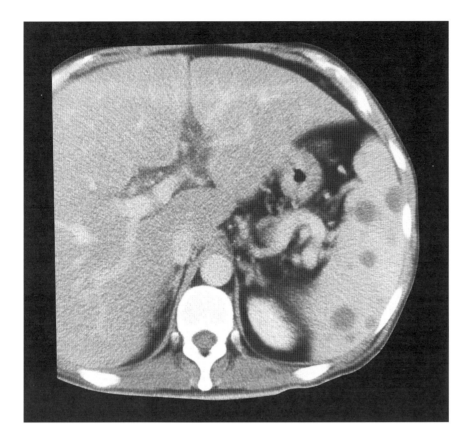

Figure 18.4. Pneumocystis carinii infection. Enhanced CT scan shows multiple hypodense lesions in the spleen.

or more. They may be the only CT evidence of *Pneumocystis* infection or they may be associated with calcifications in the spleen and other viscera. Follow-up CT examination may show a decrease in size or resolution of the focal hypodense lesions and development or progression of calcifications [11].

Although abdominal visceral and nodal calcifications in a patient with AIDS are usually the result of *Pneumocystis* infection, these findings are not specific. Visceral calcifications have also been reported due to disseminated infections by MAI and cytomegalovirus [12].

Fungal infections

Foremost among fungal infections that are normally contained by cell-mediated immunity are disseminated histoplasmosis, coccidioidomycosis, and cryptococcosis, and mucocutaneous candidiasis. Thus, it is not surprising that one of these mycoses is the first opportunistic infection in a significant proportion of patients with T-cell dysfunction owing to HIV infection [13]. However, disseminated candidiasis is uncommon, particularly early in the course of AIDS,

because it is usually associated with profound neutropenia or neutrophil dysfunction rather than with T-cell dysfunction.

Although most cases of disseminated histoplasmosis in patients with AIDS are thought to be due to endogenous reactivation rather than primary infection [13], radiologic evidence of previous infection (i.e. calcified granulomas in lungs, lymph nodes, liver, and spleen) is usually absent [14]. In a series of 18 patients with AIDS and disseminated histoplasmosis seen at our hospital [14, and unpublished data], hepatomegaly was seen in two-thirds of cases but was moderate or marked (cephalocaudal span >21 cm) in only 17%. Splenomegaly was seen in one-half of the patients, and was almost always marked or massive (cephalocaudal span of 16–26 cm). An uncommon but striking CT finding is diffuse low density of the spleen, which is not due to infarction (Figure 18.5). Multiple small hypodense lesions were seen in the liver and spleen in only one of 18 patients. Abdominal lymph node enlargement occurs in about 75% of cases. In half of the patients with enlarged nodes, all of the nodes have homogeneous soft-tissue density. In the other half, some or all of the nodes have central or diffuse low density.

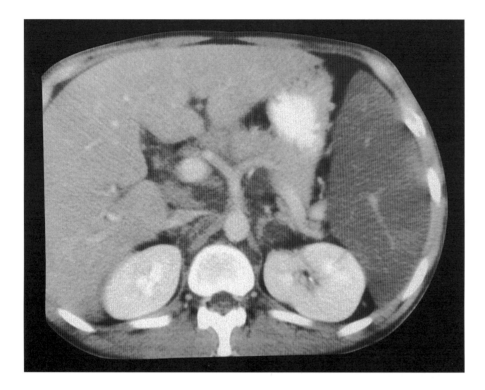

Figure 18.5. Histoplasmosis. Enhanced CT scan shows enlarged celiac lymph nodes and spleen with diffuse low density. Enhancing vessels are seen in the spleen.

The occurrence of disseminated coccidioidomycosis in patients with AIDS is usually due to reactivation of quiescent infection acquired during residence or travel in an endemic region, such as the southwestern USA or Latin America [15]. In our experience, abdominal CT findings in these patients include mild enlargement of the liver and spleen, small hypodense splenic lesions, and lymph node enlargement. Enlarged lymph nodes may have homogeneous soft-tissue density or central low density.

Although most patients with AIDS and cryptococcosis present with symptoms and signs owing to involvement of the central nervous system or lungs, widespread dissemination may also occur on occasion [13]. In the experience of others [16] and ourselves, abdominal CT findings include mild hepatomegaly, marked splenomegaly, and enlargement of lymph nodes.

In patients with AIDS, oral candidiasis is almost universal, and esophageal and vaginal involvement are common. However, disseminated infection is unusual [13]. In our experience, abdominal CT findings in patients with AIDS and systemic candidiasis are similar to those reported in patients with candidiasis related to immunosuppression by chemotherapy [17] and include small hypodense lesions in the liver, spleen, and kidneys without lymph node enlargement.

AIDS-related cholangiopathy

AIDS-related cholangiopathy may be manifested by one or more of the following: papillary stenosis, cholangitis, and cholecystitis [18]. The etiology of the biliary tract disease is uncertain. In many patients, an opportunistic infection, usually due to *Cryptosporidium* or cytomegalovirus, is implicated. In some cases, however, no pathogen is identified. Although sonography and cholangiography are probably more sensitive and specific studies in patients with AIDS-related cholangiopathy, the diagnosis can often be suggested on the basis of CT findings. These findings include common duct wall thickening (Figure 18.6), gallbladder wall thickening, and biliary dilatation, which may be asymmetric in distribution [19,20].

Kaposi's sarcoma

In the USA, the onset of the AIDS epidemic was heralded by Kaposi's sarcoma and *Pneumocystis carinii* pneumonia. Radiologic features of pulmonary and gastrointestinal involvement by Kaposi's sarcoma have been well documented. However, even though disseminated disease is common at autopsy, reports of radio-

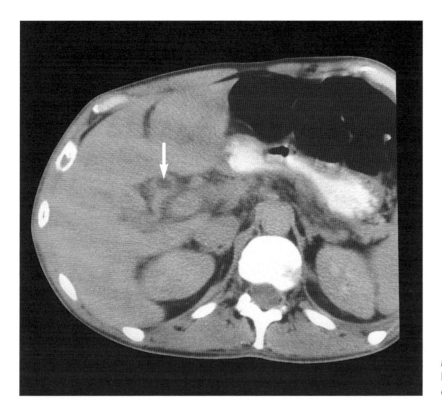

Figure 18.6. AIDS-related cholangiopathy. Enhanced CT scan shows wall thickening of the common bile duct (arrow).

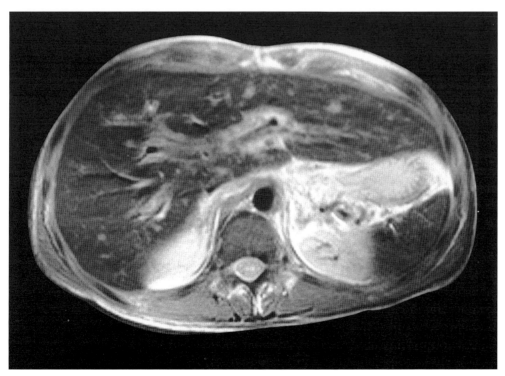

Figure 18.7. Kaposi's sarcoma. Transverse magnetic resonance image (TR 2500/TE 40) shows hyperintense periportal tissue and several small hyperintense hepatic parenchymal nodules.

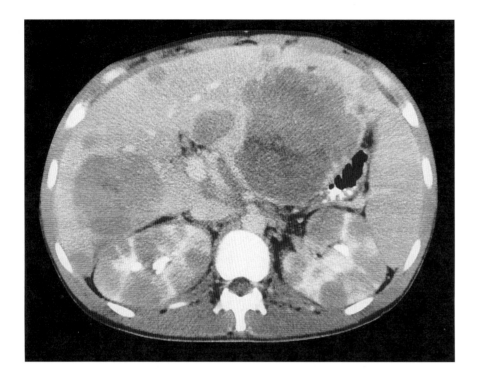

Figure 18.8. AIDS-related non-Hodgkin lymphoma. Enhanced CT scan shows multiple hypodense lesions in the liver and kidneys.

logic evidence of solid abdominal visceral involvement are few. This may be due to the greater tendency of the lesion to spread along blood vessels than to distort the architecture of the organ involved [21]. CT findings of hepatic Kaposi's sarcoma include periportal bands and small parenchymal nodules that are hypodense on unenhanced and dynamic CT, and isodense or hyperdense on delayed scans [22,23]. In our experience, sonography and magnetic resonance imaging (MRI) are more sensitive than CT for the detection of hepatic Kaposi's sarcoma. The periportal bands of tissue and the small parenchymal nodules appear hyperechoic on sonography and hyperintense on proton-density and T_2-weighted MRI (Figure 18.7). In one reported case [23], sonography showed small hyperechoic nodules in a huge spleen, but CT showed no focal splenic lesion.

AIDS-related non-Hodgkin lymphoma

After Kaposi's sarcoma, non-Hodgkin lymphoma is the most common malignancy in patients with AIDS. In a series of 112 patients with HIV infection and high-grade or intermediate-grade B-cell lymphoma, abdominal CT examination showed evidence of focal lymphomatous involvement in 64% of the patients at presentation [24]. In the 72 patients with abnormal CT findings, lymph node enlargement, usually with homogeneous soft-tissue density, was seen in 56% and extranodal disease was seen in 86%. The most common sites of extranodal involvement were the gastrointestinal tract (54%), liver (29%), kidney (11%), and adrenal gland (11%). Focal lesions were seen in the spleen and pancreas in 7% and 5% of patients, respectively. However, in an earlier series of 19 patients with AIDS-related lymphoma, focal splenic lesions were seen in 26% of patients [25].

In patients with AIDS-related lymphoma, hepatic involvement is manifested by hypodense lesions that vary from solitary to innumerable and range from less than 1 cm to greater than 15 cm in diameter (Figure 18.8) [24]. Although smaller lesions tend to be homogeneous, masses greater than 4 cm in diameter are often heterogeneous. A thin enhancing rim may be seen in one-third of patients with hepatic lesions. In patients with splenic involvement, CT may show single or multiple hypodense lesions from less than 1 cm to 6 cm in diameter. Evidence of pancreatic involvement includes single or multiple hypodense lesions and diffuse infiltration of the gland [24].

In most patients with CT evidence of abdominal involvement by AIDS-related lymphoma, the liver and

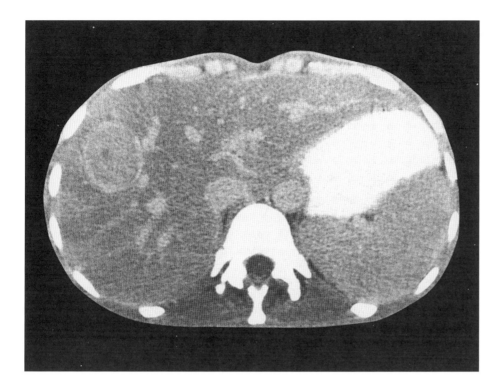

Figure 18.9. Smooth muscle tumor. Enhanced CT scan shows solitary mass with thin enhancing rim in the right lobe of the liver. (Courtesy: Ronald H. Wachsberg, M.D., Newark, NJ, USA.)

spleen are normal in size or only mildly enlarged [24]. In the minority of patients with moderate or marked enlargement of the liver (cephalocaudal span >20 cm) or spleen (cephalocaudal span >15 cm), focal hypodense lesions are usually seen in the liver.

Smooth muscle tumors

Since 1990, smooth muscle tumors have been reported in several children and at least three adults with HIV infection [26–28]. In addition to the fact that smooth muscle tumors are rare in childhood, these cases have been remarkable for the location and/or multiplicity of the tumors. Sites of involvement have included the lungs, gastrointestinal tract, liver, spleen and adrenal gland. Both benign and malignant tumors have been reported. The multiplicity of benign or low-grade malignant tumors in some cases suggests a multicentric origin. In patients with HIV infection and hepatic or splenic involvement by smooth muscle tumors, CT examination has shown single or multiple round, well-circumscribed masses ranging from 1 cm to 6 cm in diameter (Figure 18.9). Central necrosis and a thin enhancing rim may or may not be seen [27, and unpublished data]. The clinical significance of smooth muscle tumors in patients with AIDS has not yet been determined.

Table 18.1.   CT abnormalities of liver, spleen, and pancreas in AIDS-related infections and tumors

Infection/tumor	CT abnormality	Differential diagnosis
Mycobacterium tuberculosis (MTb)	Hypodense nodules <2 cm (liver spleen, pancreas)	MAI, bacillary peliosis, Pneumocystis, fungus, Kaposi's sarcoma, lymphoma
Mycobacterium avium-intracellulare (MAI)	Hypodense nodules <2 cm (liver, spleen)	MTb, bacillary peliosis, Pneumocystis, fungus, Kaposi's sarcoma, lymphoma
	Hepatosplenomegaly	Fungus, Kaposi's sarcoma
Bacillary peliosis	Hypodense nodules <2 cm (liver, spleen) Hypodense masses ≥2 cm (liver, spleen)	MTb, MAI, Pneumocystis, fungus Kaposi's sarcoma, lymphoma Pneumocystis, lymphoma, smooth muscle tumor
Pneumocystis	Calcifications (liver, spleen) Hypodense nodules <2 cm (spleen) Hypodense masses ≥2 cm (spleen)	MAI, cytomegalovirus MTb, MAI, bacillary peliosis, fungus, Kaposi's sarcoma, lymphoma Bacillary peliosis, lymphoma, smooth muscle tumor
Fungus: Histoplasma, Coccidioides, Cryptococcus, Candida	Hypodense nodules <2 cm (liver, spleen) Hepatosplenomegaly	MTb, MAI, bacillary peliosis, Pneumocystis, Kaposi's sarcoma, lymphoma MAI, Kaposi's sarcoma
Kaposi's sarcoma	Hypodense periportal bands (liver) Hypodense nodules <2 cm (liver, spleen) Hepatosplenomegaly	— MTb, MAI, bacillary peliosis, Pneumocystis, fungus, lymphoma MAI, fungus
AIDS-related lymphoma	Hypodense nodules <2 cm (liver spleen, pancreas) Hypodense masses ≥ 2 cm (liver, spleen)	MTb, MAI, bacillary peliosis, Pneumocystis, fungus, Kaposi's sarcoma Bacillary peliosis, Pneumocystis, smooth muscle tumor
Smooth muscle tumor	Hypodense mass(es) ≥2 cm (liver, spleen)	Bacillary peliosis, Pneumocystis, lymphoma

References

1   Aronchick JM, Miller WT Jr. Disseminated nontuberculous mycobacterial infections in immunosuppressed patients. *Semin Roentgenol* 1993; **28**: 150–157.

2   Kotloff RM. Infection caused by nontuberculous mycobacteria: clinical aspects. *Semin Roentgenol* 1993; **28**: 131–138.

3   MacGregor RR. Tuberculosis: from history to current management. *Semin Roentgenol* 1993; **28**: 101–108.

4   Modilevsky T, Sattler FR, Barnes PF. Mycobacterial disease in patients with human immunodeficiency virus infection. *Arch Intern Med* 1989; **149**: 2201–2205.

5   Radin DR. Intraabdominal *Mycobacterium tuberculosis* vs *Mycobacterium avium-intracellulare* infections in patients with AIDS: distinction based on CT findings. *AJR* 1991; **156**: 487–491.

6   Nyberg DA, Federle MP, Jeffrey RB, Bottles K, Wofsy CB. Abdominal CT findings of disseminated *Mycobacterium avium-intracellulare* in AIDS. *AJR* 1985; **145**: 297–299.

7   Radin DR, Kanel GC. Peliosis hepatis in a patient with human immunodeficiency virus infection. *AJR* 1991; **156**: 91–92.

8   Slater LN, Welch DF, Min KW. Rochalimaea henselae causes bacillary angiomatosis and peliosis hepatis. *Arch Intern Med* 1992; **152**: 602–606.

9   Goodman P, Balachandran S. Bacillary angiomatosis in a patient with HIV infection [letter]. *AJR* 1993; **160**: 207–208.

10 Radin DR, Baker EL, Klatt EC et al. Visceral and nodal calcification in patients with AIDS-related *Pneumocystis carinii* infection. *AJR* 1990; **154**: 27–31.

11 Lubat E, Megibow AJ, Balthazar EJ, Goldenberg AS, Birnbaum BA, Bosniak MA. Extrapulmonary P*neumocystis carinii* infection in AIDS: CT findings. *Radiology* 1990; **174**: 157–160.

12 Towers MJ, Withers CE, Hamilton PA, Kolin A, Walmsley S. Visceral calcification in patients with AIDS may not always be due to *Pneumocystis carinii*. *AJR* 1991; **156**: 745–747.

13 Diamond RD. The growing problem of mycoses in patients infected with the human immunodeficiency virus. *Rev Infect Dis* 1991; **13**: 480–486.

14 Radin DR. Disseminated histoplasmosis: abdominal CT findings in 16 patients. *AJR* 1991; **157**: 955–958.

15 Minamoto G, Armstrong D. Fungal infections in AIDS: histoplasmosis and coccidioidomycosis. *Infect Dis Clin North Am* 1988; **2**: 447-456.

16 Scalfano FP Jr, Prichard JG, Lamki N, Athey P, Graves RC. Abdominal cryptococcoma in AIDS: a case report. *J Comput Tomogr* 1988; **12**: 237–239.

17 Shirkhoda A. CT findings in hepatosplenic and renal candidiasis. *J Comput Assist Tomogr* 1987; **11**: 795–798.

18 Cello JP. Acquired immunodeficiency syndrome cholangiopathy: spectrum of disease. *Am J Med* 1989; **86**: 539–546.

19 Dolmatch BL, Laing FC, Federle MP, Jeffrey RB, Cello J. AIDS-related cholangitis: radiographic findings in nine patients. *Radiology* 1987; **163**: 313–316.

20 Radin DR, Cohen H, Halls JM. Acalculous inflammatory disease of the biliary tree in acquired immunodeficiency syndrome: CT demonstration. *J Comput Assist Tomogr* 1987; **11**: 775–778.

21 Niedt GW, Schinella RA. Acquired immunodeficiency syndrome: clinicopathologic study of 56 autopsies. *Arch Pathol Lab Med* 1985; **109**: 727–734.

22 Luburich P, Bru C, Ayuso MC, Azón A, Condom E. Hepatic Kaposi sarcoma in AIDS: US and CT findings. *Radiology* 1990; **175**: 172–174.

23 Valls C, Cañas C, Turell LG, Pruna X. Hepatosplenic AIDS-related Kaposi's sarcoma. *Gastrointest Radiol* 1991; **16**: 342–344.

24 Radin DR, Esplin JA, Levine AM, Ralls PW. AIDS-related non-Hodgkin's lymphoma: abdominal CT findings in 112 patients. *AJR* 1993; **160**: 1133–1139.

25 Nyberg DA, Jeffrey RB Jr, Federle MP, Bottles K, Abrams DI. AIDS-related lymphomas: evaluation by abdominal CT. *Radiology* 1986; **159**: 59–63.

26 Radin DR, Kiyabu M. Multiple smooth-muscle tumors of the colon and adrenal gland in an adult with AIDS. *AJR* 1992; **159**: 545–546.

27 Wachsberg RH, Cho KC, Adekosan A. Two leiomyomas of the liver in an adult with AIDS: CT and MR appearance. *J Comput Assist Tomogr* 1994; **18**: 156–157.

28 Dahan H, Bèges C, Weiss L et al. Leiomyoma of the adrenal gland in a patient with AIDS. *Abdom Imaging* 1994; **19**: 259–261.

19 IMAGING OF THE RETROPERITONEUM

Robert L. Lavayssière
Muriel Eliaszewicz
Anne-Elizabeth Cabée
Pierre M. Trotot

Introduction

In the early stages of human immune deficiency virus (HIV) infection, retroperitoneal involvement is not frequent and is usually asymptomatic. Benign lymphadenopathy associated with numerous lymph nodes, normal or slightly enlarged, can be found during routine abdominal exploration with computed tomography (CT) or ultrasound (US) examinations.

At the time of clinical presentation, patients with acquired immune deficiency syndrome (AIDS)-related diseases of the retroperitoneum have frequently advanced disease involving multiple involvements (e.g. nodes, digestive tract, liver, spleen, chest, or brain), but some diseases may be clinically silent and discovered only at autopsy [1–3].

Imaging procedures are requested because many of these patients present with abdominal symptoms, upper abdominal pain, or evidence of hepatobiliary dysfunction, palpable mass or general symptoms, weight loss or fever. All modern imaging methods are highly sensitive but are not specific in most cases. Their results must be interpreted in the light of clinical and biological information as well as the results of other procedures. Good clinical practice includes close cooperation between clinicians and radiologists. Imaging procedures should be used to suggest diagnoses, assist with the diagnostic work-up, and monitor the effectiveness of treatment. In some cases, fine-needle aspiration biopsy (FNAB) can be performed under imaging guidance with US or CT.

Definition of the retroperitoneum

The retroperitoneum lies behind the abdominal peritoneum and contains the kidneys, the ureters, the adrenal glands, the distal duodenum, the ascending and descending colon, the pancreas, the great vessels (aorta and inferior vena cava), and the lymph nodes, all elements being surrounded by fat. It communicates with the thorax through the inframediastinal space and below with the pelvis. The kidneys and pancreas are discussed in detail in Chapters 17, 18 and 20.

Retroperitoneal imaging, benefits, and limitations

Plain film study of the abdomen is used routinely to investigate the osseous component, and the bowels (air/fluid/repartition), and to look for calcification(s) and ascites.

Lymphangiography is not used routinely. At the beginning of the AIDS epidemic, we performed lymphangiography on a few cases of AIDS-related lymphoma without finding any particularly helpful features [4].

Ultrasound

Real-time ultrasonography can be performed quite easily under any circumstances, even at the bedside,

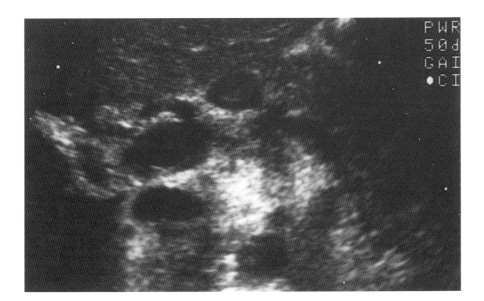

Figure 19.1. A 28-year-old man (T4 <50) with general progressive deterioration and fever. US: multiple hypoechoic nodes. Autopsy: *Mycobacterium avium intracellulare.*

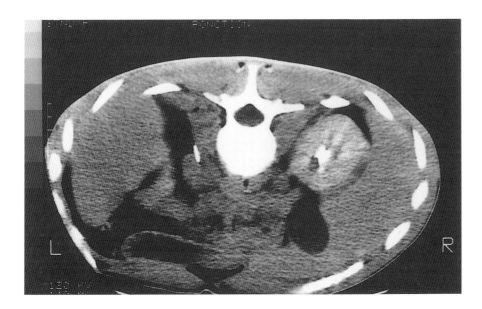

Figure 19.2. A CT-guided FNAB of a retroperitoneal lymph node: *Mycobacterium tuberculosis* with the patient in prone position.

to explore the retroperitoneum as well as the adjacent organs. A general survey of the abdomen and the pelvis should be done using 3.5 or 5 MHz transducers.

Because small reactive lymphadenopathy is common in HIV-positive patients, only adenopathy greater than 1.5 cm at its largest dimension should be reported as pathological. Hepatosplenomegaly is also quite frequent in HIV-positive patients and careful attention must be paid to the liver, the biliary system, the spleen, and the kidneys.

Despite its high sensitivity, US is lacking in specificity and additional procedures may be needed. Ultrasound needs an experienced sonographer and may

be difficult to perform in some cases, such as unco-operative patients, ileus, and deep lesions, especially in the retroperitoneum.

Computed tomography

CT comes second to US in exploring the retroperitoneum as it is more expensive and needs contrast injection in most cases as well as digestive opacification. A CT scanner is a powerful tool if properly used to survey the abdomen as a whole, including the retroperitoneum.

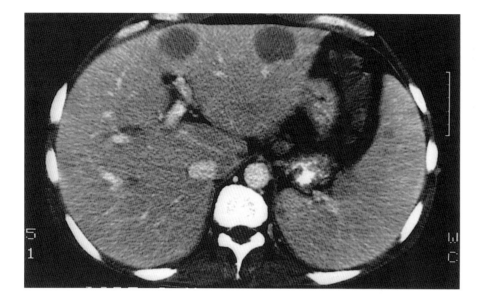

Figure 19.3 A 48-year-old man (T4 <50) with poor general condition and diffuse abdominal pain. He was previously treated for MAI and *Rhodococcus equi* lung infections. BDCT showed NHL (B L), stage IV with hepatic, splenic, renal and retroperitoneal nodes involvement.

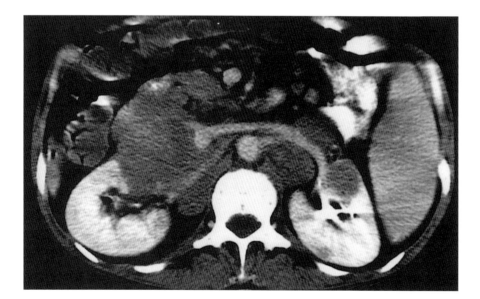

Figure 19.4 A 48-year-old male (T4 <50) with poor general condition and diffuse abdominal pain. He was previously treated for MAI and *Rhodococcus equi* lung infections. BDCT showed NHL (B L), stage IV with hepatic, renal, splenic, and retroperitoneal nodes involvement.

It can be helpful to perform studies both with and without contrast injection. The first step, without injection, is useful because some lesions may be obscured by contrast opacification, especially in the liver and the spleen. The best way to explore the liver after contrast injection is the bolus dynamic CT (BDCT) using a fast CT, conventional or helicoidal CT, and an injector [5]. There is no significant difference between ionic and non-ionic contrast agents regarding the degree of enhancement. Non-ionic contrast agents are better tolerated but they are far more expensive.

With up-to-date CT scanners, a complete survey of the retroperitoneum can be performed within minutes with good contrast resolution, especially between the retroperitoneal great vessels and the lymph nodes.

CT scanning also has its drawbacks. Use of contrast media must be limited in patients with renal insufficiency, lack of retroperitoneal fat can make difficult the detection and differentiation of the nodes from vessels and/or the bowels. In some patients with diarrhea, opacification of the bowels may be inefficient. CT has several advantages, including being less

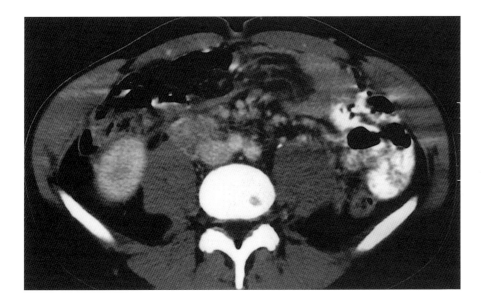

Figure 19.5. 32-year-old man (T4: 200) with cutaneous Kaposi's sarcoma. BDCT: retroperitoneal nodes. FNAB: KS.

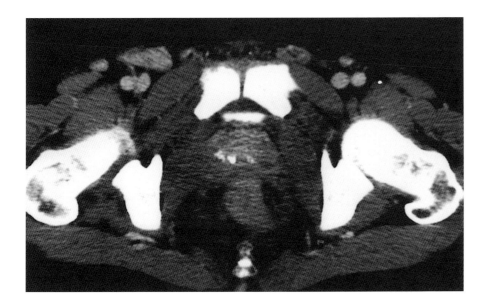

Figure 19.6. A 32-year-old man (T4: 200) with cutaneous Kaposi's sarcoma. BDCT: inguino-femoral nodes.

operator-dependent and more easily reproducible than ultrasound, allowing follow-up studies and comparisons under treatment.

Magnetic resonance imaging

Magnetic resonance imaging (MRI) is probably not a routine method to explore the abdomen and the retroperitoneum in AIDS patients. Imaging of the abdomen accounts for 1 or 2% of the total imaging

procedures using MRI in most centers despite its advantages: no ionizing radiation, high contrast and multiparametric images, and multiplanar imaging.

MRI is theoretically useful to explore the retroperitoneum using a frontal/coronal T_1-weighted sequence, and T_1- and T_2-weighted sequences in the axial plane. T_1-weighted contrast sequences are useful in some cases to study the limits of a mass and patterns of enhancement. Fast T_2 sequences, turbo or fast–spin echo (TSE or FSE), can be used routinely with no major difference in results when compared to conven-

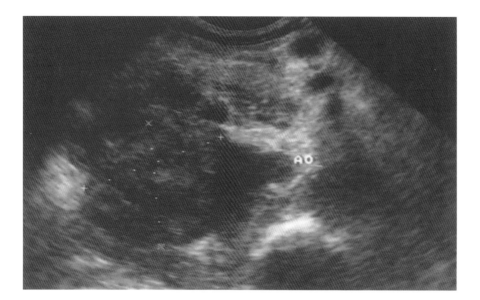

Figure 19.7 A 35-year-old woman intravenous drug abuser, showing multiples nodes. US: paraortic mass. FNAB: NHL (B lymphoma).

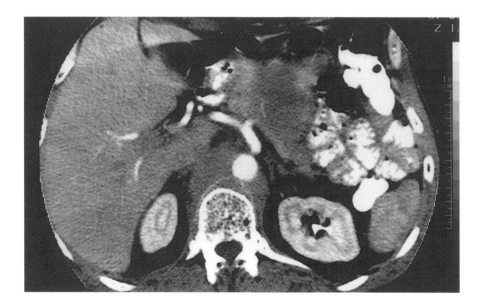

Figure 19.8. A 68-year-old man (T4: 150) with right hip pain, epigastric mass and abdomen swelling. BDCT showed NHL (B L), stage IV with mesenteric and retroperitoneal infiltration.

tional spin echo (SE) sequences, especially in patients who are very ill. Breath-hold imaging often gives poor images and echo-planar imaging is still under development.

MRI is mostly sensitive to slight modifications of tissue composition and, therefore, is highly sensitive to disease. However, motion (breathing, peristalsis) and susceptibility artefacts can degrade the quality. Beside its high cost, the major drawback is the length of examination (between 20 and 45 minutes), which requires good patient cooperation [6].

Nuclear medicine

Radionuclide imaging, if applied with an organ system approach, is useful in the diagnosis of AIDS [7]. Specific pathologic processes can be suspected on the basis of uptake patterns. For example, patterns of spleen uptake of technetium-99 and gallium-67 allow differentiation between neoplasm, Kaposi's sarcoma (KS), and infection by mycobacteria (MB). Gallium-67 [8] may be a practical diagnosis tool in HIV-infected patients with lymphadenopathy as grade 0 or 1 uptake

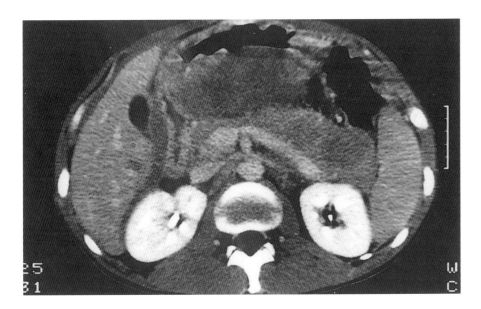

Figure 19.9. A 31-year-old man (T4 <500) with an epigastric mass with diffuse swelling of the abdomen. NHL (B L), stage IV with gastric, mesenteric, and retroperitoneal involvement. Ascites.

suggests the presence of hyperplasia instead of KS, lymphoma, MB, or Castleman disease in which uptake is 2 or 3 (≥the liver).

Imaging of AIDS-related diseases of the retroperitoneum

It has already been stated that retroperitoneal involvement in AIDS is, in most cases, part of a more general involvement implying a general survey of the body. US should be used first as it is highly sensitive to parenchymal modification. However, CT is to be preferred for exploring the retroperitoneum itself and looking for lymph nodes, paraspinous or spinous masses, or adrenal involvement which is rarely documented, although it is frequently found at autopsy. The initial imaging modality is clearly dependent upon the clinical presentation.

FNAB can be performed under CT or US guidance, but false-negative results can occur [9] and cytologic diagnosis of hyperplasia should lead to open surgical biopsy, if there is clinical suspicion of lymphoma or MB. Cytology of lymphomas is quite difficult even in the hands of an experienced pathologist and histological staging of Hodgkin's disease may require surgical biopsies. FNAB can be used as a differential diagnosis tool in questionable cases involving infectious diseases.

Comparison of US and CT: the imaging couple

Smith and Mathieson [10] attempted to establish the population incidence of abnormalities using abdominal US in AIDS patients, to study changes over time in both the prevalence of abdominal abnormalities and the usage of US, and to correlate clinical indications with the abnormalities found. From 1983 to 1991, 899 AIDS patients were seen in their hospital, representing 89.4% of the 1006 AIDS patients in the Province of British Columbia during that time. Of these, 414 (46%) underwent 684 abdominal US studies, 96% of which were available for review. US scans were abnormal in 264 patients (66%), showing splenomegaly (124; 31%), lymphadenopathy (83; 21%), gallbladder and bile duct abnormalities (80; 20%), hepatomegaly (77; 19%), and ascites (54; 14%). Clinical indications with the highest frequency of abnormal findings were hepatosplenomegaly (85%) and abnormal liver function test results (70%). Gallbladder wall thickening was usually incidental, with only 3 out of 30 (10%) cases representing cholecystitis. Lymph nodes >3 cm (10 out of 83 patients with enlarged nodes) always represented an abnormality other than reactive hyperplasia. The percentage of abnormal studies grew from 25% to 80%. They concluded that US is useful and is increasingly used in AIDS patients, and the prevalence of abdominal abnormalities in AIDS patients has increased since 1983.

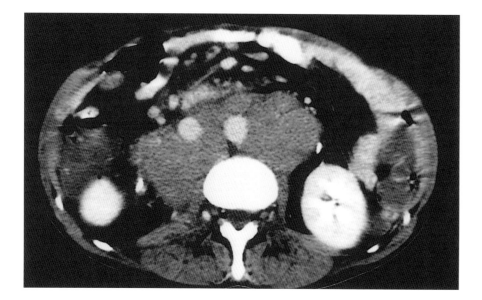

Figure 19.10. A 31-year-old man (T4 <500) with an epigastric mass with diffuse swelling of the abdomen. NHL (B L), stage IV with gastric, mesenteric, and retroperitoneal involvement. Ascites.

According to Townsend [11], in a series of 38 patients with abdominal AIDS-related lymphoma, abnormal masses were detected in 33 patients (87%). In 20 patients, no significant differences between US and CT findings were identified, but in 14 cases CT was considered to be superior to US. In three of these cases, the US examination was normal but CT depicted lymphomatous masses: one case of retroperitoneal adenopathy, one case of psoas mass and retroperitoneal adenopathy and one of paraspinous/epidural mass. In six other cases, CT showed lesions additional to those identified at the US, mainly extraretroperitoneal lesions (liver, bowel, omentum, bone). Of course, additional information offered by CT may not affect prognosis or treatment. US resolved abnormalities in two cases better than CT by identifying liver lesions not seen on CT. In two cases, neither CT nor US depicted lesions (bile duct, anus). Twenty-one patients underwent US-guided fine needle biopsy (22 G) with immediate success in 17 patients. Farizo et al. [12] found significant infection complications in only 7% of patients with a CD4 count >200 but, when the CD4 count was less than 200, over 16% developed serious infections in a 1 year period.

AIDS-related infections

These infections are often associated, and the frequency of one or more other major infectious diseases (pneumonia, bacterial sepsis, pulmonary tuberculosis) ranged from 6% to 16% in function of the CD4+ lymphocyte count [12]. This means that the frequency of multiple infections (associated) increases as long as the CD4/lymphocyte count decreases. The nodal features in retroperitoneal AIDS-related disease are summarized in Table 1.1.

Bacteria

Mycobacterium in nodes and adrenals

The distinction between *Mycobacterium tuberculosis* (MTb) and *Mycobacterium avium-intracellulare* (MAI) can be achieved with CT scanning as reported by Radin [13] in a series of 71 patients. The presence of focal visceral lesions and low-attenuation lymph nodes suggest MTb, and marked hepatic and splenic enlargement with enlarged soft density nodes (density > muscle) suggest MAI (see Table 19.2). Distinction is important because of the therapeutic implications and thus prognosis, because antimycobacterial therapy is far more effective in MTb. Definitive diagnosis requires positive culture, taking at least two weeks, with fine-needle percutaneous aspiration (FNPA) products.

The differences between MAI and MTb in the course of AIDS has been stressed by several authors [13–15]. MAI is more frequently encountered with other AIDS-defining illnesses (82%), such as KS or *Pneumocystis* infection, than MTb, which is the AIDS-defining illness in 85% of the cases [13], probably

Table 19.1. Nodal features in retroperitoneal AIDS-related diseases.

	Particular features	CT/US
AIDS-related infections		
Bacterial		
MTB	Extranodal disease liver +, spleen ++, lung) Treatable disease Often first AIDS-defining illness 300 < CD 4 < 400	CT: Central or diffuse low density US: Mostly hypoechogenic nodes
MAI	Extranodal disease (liver +, spleen +, diffuse bowel thickening) Often associated with other AIDS illnesses CD 4 < 100	CT: Homogeneous soft-density more common than low density (diffuse or central)
Viral	CMV *Varicella zoster* virus	Not described
Protozoan		
P. carinii	Extranodal disease: lung +++ Often associated with other opportunistic infections and pentamidine aerosol therapy + AZT Calcifications in other viscera (spleen, liver, kidney, adrenals)	CT: Hypodense nodes containing calcifications
Fungal		
Histoplasmosis	Previous exposure (calcium deposits) Multifocal, extranodal disease	CT: Homogeneous soft density More common than low density (lungs, liver, bone marrow) (diffuse or central)
Cryptococcosis	Often associated with meningitis	Adrenal enlargement
Malignancies		
NHL and HD	Extranodal disease (liver +, spleen +, digestive tract) Bone marrow involvement (MRI)	CT: Homogeneous soft density More common than low density US: Mostly hypoechogenic nodes Highly suspicious if diameter >1.5 cm
KS	Two main forms: Generalized form, 'epidemic', with extranodal involvement Classic form: skin and mucosa	Hyperattenuating nodes on BDCT retroperitoneum +++) Extranodal sites

reflecting a different immunity status (MT 300 <CD4 <400, MAI CD4 <100).

Virtually any other bacteria can be found in abscesses, particularly in the lumbar paraspinal location [16], where MRI is extremely useful. A few cases of bacterial myositis, due to *Staphyloccocus aureus* or *pyogenes* as well as MTb, have been reported but they did not involve retroperitoneal muscles [17].

Viruses

Cytomegalovirus

In a series of 100 autopsies performed on AIDS patients [1], inflammatory enlargement of the adrenal glands was found in 61 cases, associated in 44 cases with cytomegalovirus (CMV)-related inclusion bodies. The infection was diagnosed in 34 out of 44 cases. However,

Table 19.2. Findings in mycobacterial infections in patients with AIDS (adapted from [13]) (percentages are shown in parentheses, multiple involvement possible).

CT findings	MTb patients (n = 27)	MAI patients (n =44)
Nodal disease		
Solid nodes only	2 (7)	38 (86)
Largest ≥ 10 mm	1 (4)	24 (55)
Largest < 10 mm	1 (4)	14 (32)
Necrotic nodes	25 (93)	6 (14)
with solid nodes ≥ 10 mm	17 (63)	5 (11)
Extranodal disease		
Hepatomegaly	5 (19)	20 (45)
Mild (19–20 cm)	5 (19)	11 (25)
Marked (21–24 cm)	0	9 (20)
Splenomegaly	7 (26)	10 (23)
Mild (14–15 cm)	7 (26)	4 (9)
Marked (16–21 cm)	0 (0)	6 (14)
Focal lesions in solid viscera	12 (44)	6 (14)
Liver	3 (11)	4 (9)
Spleen	8 (30)	3 (7)
Kidney	5 (19)	1 (2)
Adrenal abnormality	0 (0)	0
Gastrointestinal tract abnormalities	4 (15) (local)	8 (18) (diffuse)
Ascites	5 (19)	5 (11)

Note. MTB: *Mycobacterium tuberculosis*; MAI: Mycobacterium avium-intracellulare.

no case of adrenal hormonal insufficiency was found, as previously mentioned [18]. CMV infection of the adrenal glands involves both the cortex and the medulla, inducing massive necrosis in the cortex [19].

Protozoa

Pneumocystis carinii

Extrapulmonary *Pneumocystis carinii* is recognized increasingly in patients being treated for *Pneumocystis carinii* pneumonia. Other typical opportunistic pulmonary pathogens are also found to involve extrapulmonary sites in patients with a low CD4 count, indicating end-stage illness. One case of a psoas abscess, probably secondary to adjacent nodal involvement, has been reported [20]. Calcifications have been described in nine patients (lung, liver, spleen, nodes, kidney, adrenals) and multiple punctuate calcifications could be seen on plain films in three patients (liver, spleen, kidney) [21]. Raviglione estimated that 1% of patients with AIDS had extrapulmonary *Pneumocystis carinii* infection [22]. It can be found in virtually all organ systems at autopsy with calcifications and granulomas [21,23]: the

majority are clinically silent. It might be more frequent in patients treated by aerosolized pentamidine for pulmonary *Pneumocystis carinii* infection as pentamidine blood level is not high enough, which could enable some organisms to survive and develop in extrapulmonary locations. Granuloma formation may be induced by improved host defense, owing to treatment by azidodideothymidine (AZT) [24].

Fungi

Histoplasmosis

The occurrence of disseminated histoplasmosis [25] in non-endemic regions is probably due to endogenous reactivation in AIDS patients with a remote history of exposure in highly endemic areas, such as Central USA or Central America [26]. In most cases, evidence of previous infection (calcification) is absent. Retroperitoneal involvement is quite infrequent and rarely reported, but when found, is often associated with other localizations [27]: the liver, the lungs, and the omentum. Enlargement of the abdominal lymph nodes is common (75% of a series of 16 patients [26]), with lymphadenopathy showing homogeneous soft-tissue density more commonly than a diffuse or central low density. Differential diagnosis includes lymphomas but, in the case of hypoattenuation, other infections, such as MTb and MAI. They are associated with marked hepatomegaly (63%) and splenomegaly (38%), with marked splenic hypoattenuation, 30 Hounsfield units under liver density post I.V. in three cases out of six. Bilateral adrenal enlargement or hypoattenuating masses were seen only in two patients [26], one of whom was seronegative. CT demonstration of adrenal masses has not been reported in large series of patients with AIDS-related lymphoma [28], KS [29], or diffuse mycobacterial infection [13]. The CT appearance is similar to that reported in patients with diffuse histoplasmosis in endemic areas [30].

Cryptococcosis

This is the first manifestation of AIDS in 45% of the cases [31], mostly dominated by meningitis (89 out of 106), and has been associated with adrenal insufficiency [32–34], with possible non-specific gland enlargement on CT, and positive aspiration biopsy [33,34].

Malignancies

While the AIDS-related infectious manifestations become more manageable, AIDS-related malignancies remain problematic. In the era of infection prophylaxis and antiretroviral therapy, the incidence of KS and aggressive non-Hodgkin lymphoma (NHL) appears to be increasing, representing more than 95% of the neoplasms in AIDS [35]. The frequency of NHLs is much greater in the AIDS population than in the general population. According to Levine et al. [36], the rate of lymphoma was 1000 times higher in HIV-positive men than expected.

Factors associated with the development of NHL were prior diagnosis of KS, *Herpes simplex* virus and CMV infection, oral hairy leukoplakia, and lower mean neutrophil count. The influence of antiretroviral therapy has also been suggested [37].

These NHLs are aggressive (high-grade histology) and initially widespread initially (stage III or IV), with frequent extranodal involvement and a poor prognosis despite improvements in treatment and follow-up.

It seems that survival in recently diagnosed KS patients is shorter than patients diagnosed with KS earlier in the epidemic [38]. The prognosis is function of three main factors: Karnofsky performance status, history of AIDS before the diagnosis of lymphoma and bone marrow involvement [39].

The relationship between AIDS and Hodgkin's disease (HD) is not clear. According to the follow-up of the San Francisco City Clinic Cohort Study [40], an excess incidence of HD was found in HIV-infected homosexual men of 19.3 cases of HD per 100 000 persons/year versus 224.9 cases of NHL per 100 000 persons/year. There are some similarities with NHL in aggressivity (type 3 or 4) and spreading (stage III or IV with general symptoms), but the rate of development of HD seems to be lower and is not included in the Centers for Disease Control (CDC) inclusion criteria for AIDS [41]. Frequent bone marrow involvement at presentation (> 50%) in a series of 24 patients [42] with HD, type 3, and in a a series of 22 patients [43], makes MRI and bone marrow biopsy necessary, especially if a spiking fever is present. In a series of Gerrano et al. [43], a high incidence of HD and intravenous drug abuse was found (86%).

Non-Hodgkin lymphoma and Hodgkin's lymphoma (Table 19.3)

Nodal involvement

In patients with AIDS or at risk of AIDS, a hypoechogenic abdominal mass is highly suggestive of lymphoma. However, because of the frequency of adenopathy, owing to reactive hyperplasia, a specific abnormality is more likely with nodes greater than 1–1.5 cm in diameter [4,10,27,28,44,45] and highly predictable if the diameter is in excess of 3 cm.

Conclusion

US and CT are the modalities of choice for exploring the retroperitoneum, depending on the clinical presentation and status. FNAB under CT or US guidance is useful when it yields positive findings (i.e. NHL or MB). In practice, CT is the most useful method [46–50] with the best cost-effectiveness ratio for the detection and the study of the retroperitoneum in AIDS patients. Figure 19.11 summarizes the diagnostic procedures to be followed in case of suspicion of retroperitoneal AIDS-related disease.

Table 19.3. Masses depicted by US in AIDS patients with abdominal lymphoma (adapted from [11]) (percentages are shown in parentheses, multiple involvement possible).

Location	Non-Hodgkin lymphoma	Hodgkin's disease	Total
Visceral	19 (58)	1 (20)	20 (53)
Liver	16 (48)	1 (20)	17 (45)
Spleen	2 (6)	0	2 (5)
Kidneys	2 (6)	0	2 (5)
Adrenals	1 (3)	0	1 (3)
Nodal	11 (33)	4 (80)	15 (39)
Retroperitoneal	9 (27)	4 (80)	13 (34)
Mesentery	4 (12)	0	4 (11)
Portal hepatis	5 (15)	1 (20)	6 (16)
Other	9 (27)	1 (20)	10 (26)
Bowel, indeterminate	7 (21)	1 (20)	8 (21)
Omentum	2 (6)	0	2 (5)

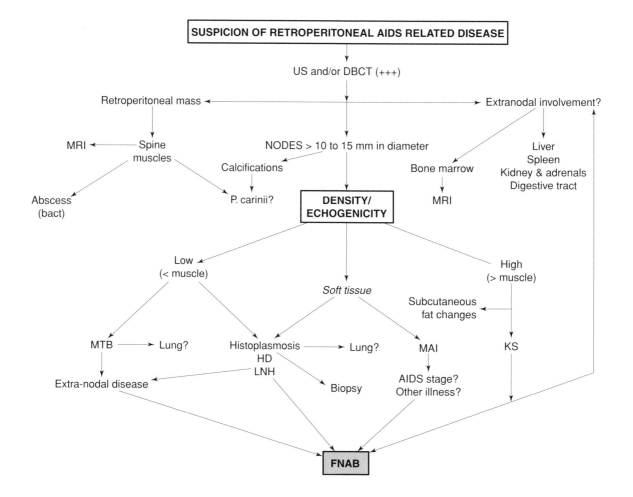

Figure 19.11

References

1   Bricaire F, Marche C, Zoubi D, Regnier B, Saimot A. Adrenocortical lesions in AIDS [letter]. *Lancet* 1988; **16**: 881.

2   Loureiro C, Gill PS, Meyer PR, Rhodes R, Rarick MU, Levine AM. Autopsy findings in AIDS related lymphoma. *Cancer* 1988; **62**: 735–739.

3   Niedt GW, Schinella RA. Acquired immunodeficiency syndrome: clinicopathologic study of 56 autopsies. *Arch Pathol Lab Med* 1985; **108**: 727–734.

4   Lavayssière RL, Cabée AE, Laissy JP, Trotot PM. Acquired immunodeficiency syndrome and retroperitoneal disease. The role of medical imaging. In: Trotot PM (ed) *Imaging of AIDS*, 1st edn. Philadelphia: BC Decker, 1991: 164–188.

5   Freeny PC. Hepatic CT: techniques, applications and results. In: JT Ferruci, DD Stark (eds) *Liver Imaging, Current Trends and New Techniques*. Boston: Andover Medical Publishers, Inc. 1990: 28–39.

6   Lavayssière RL, Cabée AE, Parienty RA. Les adénopathies rétropéritonéales. In: D Vanel (ed.) *IRM Corps Entier*, 1st edn. Paris, Berlin: Springer Verlag, 1988: 219–222.

7   Vanarthos WJ, Ganz WI, Vanartho JC, Serafini AN, Tehranzadeh J. Diagnosis ise of nuclear medicine in AIDS. *Radiographics* 1992: **12**: 731–749.

8   Podzamczer D, Ricart I, Bolao F, Romagosa V, Bonnin D, Gudiol F. Gallium 67 scan for distinguishing follicular hyperplasia from other AIDS associated diseases in lymph nodes. *AIDS* 1990; **4**: 683–685.

9   Bottles K, McPhaul LW, Volberding P. Fine needle aspiration biopsy of patients with acquired immunodeficiency syndrome (AIDS): experience in outpatient clinic. *Ann Intern Med* 1988; **108**: 42–45.

10 Smith FJ, Mathieson. Abdominal US in AIDS patients: prevalence of abnormalities in a large population. *Radiology* 1994; **192**: 691–695.

11 Townsend RR, Laing FC, Jeffrey RB Jr, Bottles K. Abdominal lymphoma in AIDS: evaluation with US. *Radiology* 1989; **171**: 719–724.

12 Farizo KM, Buehler JW, Chamberland ME et al. Spectrum of disease in person with immunodeficiency virus infection in the United States. *JAMA* 1992; **267**: 1798–1805.

13 Radin DR. Intraabdominal *Mycobacterium tuberculosis* vs *Mycobacterium avium-intracellulare* infections in patients with AIDS: distinction based on CT findings. *AJR* 1991; **156**: 487–491.

14 Modilevsky T, Sattler FR, Barnes PF. Mycobacterial disease in patients with human immunodeficiency virus infection. *Arch Intern Med* 1989; **149**: 2201–2205.

15 Pitchenik AE, Cole C, Russell BW, Fischl, Spira TJ, Snider DE Jr. Tuberculosis, atypical mycobacteriosis, and the acquired immuno deficiency syndrome among Haitian and non-Haitian patients in South Florida. *Ann Intern Med* 1984; **101**: 641–645.

16 Steinbach LS, Tehranzadeh J, Fleckentsein JL, Vanarthos WJ, Pais MJ. Human immmunodeficiency virus Infection: musculoskeletal manifestations. *Radiology* 1993; **186**: 833–838.

17 Fleckenstein JL, Burns DK, Murphy FK, Jayson HT, Bonte F. Differential diagnosis of bacterial myositis in AIDS: evaluation with MR imaging. *Radiology* 1991; **179:** 653–658.

18 Dobs A, Dempsey M, Ladenson P, Polk B. Endocrine disorders in men infected with human immunodeficiency virus. *Am J Med* 1988; **84**: 611–615.

19 Giampalmo A, Ardoino S, Borghesi MR et al. Rilievi anatomopatologici in 25 casi autopsici di AIDS. *Pathologica* 1989; **81**: 1–46.

20 Eagar GM, Friedland JA, Sagel SS. Tumefactive *Pneumocystis carinii* infection in AIDS: report of three cases. *AJR* 1993; **160**: 1197–1198.

21 Radin DR, Baker EL, Klatt EC et al. Visceral and nodal calcification in patients with AIDS related *Pneumocystis carinii* infection. *AJR* 1990; **154**: 27–31.

22 Raviglione MC. Extrapulmonary pneumocystis: the first 50 cases. *Rev Infect Dis* 1990; **12**: 1127–1138.

23 Cohen OJ, Stoeckle MY. Extrapulmonary *Pneumocystis carinii* infections in the acquired immunodeficiency syndrome. *Arch Intern Med* 1991; **151**: 1205–1214.

24 Klein JS, Warnock M, Webb WR, Gamsu G. Cavitating and non cavitating granuloma in AIDS patients with *Pneumocystis* pneumonitis. *AJR* 1989; **152**: 753–754.

25 Davies SF. Histoplasmosis: update 1989. *Semin Resp Infect* 1990; **5**: 93–104.

26 Radin DR. Disseminated histoplasmosis: abdominal CT findings in 16 patients. *AJR* 1991; **157**: 955–958.

27 Megibow AJ, Balthazae EJ, Hulnick DH. Radiology of nonneoplastic gastrointestinal disorders in acquired immuno deficiency syndrome. *Semin Roentgenol* 1987; **22**: 31–41.

28 Nyberg SA, Jeffrey RB Jr, Federle MP, Bottles K, Abrams DI. AIDS related lymphomas: evaluation by abdominal CT. *Radiology* 1986; **159**: 59–63.

29 Moon KL Jr, Federle MP, Abrams DI, Volberding P, Lewis BJ. Kaposi sarcoma and lymphadenopathy syndrome: limitations of abdominal CT in acquired immuno deficiency syndrome. *Radiology* 1984; **150**: 479–483.

30 Wilson DA, Muchmore HG, Tisdal RG, Fahmy A, Pitha JV. Histoplasmosis of the adrenal glands studied by CT. *Radiology* 1984; **150**: 779–783.

31 Chuck SL, Sande MA. Infection with cryptococcus neoformans in the Acquired immunodeficiency syndrome. *N Engl J Med* 1989, **321:** 794–799.

32 Shah B, Taylor HC, Pillay I, Chunk Park M, Dobrinich R. Adrenal insufficiency due to Cryptococcosis. *JAMA* 1986; **256**: 3247–3249.

33 Walker BF, Gunthel CJ, Bryan JA, Watts NB, Clark RV. Disseminated cryptococcosis in an apparently normal host presenting as primary adrenal insufficiency: diagnosis by fine needle aspiration. *Am J Med* 1989, **86:** 715–717.

34 Takeshita A, Nakazawa H, Akiyama H et al. Disseminated cryptococcosis presenting with adrenal insufficiency and meningitis: resistant to prolonged antifungal therapy but responding to bilateral adrenalectomy. *Intern Med (Japan)* 1992; **31**: 1401–1405.

35 Levine AM. Non Hodgkins's lymphoma and other malignancies in the acquired immunodeficiency syndrome. *Semin Oncol* 1987; **14**: 34–39.

36   Levine AM, Gill PS, Krailo M et al. Natural history of persistent generalized lymphadenopathy (PGL) in gay men: risk of lymphoma (NHL) and factors associated with development of lymphoma (abstr). *Blood* 1986; **68:** 130A.

37   Moore RD, Kessler H, Richmann DD, Flexner C, Chaisson RE. Non Hodgkin's lymphoma in patients with advanced HIV infection treated with zidovudine. *JAMA* 1991: **265:** 2208–2211.

38   Abrams DI. Acquired immunodeficiency syndrome and related malignancies: a topical overview. *Semin Oncol* 1991; **18:** 41–45.

39   Levine AM, Sullivan-Halley J, Pike MC et al. Human immunodeficiency virus related lymphoma. Prognosis factors predictive of survival. *Cancer* 1993; **71:** 2466-2472.

40   Hessol NA, Katz MH, Liu JY, Buchbinder SP, Rubino CJ, Holmberg SD. Increased incidence of Hodgkin disease in homosexual men with HIV infection. *Ann Intern Med* 1992; **117:** 309–311.

41   Le Sida et la Société Française. v Décembre 1993. *Rapport au Premier Ministre.* L. Montagnier, PM Trotot (eds). Paris: La Documentation Française, 1994.

42   Ree HJ, Strauchen JA, Khan AA et al. Human immunodeficiency virus associated Hodgkin's disease. Clinicopathologic studies of 24 cases and preponderance of mixed cellularity type characterized by the occurrence of fibrohistiocytoid stroma cells. *Cancer* 1991; **67:** 1614–1621.

43   Serrano M, Bellas C, Campo E et al. Hodgkin's disease in patients with antibodies to human immunodeficiency virus. A study of 22 patients. *Cancer* 1990; **65:** 2248–2254.

44   Jeffrey RB, Nyberg DA, Bottles K et al. Abdominal CT in acquired immunodeficiency syndrome. *AJR* 1986; **146:** 7–13.

45   Geoffray A, Binet A, Cassuto JP, Dujardin P, Coussement A. Sonography of abdominal adenopathies in patients with anti-HIV positive serology. In: Trotot PM (ed.) *Imaging of AIDS,* 1st edn. Philadelphia: BC Decker, 1991: 189–194.

46   Townsend RR. CT of AIDS related lymphoma. *AJR* 1991; **156:** 969–974.

47   Federle MP. A radiologist looks at AIDS: imaging evaluation based on symptom complexes. *Radiology* 1988; **165:** 553–562.

48   Dodd GD, Greenler DP, Confer SR. Thoracic and abdominal manifestations in lymphoma occuring in the immunocompromise patient. *Radiol Clin North Am* 1992; **30:** 597–610.

49   Herts BR, Megibow AJ, Birnbaum BA, Kanzer GK, Noz ME. High attenuation lymphadenopathy in AIDS patients: significance of findings at CT. *Radiology* 1992; **185:** 777–781.

50   Kuhlman JE, Browne D, Shermak M, Hamper UM, Zerhouni EA, Fishman EK. Retroperitoneal and pelvic CT of patients with AIDS: primary and secondary involvement of the genitourinary tract. *Radiographics* 1991; **11:** 473–483.

20 RENAL MANIFESTATIONS

Frank H. Miller
Richard M. Gore

Introduction

Parenchymal involvement of the solid abdominal organs has become increasingly common since the acquired immunodeficiency syndrome (AIDS) was first described in 1981 [1]. Renal complications are becoming more prevalent, owing to prolonged patient survival and an increased incidence of AIDS transmission in intravenous drug abusers [2,3]. The kidneys in AIDS patients are subject to a wide variety of infectious, neoplastic, immunologic, vascular, and drug-related insults (Table 20.1), which can produce a number of often confusing abnormalities on cross-sectional renal imaging studies [4–8]. Since plain abdominal radiographs and intravenous urography do not play a major role in the evaluation of these complications, the computed tomography (CT) and ultrasound findings (Table 20.2) of the more important renal complications of AIDS and their pathological basis are emphasized in this chapter.

HIV-associated nephropathy

In 1984, a specific disease entity in human immune deficiency virus (HIV)-positive patients was described: HIV-associated nephropathy (HIVAN) [9,10]. This disorder is characterized by a focal and segmental glomerulosclerosis with marked hypertrophy of the visceral epithelial cells with coarse cytoplasmic vacuoles, microcystic dilatation of tubules containing protein casts, Bowman's space dilatation, and edema and inflammatory changes. Grossly, the kidneys, cortex, and medulla are widened and edematous [11,12]. Less common histological findings include minimal change glomerulopathy, focal to diffuse mesangial hypercellularity, diffuse proliferative glomerulonephritis, and membranous and membranoproliferative glomerulonephritis [9–13].

Patients characteristically have heavy proteinuria (>3.5 g/day), large kidneys, and mild hypertension. Renal disease may be an early, unsuspected manifestation of HIV infection. Indeed, in one study almost half of the patients with HIVAN were asymptomatic or showed only early signs of AIDS-related complex [12]. Renal involvement is more prevalent in AIDS patients with multiple risk factors and intravenous drug abusers than in the homosexual population with AIDS [8].

The sonographic findings (Figure 20.1) of HIVAN include enlarged echogenic kidneys with poor corticomedullary differentiation. They are most likely to be the result of focal and segmental glomerulosclerosis, and dilated renal tubules filled with proteinaceous material [14–16]. The degree of echogenicity does not directly correlate with the extent of renal disease. With progression to end-stage renal disease, the kidneys remain large. The major CT abnormalities in HIVAN are enlarged kidneys (Figure 20.2) and, occasionally, increased attenuation of the medulla on non-contrast scans [7,8,17]. The cause of the increased medullary attenuation is not known, but may be the result of the tubular abnormalities of HIVAN. The CT findings are usually less dramatic than those seen sonographically [8].

The prognosis of HIVAN is poor with isolated reports demonstrating beneficial effects of zidovudine (AZT) in some patients [18,19]. Some nephrologists aggressively biopsy HIV-infected patients with glomerular diseases because of the poor prognosis associated with HIVAN and concern over treating HIV-infected patients with steroids or immunosuppressive drugs [20].

Infections

The prevalence of acute and recurrent urinary tract infections has been reported as high as 50% in AIDS

Table 20.1. Renal lesions associated with HIV infection.

Disseminated infections	Glomerular lesions
Cytomegalovirus	Focal and segmental glomerulosclerosis (HIV-associated nephropathy)
Mycobacterium tuberculosis	
Mycobacterium avium intracellulare	Mesangial proliferative glomerulonephritis
Cryptococcus	Minimal change disease
Candida	Membranoproliferative glomerulonephritis
Pneumocystis carinii	Membranous glomerulonephritis
Histoplasmosis	Acute postinfectious glomerulonephritis

Neoplasms	Vascular lesions
Kaposi's sarcoma	Hemolytic–uremic syndrome
Lymphoma	Infarcts
Renal cell carcinoma	Renal cortical necrosis
	Vasculitis

Acute tubular necrosis	Allergic interstitial nephritis
Toxic	Drug-induced
Ischemic	

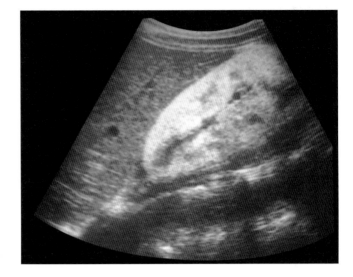

Figure 20.1. HIV-associated nephropathy: sonographic findings. Sagittal sonogram of the right kidney demonstrates nephromegaly, a strikingly echogenic renal cortex and poor corticomedullary differentiation. Increased cortical echogenicity is due to focal and segmental glomerulosclerosis and dilated tubules filled with proteinaceous material.

common ones that affect the urinary tract of immuno-competent individuals [4–6].

Pyogenic infections

Owing to a deficiency in humoral-mediated immunity, AIDS patients are at increased risk for serious bacterial urinary tract infections, including pyelonephritis and renal abscesses. Intravenous drug abusers may develop septic emboli and *Staphylococcus*

patients [4–6]. The HIV causes progressive depletion of T-helper lymphocytes, which serve a major role in cell-mediated immunity. Consequently, these patients are extremely susceptible to a variety of infections due to viruses, mycobacteria, fungi, and protozoa. In most cases, however, the causative organisms are the

Table 20.2. Imaging findings in common renal lesions of AIDS patients

	US	CT
HIVAN	Hyperechoic, enlarged kidneys	Enlarged kidneys, hyperdense medulla
Pneumocystis carinii	Small echogenic foci; hepatosplenic involvement	Low-attenuation lesions; calcifications
Mycobacterium tuberculosis	Low-attenuation lymphadenopathy; focal liver/spleen/renal lesions	
Mycobacterium avium-intracellulare	Hepatosplenomegaly; diffuse jejunal wall thickening/soft-tissue-density lymph nodes; may mimic *Pneumocystis* (renal calcifications)	
Candidiasis	Focal renal lesions; associated liver/spleen lesions	
AIDS-related lymphoma	Hypoechoic masses; adenopathy	Low-attenuation masses; hydronephrosis may result from obstructing lymph nodes
Kaposi's sarcoma	Microscopic involvement; may be obstructive uropathy due to lymphadenopathy; associated skin findings	

US, ultrasound; CT, computed tomography.

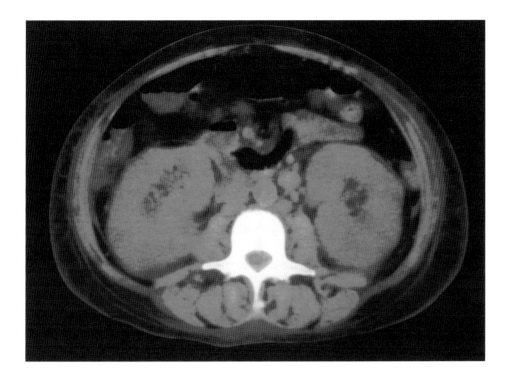

Figure 20.2. HIV-associated nephropathy: CT findings. Non-contrast CT scan demonstrates bilateral, global nephromegaly with several subtle areas of increased medullary attenuation in the left kidney.

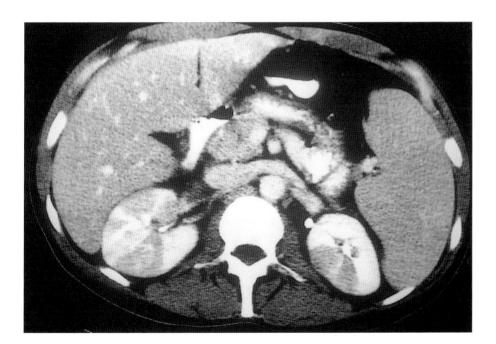

Figure 20.3. Pyelonephritis due to *Klebsiella*: CT findings. Bilateral wedge-shaped areas of decreased attenuation and striated nephrograms are demonstrated on this contrast-enhanced scan. There is splenomegaly.

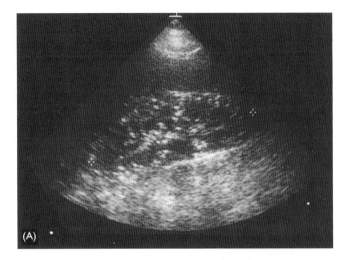

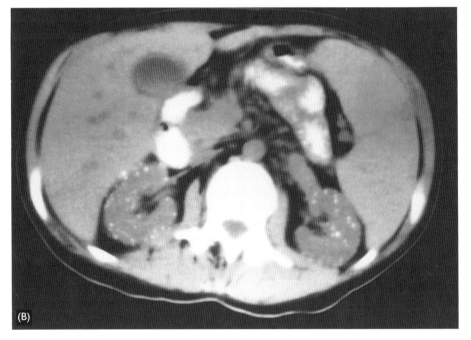

Figure 20.4. Renal *Pneumocystis carinii* infection. (A) Longitudinal sonogram of the right kidney reveals multiple scattered echogenic foci due to calcifications resulting from the infection. (B) Non-contrast enhanced CT scan in the same patient documents the presence of multiple punctate calcifications.

aureus microabscesses [5]. The cross-sectional imaging findings of bacterial pyelonephritis (Figure 20.3), lobar nephronia, and pyogenic abscess in AIDS patients are identical to those seen in immunocompetent individuals. In AIDS patients, however, these findings can be difficult to distinguish from non-bacterial infections and even neoplasms, such as AIDS-related lymphoma. Consequently, needle aspiration is often required to establish the diagnosis of renal abscess.

Pneumocystis carinii

Extrapulmonary *Pneumocystis carinii* is being documented more frequently in AIDS patients owing to

their increasing life span, change in *P. carinii* virulence factors, and the use of prophylactic aerosolized pentamidine [21–23]. Although this route of delivery prevents the development of pneumonia, serum levels are not sufficient to prevent systemic spread. Extrapulmonary involvement most often involves the lymph nodes followed by the spleen, liver, bone marrow, gastrointestinal tract, eyes, thyroid, adrenal glands, and kidneys. Fortunately, systemic spread occurs in fewer than 1% of patients, although many cases are probably not diagnosed because they are clinically silent or diagnostic imaging or an autopsy is not performed [21–23]. Disseminated disease has an extremely poor prognosis unless systemic therapy is instituted, or if only one site is involved and *P. carinii* pneumonia is not present.

In patients with renal *Pneumocystis* infection, CT scans may demonstrate low-attenuation lesions and punctate calcifications [24–27]. Low-attenuation lesions are not specific and can be seen in lymphoma, bacterial, mycobacterial, and *Candida* microabscesses, and Kaposi sarcoma [25]. Calcifications are typical of *Pneumocystis* infection and may be present in active disease, unlike candidiasis or lymphoma, where they are classically seen in treated or inactive infection [26]. These calcifications were initially believed to be specific for *Pneumocystis* infection but have also been described in *Mycobacterium avium-intracellulare* (MAI) and cytomegalovirus infection [28,29]. Ultrasound may demonstrate multiple tiny echogenic foci (Figure 20.4A), with or without shadowing in the involved organs [8]. These echogenic foci are secondary to calcifications which may be identified on CT scans (Figure 20.4B) or granulomas, which are not demonstrable on CT [30]. Non-contrast CT scans should initially be obtained in patients with AIDS to assess for calcifications which might be obscured by contrast medium.

Mycobacterium avium-intracellulare

Infection with *Mycobacterium avium* and *Mycobacterium intracellulare* have been reclassified under the name of *Mycobacterium avium-intracellulare* because of the difficulty of distinguishing the two organisms clinically and in the laboratory [31]. Prior to the AIDS epidemic, MAI was isolated to elderly patients with chronic disease who developed an indolent infection mimicking *Mycobacterium tuberculosis* [32]. In 5.5% of patients with AIDS, MAI disseminates hematogenously to involve multiple organs, especially the reticuloendothelial system [33]. Most commonly, the lymph nodes, liver, spleen, bone marrow, and gastrointestinal tract are involved. Other organs affected by systemic spread include the kidneys, thyroid, pancreas, adrenal glands, muscle, and brain [33,34]. Solitary organ involvement is rare.

When attempting to make the diagnosis of MAI, a high index of suspicion is required and biopsy specimens should be routinely stained for acid-fast bacilli and cultured for MAI. Acid-fast stains usually demonstrate a large number of organisms within macrophages, without evidence of granuloma formation or inflammatory reaction, unlike *Mycobacterium tuberculosis* [33].

The most common abdominal CT finding in patients with MAI infection is lymphadenopathy. Radiological evidence of parenchymal organ disease is often absent despite pathological involvement. Case reports have described multiple tiny echogenic foci in the liver and kidneys [25,29]. Abscesses, which are usually hypodense on CT (Figure 20.5) and hypoechoic on ultrasound, may be seen in the kidneys, spleen, or liver. MAI is usually resistant to standard antituberculosis medications and often multiple investigational drugs are required for therapy.

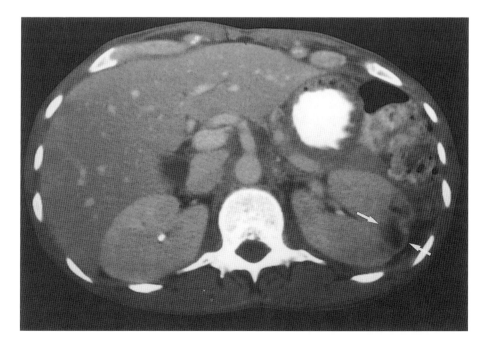

Figure 20.5. Mycobacterium avium-intracellulare abscess: CT features. A low-density left renal mass (arrows) is identified on this CT scan.

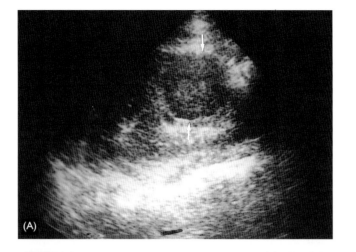

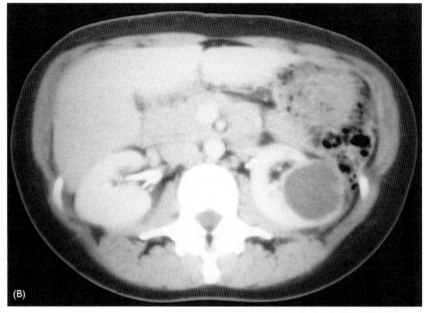

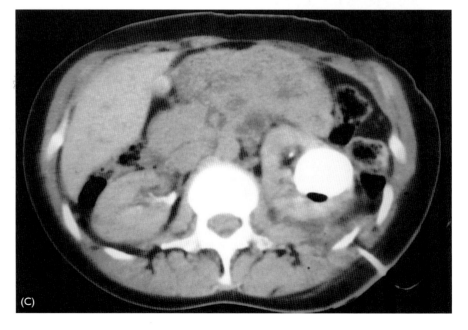

Figure 20.6. Mycobacterium tuberculosis abscess: ultrasound and CT features. (A) Longitudinal sonogram demonstrates a hypoechoic mass (arrows) at the lower pole of the left kidney. (B) Corresponding CT scan demonstrates a hypodense mass with a thick wall in the same region. (C) This mass was percutaneously drained and contrast material was injected showing filling of the abscess cavity. Cultures were positive for M. tuberculosis.

Mycobacterium tuberculosis

After decades of decreasing incidence, a resurgence of *Mycobacterium tuberculosis* (MTb) has accompanied the AIDS epidemic [34]. MTb may develop during the course of HIV infections before other opportunistic infections indicative of AIDS [35]. The immunosuppressed state associated with AIDS predisposes patients with latent tuberculosis to reactivate their disease. Less typical presentations of tuberculosis are becoming more prevalent. Extrapulmonary involvement in patients with AIDS is identified in up to 70% of patients with MTb: central nervous system, bone, gastrointestinal, renal, and soft tissue involvement [36]. Indeed, extrapulmonary disease is now being used as an index infection for the diagnosis of AIDS in HIV-infected patients [37].

There are several CT findings that can help differentiate MTb from MAI infection. Focal hepatic, splenic, and renal lesions associated with low-attenuation lymph nodes are more suggestive of disseminated MTb than MAI [38]. MTb abscesses are generally low density on CT and hypoechoic on ultrasound (Figure 20.6). Marked hepatosplenomegaly, diffuse jejunal wall thickening, and enlarged soft-tissue-density lymph nodes are typically found in disseminated MAI infection. Additionally, 82% of patients with MAI have prior AIDS-defining illnesses, while MTb infection may be an initial manifestation of the disease.

Candidiasis

Disseminated candidiasis can cause focal abscesses in the kidneys, and is usually associated with splenic and hepatic involvement. The diagnosis is often difficult because there is no classic presentation, and *Candida* is difficult to culture following needle biopsy [39]. Patients usually have fevers and chills that are unresponsive to antibiotics. *Candida* microabscesses are typically hypoechoic, often with a 'bull's-eye' appearance on ultrasound. On CT, they appear as multiple, small, low-attenuation masses that are better demonstrated following intravenous contrast (Figure 20.7). After treatment, calcifications of the lesions may develop [7,8].

Neoplasms

Lymphoma

AIDS-related lymphoma (ARL) consists of a variety of relatively aggressive undifferentiated forms of non-Hodgkin lymphoma (NHL), including small non-cleaved, large, immunoblastic, and undifferentiated cell types [40]. These lymphomas fulfill the criteria of the Centers for Disease Control (CDC) for the diagnosis of AIDS, whereas it remains controversial whether Hodgkin's lymphoma constitutes a manifestation of AIDS [41,42]. The patient with AIDS-related NHL or Hodgkin's disease tends to have a more advanced grade

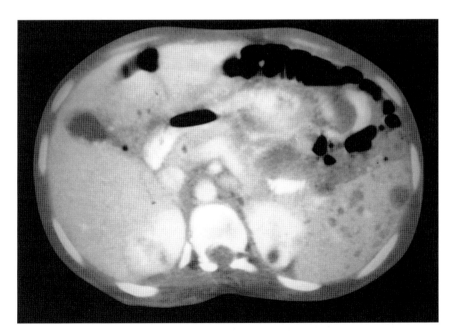

Figure 20.7. Renal and splenic candidiasis: CT findings. Multiple low-density masses are seen in the kidneys and spleen on this contrast-enhanced scan.

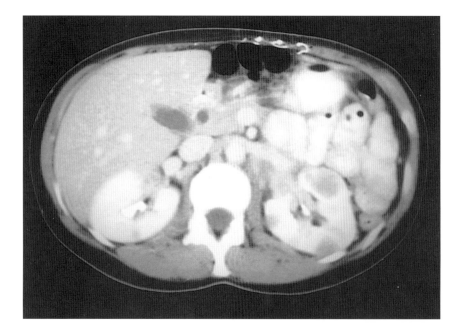

Figure 20.8. AIDS-related non-Hodgkin's lymphoma: CT findings. Multiple low-density renal masses are identified. Ultrasound directed biopsy was needed to establish the diagnosis. Adenopathy is present in the left renal hilum.

of tumor when compared to patients with lymphoma without AIDS. ARL is associated with aggressive growth and involvement of extranodal sites, especially the brain, bone marrow, and abdominal organs [42]. Additionally, mesenteric and retroperitoneal adenopathy are relatively more common in patients with ARL. Focal renal masses are less common than hepatic or splenic involvement. Six to twelve per cent of patients with ARL have renal involvement on imaging studies [41,42].

Renal involvement by ARL usually manifests as bilateral low-density lesions on CT (Figure 20.8). This is in contrast to the diffuse renal enlargement that characterizes renal lymphoma in patients without AIDS [41–43]. On ultrasound the lesions are typically hypoechoic. Other renal findings in patients with ARL include direct renal invasion or hydronephrosis (Figure 20.9) from obstruction of the ureter by enlarged lymph nodes [17,42].

Adenopathy is a common manifestation of ARL, reactive hyperplasia, MAI and Kaposi's sarcoma. Unlike mycobacterial infections, low-attenuation regions are not typically seen within nodal masses of ARL. When

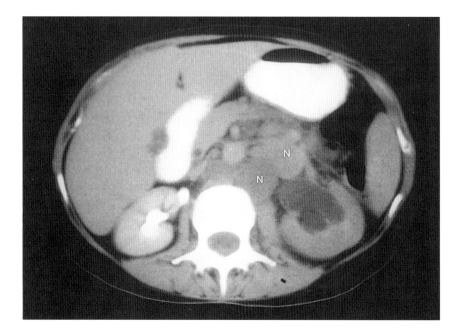

Figure 20.9. Hydronephrosis due to AIDS-related lymphoma. Multiple enlarged retroperitoneal lymph nodes (N) cause hydronephrosis of the left kidney.

extensive lymphadenopathy is detected, ARL, MAI, and Kaposi's sarcoma should be considered [17,44]. Biopsy is required for definitive diagnosis and can be performed with CT or sonographic guidance [45].

Kaposi's sarcoma

Kaposi's sarcoma (KS) is a common complication in sexually transmitted AIDS. It is less commonly seen in intravenous drug abusers, and AIDS transmitted through blood and blood products [46]. The KS lesion histologically consists of irregularly dilated vascular spaces coated with swollen endothelial cells, with an inflammatory response containing lymphocytes and neutrophils [47–49]. The lymph nodes are the third most common site of involvement in KS patients following cutaneous and oral mucosal disease, which is noted in 95% of cases [48]. With extensive retroperitoneal tumor, ureteral obstruction may occur [17]. Mild splenomegaly is common. Although involvement of the kidney, spleen, and liver is often noted at autopsy, focal lesions are seldom identified on cross-sectional imaging because the neoplasm spreads via microscopic infiltration along established vascular tracts [49]. Retroperitoneal and pelvic adenopathy, which often demonstrates striking contrast enhancement, can be quite prominent.

Renal cell carcinoma

Reports have demonstrated a suspected association between the immunosuppression associated with HIV infection and the development of solid genitourinary tumors. Renal cell carcinoma, angiosarcoma, and testicular seminomas and embryonal cell tumors have been identified in patients with AIDS. At present, one can only speculate whether these cancers are related to HIV infection or are a chance association [50,51]. The development of renal cell carcinoma in relatively young patients raises the possibility that the immunosuppression associated with AIDS may contribute to the development or at least earlier manifestation of these tumors.

Hydronephrosis

Hydronephrosis in AIDS patients may be due to extrinsic causes, such as adenopathy from ARL or KS, a large abscess, or from obturation due to a fungus ball (Figure 20.10), blood clot, or stone [6,17].

Conclusion

Cross-sectional imaging is very useful in detecting and in some instances characterizing the many infectious and neoplastic disorders that involve the kidney in AIDS patients. Ultrasound has the advantages of lower cost, and portability, and does not require intravenous contrast media that have the potential to be nephrotoxic. Ultrasound may demonstrate striking abnormalities of HIVAN while CT scans are normal or demonstrate only enlarged kidneys. In addition, diffuse echogenic foci may be noted in infections such as *Pneumocystis* and MAI, while CT scans remain unremarkable. CT scans and magnetic resonance imaging may be required to demonstrate focal masses that are not well visualized on ultrasound. In addition, associated findings including lymphadenopathy, other organ involvement, and bowel pathology are often better appreciated on CT.

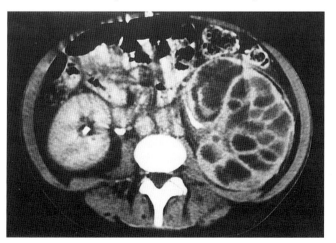

Figure 20.10. Hydronephrosis: cysts and calyceal displacement of left kidney, due to AIDS-related Renal Aspergilloma (courtesy: V. Guadano, MD, Madrid, Spain)

References

1   Frassetto L, Schoenfeld PY, Humphreys MH. Increasing incidence of human immunodeficiency virus-associated nephropathy at San Francisco General Hospital. *Am J Kidney Dis* 1991; **18**: 655–659.

2   Schacker T, Collier AC, Hughes J et al. Clinical and epidemiologic features of primary HIV infection. *Ann Intern Med* 1996; **125**: 257–269.

3   Moore RD, Chiasson RE. Natural history of opportunistic disease in an HIV-infected urban clinical cohort. *Ann Intern Med* 1996; **124**: 663–642.

4   Bourgoignie JJ, Meneses R, Ortiz C et al. The clinical spectrum of renal disease associated with human immunodeficiency virus. *Am J Kidney Dis* 1988; **12**: 131–137.

5   Vaziri ND, Barbari A, Licorish K et al. Spectrum of renal abnormalities in acquired immunodeficiency syndrome. *J Natl Med Assoc* 1985; **77**: 369–375.

6   Miles BJ, Meiser M, Farah R et al. The urological manifestations of acquired immunodeficiency syndrome. *J Urol* 1989; **142**: 771–773.

7   Jeffrey RB. Abdominal imaging in the immunocompromised patient. *Radiol Clin North Am* 1992; **30**: 579–596.

8   Miller FH, Parikh S, Gore RM et al. Renal manifestations of AIDS. *RadioGraphics* 1993; **13**: 587–596.

9   Rao TKS, Fillippone EJ, Landesman SH et al. Acquired immunodeficiency syndrome (AIDS)-associated nephropathy; focal and segmental glomerulosclerosis: a new entity. *Kidney Int* 1984; **25**: 174.

10 Rao TKS, Fillippone EJ, Nicastri AD et al. Associated focal and segmental glomerulosclerosis in the acquired immunodeficiency syndrome. *N Engl J Med* 1984; **310**: 669–673.

11 Rao TKS, Friedman EA. AIDS (HIV)-associated nephropathy; does it exist? *Am J Nephrol* 1989; **9**: 441–453.

12 Rao TKS. Human immunodeficiency virus (HIV)-associated nephropathy. *Annu Rev Med* 1991; **42**: 391–401.

13 Glassock RJ, Cohen AH, Danovitch G et al. Human immunodeficiency virus (HIV) infection and the kidney. *Ann Intern Med* 1990; **112**: 35–49.

14 Hamper UM, Goldblum LE, Hutchins GM et al. Renal involvement in AIDS: sonographic-pathologic correlation. *AJR* 1988; **150**: 1321–1325.

15 Schaffer RM, Schwartz GE, Becker JA et al. Renal ultrasound in acquired immunodeficiency syndrome. *Radiology* 1984; **153**: 511–513.

16 Kay CJ. Renal diseases in patients with AIDS: sonographic findings. *AJR* 1992; **159**: 551–554.

17 Kuhlman JE, Browne D, Shermak M. et al. Retroperitoneal and pelvic CT of patients with AIDS: primary and secondary involvement of the genitourinary tract. *RadioGraphics* 1991; **11**: 473–483.

18 Babut-Gay ML, Echard M. Zidovudine and nephropathy with human immunodeficiency virus (HIV) infection. *Ann Intern Med* 1989; **111**: 856–857.

19 Cook PP, Appel RG. Prolonged clinical improvement in HIV-associated nephropathy with zidovudine therapy. *J Am Soc Nephrol* 1990; **1**: 842.

20 Korbet SM, Schwartz MM. Human immunodeficiency virus infection and nephrotic syndrome (clinical conference). *Am J Kidney Dis* 1992; **20**: 97–103.

21 Bernard EM, Sepkowitz KA, Telzak EE et al. Pneumocystis. *Med Clin North Am* 1992; **76**: 107–120.

22 Raviglione MC. Extrapulmonary pneumocystosis: the first 50 cases. *Rev Infect Dis* 1990; **12**: 1127–1138.

23 Witt K, Nielsen TN, Junge J. Dissemination of *Pneumocystis carinii* in patients with AIDS. *Scand J Infect Dis* 1991; **23**: 691–695.

24 Lubat E, Megibow AJ, Balthazar EJ et al. Extrapulmonary *Pneumocystis carinii* infection in AIDS: CT findings. *Radiology* 1990; **174**: 157–160.

25 Falkoff G, Rigsby CM, Rosenfield AT. Partial, combined cortical and medullary nephrocalcinosis: US and CT patterns in AIDS-associated MAI infection. *Radiology* 1987; **162**: 343–344.

26 Radin DR, Baker EL, Klatt EC et al. Visceral and nodal calcification in patients with AIDS-related *Pneumocystis carinii* infection. *AJR* 1990; **154**: 27–31.

27 Feuerstein JM, Francis P, Raffeld M et al. Widespread visceral calcifications in disseminated *Pneumocystis carinii* infection: CT characteristics. *J Comput Assist Tomogr* 1990; **14**: 149–151.

28 Bray HJ, Lail VJ, Cooperberg PL. Tiny echogenic foci in the liver and kidney in patients with AIDS: not always due to disseminated *Pneumocystis carinii*. *AJR* 1992; **158**: 81–82.

29 Towers MJ, Withers CE, Hamilton PA et al. Visceral calcification in patients with AIDS may not always be due to *Pneumocystis carinii*. *AJR* 1991; **156**: 745–747.

30 Spouge AR, Wilson ST, Gopinath N et al. Extrapulmonary *Pneumocystis carinii* in a patient with AIDS: sonographic findings. *AJR* 1990; **155**: 76–78.

31 Horsburgh CR Jr, Selik RM. The epidemiology of disseminated nontuberculous mycobacterium infection in acquired immunodeficiency syndrome (AIDS). *Am Rev Respir Dis* 1989; **139**: 4–7.

32 Pitchenik AE, Fertel D. Tuberculosis and nontuberculous mycobacterial disease. *Med Clin North Am* 1992; **76**: 121–172.

33 Ellner JJ, Goldberger MJ, Parenti DM. Mycobacterium avium infection and AIDS: a therapeutic dilemma in rapid progression. *J Infectious Dis* 1991; **163**: 1326–1335.

34 Buckner CB, Leithiser RE, Walker CW et al. The changing epidemiology of tuberculosis and other mycobacterial infections in the United States: implications for the radiologist. *AJR* 1991; **156**: 255–264.

35 Markowitz N, Hansen NI, Hopewell, PC et al. Incidence of tuberculosis in the United States among HIV-infected persons. *Ann Intern Med* 1997; **126**: 123–132.

36 Sanderman G, McDonald RJ, Maniatis T et al. Tuberculosis as a manifestation of the acquired immunodeficiency syndrome (AIDS). *JAMA* 1986; **256**: 362–366.

37 Sathe SS, Reichman LB. Mycobacterial disease in patients infected with the human immunodeficiency virus. *Clin Chest Med* 1989; **10**: 445–463.

38 Radin DR. Intraabdominal mycobacterium tuberculosis v. Mycobacterium avium-intracellulare infections in patients with AIDS: distinction based on CT findings. *AJR* 1990; **156**: 487–491.

39 Shirkhoda A. CT findings in hepatosplenic and renal candidiasis. *J Comput Assist Tomogr* 1987; **11**: 795–798.

40 Levine AM. AIDS-associated lymphoma. *Med Clin North Am* 1992; **76**: 253–268.

41 Townsend RR, Laing FC, Jeffrey RB et al. Abdominal lymphoma in AIDS: evaluation with US. *Radiology* 1989; **171**: 719–724.

42 Townsend RR. CT of AIDS-related lymphoma. *AJR* 1991; **156**: 969–974.

43 Ferrozzi F, Bova D, Campodonico F et al. AIDS-related malignancies: clinico-radiological correlation. *Eur Radiol* 1995; **5**: 477–485.

44 Nyberg DA, Federle MP. AIDS-related Kaposi sarcoma and lymphoma. *Semin Roentgenol* 1987; **22**: 54–65.

45 Strigle SM, Martin SE, Levine AM et al. The use of fine needle aspiration cytology in the management of human immunodeficiency virus-related non-Hodgkin's lymphoma and Hodgkin's disease. *J Acquir Immune Defic Syndr* 1993; **6**: 1329–1334.

46 Friedman-Kien AE, Laubenstein LJ, Rubinstein PI et al. Disseminated Kaposi's sarcoma in homosexual men. *Ann Intern Med* 1982; **96**: 693.

47 Krown SE, Myskowski PL, Paredes J. Kaposi's sarcoma. *Med Clin North Am* 1992; **76**: 239–252.

48 Longo DL. Kaposi's sarcoma and other neoplasms. *Ann Intern Med* 1984; **100**: 92–96.

49 Luburich P, Bru C, Ayuso MC et al. Hepatic Kaposi sarcoma in AIDS: US and CT findings. *Radiology* 1990; **175**: 172–174.

50 Adjiman S, Zerbib M, Flam T et al. Genitourinary tumors and HIV-1 infection. *Eur Urol* 1990; **18**: 56–60.

51 Azon-Masoliver A, Moreno A, Gatell JM et al. Renal cell adenocarcinoma associated with AIDS-related Kaposi's sarcoma. *AIDS* 1990; **4**: 818–819.

21 DERMATOLOGIC AND VENEREAL MANIFESTATIONS

Hendrik J. Hulsebosch

Introduction

Since the start of the human immune deficiency virus (HIV) epidemic in the early 1980s, many dermatologic and venereal diseases have been described in association with the HIV infection. The reasons for these associations were that well-known dermatological and venereal diseases were seen in a higher frequency in HIV-infected patients, or that unusual expressions of these diseases were seen as a result of HIV-induced immunodeficiency. Moreover, otherwise rare dermatoses could be diagnosed in these patients, and even new skin and mucous membrane diseases occurred.

Gradually what may be called HIV dermato-venereology has come into being. This chapter aims to present an overview of this subject. For further reading, *Skin Manifestations of AIDS* [1], with attention paid to histopathologic findings, and *A Colour Atlas of AIDS in the Tropics* [2] are advised. It is to be expected that other diseases will be added to the list because of the increasing survival time of patients as a result of therapeutic regimens. Epidemiological aspects, concerning the interaction of sexually transmitted HIV infection with other venereal diseases, especially genital ulcer disease, have been left aside. They are beyond the scope of this chapter.

Skin and mucous membrane involvement occurs in two phases of the HIV infection: (I) as part of the primary HIV infection; and (II) associated with HIV-induced immune deficiency, or the acquired immunodeficiency syndrome (AIDS).

Primary HIV infection

Primary infection with HIV-1 is symptomatic in the majority of cases, with an incubation time of 1–4 weeks and a duration of about 2 weeks. The clinical picture of acute HIV infection varies from influenza-like symptoms to an illness with as its main clinical features, fever ranging from 38 to 40° C, malaise, diarrhea, myalgia, arthralgia, sore throat, headache, lymphadenopathy, and a skin rash. The exanthem consists of maculopapular, roseola-like lesions, sometimes with a central crust, disseminated over the upper part of the body, or generalized, palms and soles included (Figure 21.1). Besides that there are is an enanthem with superficial ulcerations. Genital and anal mucosal ulcerations may be present. During the early stages of primary HIV infection, HIV p24 antigen can be demonstrated in plasma, usually before seroconversion to HIV antibodies occurs. Coinciding with clinical improvement, p24 antigen decreases to undetectable levels, while antibody tests become positive. A window-phase may occur, in which HIV antigenemia has disappeared prior to the appearance of HIV antibodies. During this period no serological markers for HIV-1 infection can be detected. As a consequence, sequential testing for HIV antibodies in the serum to document seroconversion is necessary. The main differential diagnosis of primary HIV infection is secondary syphilis, because of similarities in skin symptoms and the sexual risk behaviour in the patients' history [3].

Dermatologic and venereal disease in HIV-induced immunodeficiency

When HIV-induced immunodeficiency develops, three groups of HIV-associated skin diseases can be distinguished: infectious dermatoses, skin tumors, and a group of non-infectious, non-tumorous skin diseases. Table 21.1 gives an overview. Systematic grouping of HIV-associated dermatologic and venereal diseases

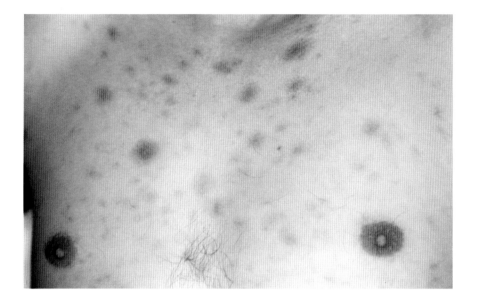

Figure 21.1. HIV exanthem, part of the primary HIV infection. Round to oval erythemato-squamous lesions, sometimes with a central crust.

Table 21.1. Grouping of HIV-associated dermatologic and venereal diseases.

Infectious dermatoses	Tumors	Non-infectious, non-tumorous skin diseases
Bacterial infections	Kaposi's sarcoma	Erythematous–squamous dermatoses
Viral infections	Lymphomas	Macular and/or papular dermatoses
Protozoan infections	Skin carcinomas	Itchy dermatoses
Fungal infections	Melanoma	Vesiculo-bullous dermatoses
Infestations		Solitary dermato-venereological conditions
		Hair disorders
		Nail disorders
		Pigment disorders
		Oral disorders

increases insight, and is of practical use when making a (differential) diagnosis.

Infectious dermatoses

Bacterial infections

Bacterial infections of the skin are seen less frequently in HIV-infected patients than viral infections, with the exception of babies and young children, where it is the other way around.

Pyodermas, caused by *Staphylococcus aureus* and *Streptococcus pyogenes*, can give unusual clinical pictures.

Examples are candidiasis-like intertriginous infection, plaque-like lesions (Figure 21.2) that can be treatment resistant, botryomycosis, and pruritic *S. aureus* folliculitis. The latter is in the differential diagnosis of itch in HIV infection.

Pseudomonas aeruginosa can be the cause of abscesses.

Mycobacterial infections caused by *Mycobacterium tuberculosis* and *M. avium intracellulare complex* in general are part of systemic disease. They appear as erythematous nodi, skin ulcers, or as miliary tuberculosis or lichen scrofulosorum. The influence of the HIV epidemic on leprosy still has to be determined.

Primary syphilis is one of the genital ulcer diseases that play an epidemiological role in HIV transmission. In the differential diagnosis, one should be aware of

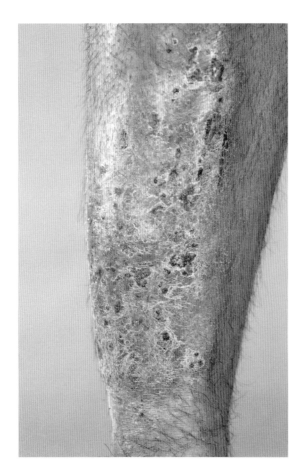

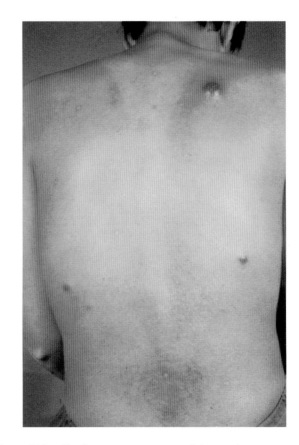

Figure 21.3. Bacillary angiomatosis, nodular erythematous lesions.

Figure 21.2. Treatment-resistant plaque-like *Staphylococcus aureus* infection on the lower leg.

ulcus molle, lymphogranuloma venereum, donovanosis, and, of course, herpes simplex. Secondary syphilis can display 'forgotten' pictures from the past, such as syphilis maligna with ulcerative skin lesions. In HIV-infected patients, the symptomatic stages of syphilis can succeed each other more quickly than usual. This especially concerns central nervous system involvement, demanding an adequate therapeutic regimen. Syphilis serology can provide unusual results, varying from false-negative to abnormally high titers [4].

Neisseria gonorrhoea and *N. meningitides* can cause disseminated infections.

Bacillary angiomatosis, initially known as epithelioid angiomatosis and cat-scratch disease in AIDS, is a disease newly recognized in HIV infection caused by *Bartonella* formerly *Rochalimaea henselae* or *B. quintana*. It is characterized by erythematous indurated nodular to tumorous skin lesions (Figure 21.3), with involvement of internal organs [5].

Viral infections

Viral skin and mucous membrane infections are frequently seen in HIV infection. The clinical picture can be atypical and the course chronic without spontaneous healing. Besides viral cultures, histopathological examination, including monoclonal antibodies, may be necessary to make the right diagnosis.

Herpes simplex virus (HSV) is often the cause of ulcerations, especially in the anogenital region. These ulcerations vary from a small fissure-like chronic defect in the anal rim to large ulcers (Figure 21.4). Besides that there is herpes simplex disseminata, with small ulcerative lesions disseminated over the body. Every ulcerative lesion in an HIV-infected individual has to be cultured routinely for viruses, especially HSV. Acyclovir resistance may cause a treatment problem.

varicella zoster virus is responsible for herpes zoster, known to be an early clinical sign of developing immunodeficiency. Later on in HIV infection varicella

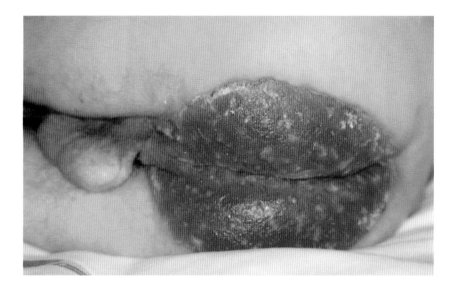

Figure 21.4. Perianal ulcer caused by *Herpes simplex* virus.

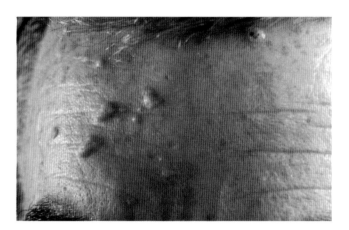

Figure 21.5. *Varicella zoster* hyperkeratoticum in the face.

zoster disseminata can be observed. Hyperkeratotic varicella zoster with wart-like lesions is a new entity in the HIV era (Figure 21.5). Here too, acyclovir resistance of the virus can be a problem.

Human papilloma virus infections, such as verrucae vulgares, verrucae planae and condylomata acuminata, generally produce familiar clinical pictures, but may deviate in seriousness and chronicity. Attention should be paid to the oncogenic potency of some of the viral strains, in view of cervical and anal cancer [6].

Oral hairy leukoplakia was first described in HIV-infected individuals. This new disease of the mucous membranes is caused by the Epstein–Barr virus. The clinical picture consists of linear or sometime more blotchy white lesions on the lateral sides of the tongue.

Mollusca contagiosa, a harmless self-limiting infection in children, can be a serious opportunistic infection in HIV-infected patients. The clinical picture varies from the well-known dome-shaped white papules with central umbilication to tumorous and cyst-like lesions, or even white macules or flat papules. They may be present in large numbers. There is a predilection for the face, especially the beard region.

Cytomegalovirus (CMV) infection of the skin as a primary disease seems to be rare. CMV can be found in histopathologic sections of known dermatoses in HIV-infected patients without giving a clear contribution to the disease, it is probably secondary to a generalized infection. CMV is sometimes cultured from skin ulcers, especially in the perianal region.

Protozoan infections

Skin manifestations due to protozoa are in general part of systemic infection. From the dermatological point of view, leishmaniasis is prominent; amoebiasis, toxoplasmosis and *Pneumocystis carinii* infection are only occasionally the cause of skin eruptions.

Leishmaniasis may appear as a primary cutaneous infection. However, inconspicuous papular skin lesions may be a symptom of visceral leishmaniasis. Venereal transmission seems possible.

Fungal infections

Candidiasis of the oral cavity can be an early symptom of HIV infection. When oesophageal candidiasis develops, this implies AIDS.

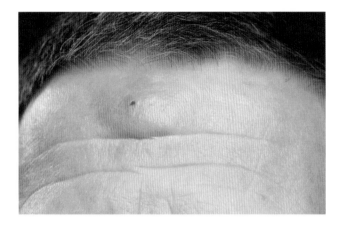

Figure 21.6. Cryptococcal plaque-like lesions with small ulcer on the forehead.

Pityrosporum ovale causes pityriasis versicolor, but more important in HIV-infected patients is pityrosporal folliculitis, which is in the differential diagnosis of itch.

Fungal infections of the feet, including the nails, are quite common in immunocompetent individuals and will, therefore, also be frequently seen in HIV-infected individuals. Fungal infections of the groins may show the familiar picture, an elevated border and central healing, but the presentation may be atypical with erythemato-squamous eczematous eruptions. White nails caused by *Trichophyton* species are a special feature in HIV infection. One should be prepared for rare fungal infections, the most important are cryptococcosis, histoplasmosis, coccidioidomycosis, and sporotrichosis.

In general, cryptococcosis is a disseminated infection. Skin lesions vary from papulopustular and plaque-like lesions (Figure 21.6) to molluscum contagiosum and herpes-like eruptions. Making the diagnosis is important in view of the recognition of internal disease, especially involvement of the central nervous system. In general, histoplasmosis of the skin is also part of a disseminated infection and may occur with a variety of skin lesions similar to those described in cryptococcosis.

Infestations

Sarcoptus scabiei infestation is one of the causes of itch in HIV infection. The clinical picture varies from the usual appearance to scabies Norvegica. *Demodex* folliculitis is also in the differential diagnosis of itch in HIV infection.

Skin tumors

Kaposi's sarcoma is the main skin tumor in HIV infection. The histopathology shows a proliferation of endothelial cells with vessel-like structures and slits containing erythrocytes. In older lesions a spindle cell component is present, representing transformed endothelial cells. Epidemiological data gave support to a sexually transmittable agent, facilitated by HIV. Recently human herpesvirus 8 (HHV8), also called Kaposi Sarcoma Herpesvirus (KSHV), by several investigators has been indicated as being the causal organism [7]. Kaposi's sarcoma of the skin is a polymorph disease The 'typical' lesion is an oval, purple-red, nodular lesion with the axis following the lines of cleavage of the skin. However, lesions can also be plaque-like, psoriatiform (Figure 21.7), or deep-seated nodules, and, on the nose, lupus pernio-like. Obstruction of the lymphatics may cause lymphoedema, especially on the legs, the genitals (Figure 21.8), and around the eyes. Internal localizations may form a serious complication. Skin lesions can be treated locally with

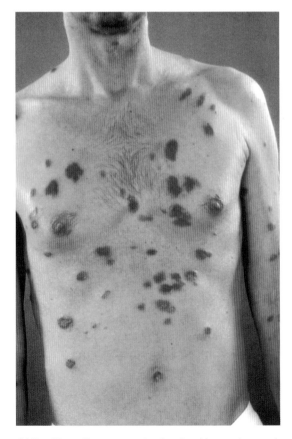

Figure 21.7. Kaposi's sarcoma, in the shoulder region oval-nodular and on the trunk plaque-like lesions, some psoriatiform.

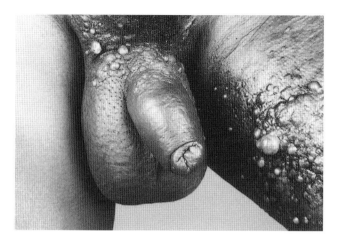

Figure 21.8. Late-stage Kaposi's sarcoma with nodular lesions, and as a complication edema of the left leg and genitals.

intralesional diluted vinblastine, radiotherapy, or cryosurgery. When the disease is extensive, systemic chemotherapy can be indicated [7].

B-cell and T-cell lymphomas are also quite common neoplasms in HIV-infected patients [8]. Skin lesions may be part of the disease and may be the revealing symptom, varying from erythematous nodules to skin ulcers.

Up to now, skin cancers and melanoma have been relatively rare in HIV infection, possibly because the patients are usually young when infected and the survival time of the patients is limited. A longer life span may result in an increase [9,10].

Non-infectious, non-tumorous skin diseases

Non-infectious, non-tumorous skin diseases in HIV infection can be subdivided according to their clinical characteristics, when necessary in conjunction with histopathological criteria.

Erythemato-squamous dermatoses

Seborrheic dermatitis is frequently seen in HIV infection, often as an early skin symptom. Being a common disease in non-HIV-infected persons, it is not to be used as an indicative for HIV infection in patients of the HIV-risk groups. HIV infection is often accompanied by a dry skin, which may develop into asteatotic eczema or even into acquired ichthyosis. Besides these, psoriasis, psoriatiform eruptions, morbus

Reiter, pityriasis rosea, pityriasis rubra pilaris, acrodermatitis enteropathica, lichen spinulosis and Kawasaki syndrome [11] have been described in HIV infection. Drug eruptions are part of the differential diagnosis. Erythroderma may be a complication of the diseases mentioned.

Macular and/or papular dermatoses

Some of the dermatoses in this group are of the interface dermatitis type with hydropic degeneration of the basal cell layer, possibly an autoimmune phenomenon. Examples are interface dermatitis in AIDS, lichenoid granulomatous papular dermatosis, and erythema dyschromicum perstans. Other skin diseases belonging to this group are granuloma annulare, erythema elevatum diutinum and Gianotti–Crosti syndrome [12]. Once again, drug eruptions are mentioned in the differential diagnosis.

Itchy skin diseases

Itch is a frequent complaint in HIV-infected patients, with a multitude of causes. A subdivision into non-follicular and follicular itchy skin diseases can be made. The first group includes the prurigo parasitaria-like eruption in HIV infection, the pruritic papular eruption of AIDS, dry skin, seborrheic dermatitis and other eczematous conditions, the hypereosinophilic syndrome, drug eruptions, scabies, prurigo and pruritus, that is, itch without perceptible skin disease. In the second group are erythematous papular or papulo-pustular follicular eruptions occur, including eosinophilic pustular folliculitis in HIV infection (Figure 21.9) (formerly thought to be analogous to Ofuji's disease but, because of a different clinical picture now separated from this disease), pityrosporal folliculitis, *Demodex* folliculitis, itchy *S. aureus* folliculitis, itchy folliculitis e.c.i., and itchy folliculitis with a combination of the causes mentioned (Figure 21.10) [13].

Vesiculo-bullous skin diseases

The main diseases in this group are erythema multiforme, toxic epidermal necrolysis and porphyria.

Solitary dermato-venereological conditions

A rest group, including diseases such as some drug eruptions and exanthemas which are infectious or

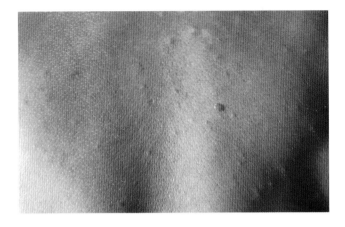

Figure 21.9.   Eosinophilic pustular folliculitis in HIV infection on the back.

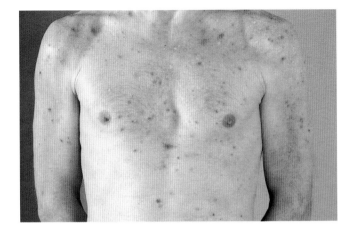

Figure 21.10.   Multicausal itching folliculitis. *Demodex folliculorum* was found, *S. aureus* was cultured. The histopathologic diagnosis was eosinophilic pustular folliculitis.

without a clear cause, Foscarnet balanitis/vulvitis, genital ulcers without a clear cause, vasculitis, and erythema nodosum.

Hair, nail, pigment and oral disorders

HIV-associated abnormalities of hair are thinning and premature greying. Nail changes comprise, beside fungal infections, the yellow nail syndrome and zidovudine pigmentation. Pigment disorders are vitiligo and hyperpigmentation caused by zidovudine. The main oral disorders, besides candidiasis, hairy leukoplakia, and Kaposi's sarcoma, are gingivitis and parodonitis, and ulcers with a multitude of causes [14].

Dermatologic/venereal diseases and immunodeficiency

The skin diseases described in this chapter are derived from the literature on HIV and may be called 'HIV-associated' diseases. This implies that, when a patient

at risk appears to have one of these diseases, HIV infection may be suspected. However, one has to be careful, because most of these skin diseases can be seen also in non-HIV-infected persons. Only a few skin diseases are defining for AIDS, and in general it is impossible to conclude that a patient has AIDS based on skin symptoms in HIV-infected patients.

Some diseases, however, can be an indication of severe immunodeficiency, represented by low CD4+ lymphocyte counts. Based on investigations in a group of HIV-infected patients seen in the Academic Medical Center in Amsterdam from the beginning of the HIV epidemic up to July 1992, concerning 530 patients with a total of 1754 dermato-venerologic diagnoses, it was concluded that herpes simplex ulcera, herpes simplex and varicella zoster disseminata, hyperkeratotic varicella zoster, mollusca contagiosa, lymphomas, asteatotic eczema, and acquired ichthyosis are skin signs of severe immunodeficiency. In spite of this, the diagnosis of AIDS, according to the definition by the Centers for Disease Control (1987), in general only had been made in about half of the patients with these diseases [15].

References

1 Penneys NS. *Skin manifestations of AIDS. Second Edition.* London: Martin Dunitz, 1995.

2 Ansary MA, Hira Sk, Bayley AC et al. *A Colour Atlas of AIDS in the Tropics.* Ipswich: Wolfe Medical Publications, 1989.

3 Jong M de, Hulsebosch HJ, Lange JMA. Clinical and immunological features of primary HIV-1 infection. *Genitourin Med* 1991; **67**: 367–373.

4 Engelkens JH, Sluis J van der, Stolz E. Syphilis in the AIDS era. *Intern J Dermatol* 1991; **30**: 254–256.

5 Cockerell CJ. Bacillary angiomatosis and related diseases caused by *Rochalimaea. J Am Acad Dermatol* 1995; **32**: 703–790.

6 Palefski JM. Anal human papillomavirus infection and anal cancer in HIV-positive individuals: an emerging problem. *AIDS* 1994; **8**: 283–295.

7 Lee F-C, Mitsuyasu RT, Miles SA. Kaposi's sarcoma: relationship to a novel herpesvirus and advances in therapy. *AIDS* 1996; **10**(suppl A): S173–179.

8 Kerschmann RL, Berger TG, Weiss LM et al. Cutaneous presentations of lymphoma in human immunodeficiency virus disease. *Arch Dermatol* 1995; **131**: 1281–1282.

9 Smith KJ, Skelton HG, Yeager J et al. Cutaneous neoplasms in a military population of HIV-1-positive patients. *J Am Acad Dermatol* 1993; **29**: 400–406.

10 McGregor JM, Newell M, Ross J et al. Cutaneous malignant melanoma and human immunodeficiency virus (HIV) infections: report of three cases. *Br J Dermatol* 1992; **126**: 516–519.

11 Bayrou O, Phlippoteau C, Artigou C et al. Adult Kawasaki syndrome associated with HIV infection and anticardiolipin antibodies. *J Am Acad Dermatol* 1993; **29**: 663–664.

12 Blauvelt A, Turner ML. Gianotti–Crosti syndrome and human immunodeficiency virus infection. *Arch Dermatol* 1994; **130**: 481–483.

13 Hulsebosch HJ. AIDS and itch. *J Europ Acad Dermatol* 1992; **1**: 311–318. [Published erratum of legends/figures appears in *J Europ Acad Dermatol* 1993; **2**: 62.]

14 Itin PH, Lautenschlager S, Flücker R et al. Oral manifestations in HIV-infected patients: diagnosis and management. *J Am Acad Dermatol* 1993; **29**: 749–760.

15 Hulsebosch HJ. *Huidziekten bij HIV-infecties.* Thesis, Amsterdam, 1993.

22 MUSCULOSKELETAL IMAGING IN AIDS

Donna Magid

Introduction

Since the recognition of human immune deficiency virus (HIV)-associated disease 17 years ago, the profile of 'typical' clinical musculoskeletal manifestations has changed. As supportive or suppressive therapy allows prolonged survival, we are seeing an expanding population manifesting the consequences of chronic immunosuppression and illness.

Most early musculoskeletal reports focused on the widespread resurgence of opportunistic infections and tumors which had been quite rare before HIV. More recent reports have explored the possible association between HIV and various inflammatory or arthritic manifestations.

Conventional radiography remains the gateway to diagnostic imaging. In an era of increasing economic limitations, it provides a readily available and economically feasible starting point for diagnostic assessment. It may suggest a diagnosis not yet considered (e.g. tumor or avascular necrosis in a patient with joint pain) (Figure 22.1), or confirm a clinical suspicion. Imaging suspected musculoskeletal disease in the HIV patients is more different in quantity than quality from other patients; both the clinical and radiographic signs may be far more subtle than usual.

Computed tomography (CT) was still relatively new and not yet routinely available during the earliest part of the epidemic and magnetic resonance imaging (MRI) became clinically available halfway into the first decade of the acquired immune deficiency syndrome (AIDS). Musculoskeletal scintigraphy became more sophisticated in the 1980s, as the development and availability of specially tagged cells or agents extended the scope and selectivity of available diagnostic tests.

In the face of increasingly complex and subtle clinical musculoskeletal problems, diagnostic imaging may play a major role in patient care and research. This chapter will review some aspects of diagnostic imaging of the spectrum of musculoskeletal involvement in the HIV patient.

Musculoskeletal involvement

Unlike the lungs, gastrointestinal tract, and central nervous system, the musculoskeletal system tends not to be involved in the early stages of HIV-related disease. In patients with more advanced HIV infection, infections are the most common musculoskeletal abnormality, but avascular necrosis, arthritis, lymphoma, and Kaposi's sarcoma may also be seen.

Soft tissue and bone infections may result from a combination of changes in host immunity and the induced risks of underlying behaviors associated with the transmission of the original virus. Some authors note an increased incidence of Kaposi's sarcoma in homosexual patients, or of septic arthritis or other rheumatoid-like arthridites in intravenous drug abusers (IVDA) infected with HIV [1]. Opportunistic infections which once were rarely identified have become increasingly common in the HIV-positive population. *Nocardia asteroides*, *Cryptococcus neoformans*, *Sporothrix schenkii*, *Campylobacter fetus*, fungal osteomyelitis, and bacillary angiomatosis due to a rickettsia-like organism have all been reported [2,3].

In approaching the HIV patient with potential musculoskeletal involvement, the only rule is to disregard the conventional rules. Infection or disease may be subtle, with subdued clinical or laboratory presentation; agents may be atypical or unpredictable in behaviour or location; and therapeutic response may be slow and difficult to document.

Cellulitis and lymphedema

Cellulitis is a readily detectable superficial manifestation of inflammation which may be diagnosed without

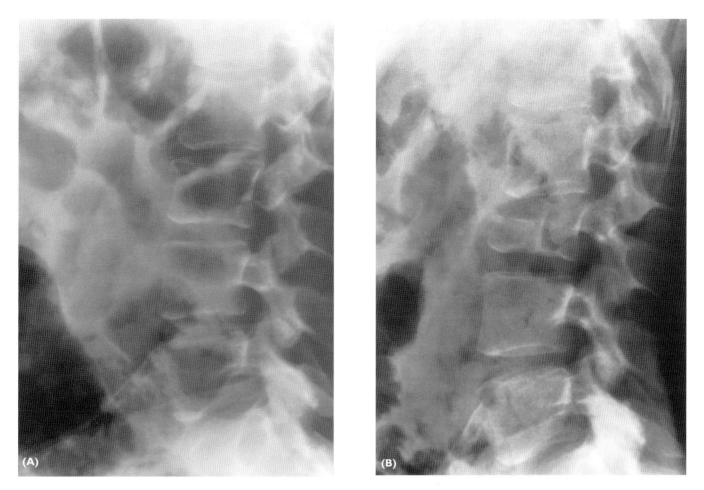

Figure 22.1. (A) A 37-year-old HIV-positive female with a previous history of steroid administration, osteopenia, and previous hip arthroplasty. Lateral lumbar spine taken for back pain showed very minimal deformity of the superior end plate of L3 with minimal disc space narrowing at L2–3. (B) Six weeks later, she returned complaining of increasing back pain. Since the earlier examination, repeat lateral lumbar spine film now shows marked compression and anterior wedging of L3 with minimal further loss of lumbar lordosis.

supporting symtomatology or laboratory evidence. However, a superficial primary cellulitis or erysipelas must be distinguished from changes representing the visible component of a deeper infection. When such an underlying process generates a mass effect or is accompanied by drainage, the need to pursue the underlying process is obvious. In the HIV patient, however, presentation may be more subtle. Conventional radiography is limited in assessing soft tissue changes; extensive soft tissue edema or distortion of fascial planes may be underestimated or missed. CT is more sensitive to subtle soft tissue attenuation or contour changes, will detect underlying abscess or fluid collection, and may suggest underlying osteomyelitis or tumor. In the extremities, cellulitis elevates the normal subcutaneous fat attenuation (–90 to –110 HU) to approximate that of surrounding soft tissue.

The change is often geographic, but homogeneous and featureless (Figure 22.2). If an underlying etiology, such as abscess or hematoma, is suggested, CT-guided aspiration may confirm the diagnosis.

The patient with chronic soft-tissue inflammation or ulceration may demonstrate periosteal or cortical changes locally. Since progression to osteomyelitis would warrant more aggressive treatment, it is desirable to distinguish between reactive hyperemia with secondary osseous changes, and true osseous infection. This can be a frustrating, expensive, and unsatisfying clinical and radiographic pursuit; specialized imaging may add to the cost and complexity of patient assessment without being definitive. In some cases, sequential plain films may still offer the simplest and most cost-effective means of following secondary bone changes (Figure 22.3).

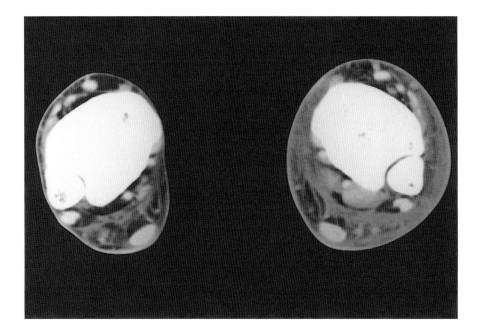

Figure 22.2. A middle-aged male with diffuse lower extremity swelling and palpable groin adenopathy and lymphedema. One transaxial CT with narrow windows, through the proximal calf, demonstrates enlargement of the left side compared to the right. The underlying muscles are symmetric in size, shape, and attenuation. The left subcutaneous tissue is diffusely engorged and reticulated, with moderate diffuse skin thickening, compatible with lymphedema.

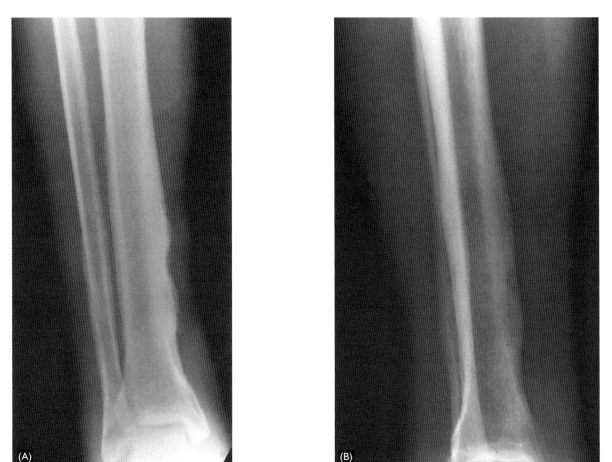

Figure 22.3. (A) A 45-year-old male lower leg. A radiograph shows acute, fluffy periositis suggesting possible active osteomyelitis. (B) Follow-up radiograph shows increasing consolidation and maturation of 10 cm of focal cortical thickening and periositis, 4 months later. There had been no significant changes in symptoms or laboratory values; the radiographic progression towards healing allowed cautious optimism that this process might be resolving.

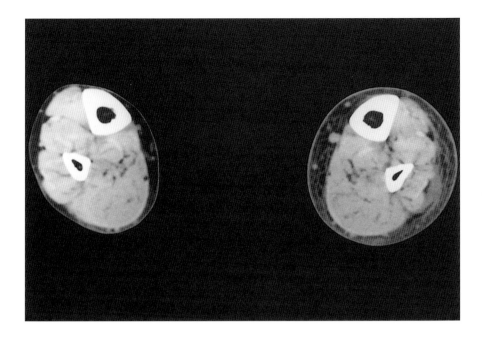

Figure 22.4. Transverse CT at narrow windows, just proximal to the ankle. There is marked, diffuse, left, soft-tissue swelling, primarily of the subcutaneous compartment. The usual subcutaneous fat density has been replaced by largely homogenous soft tissue or fluid attenuation, without definite focal abscess or fluid. There is no definite skin thickening or asymmetry compared to the normal right side. These changes are compatible with cellulitis.

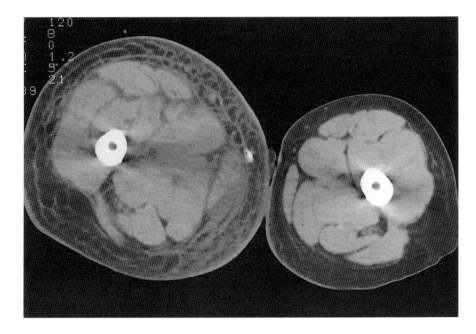

Figure 22.5. A 40-year-old HIV-positive IVDA female, with marked swelling of the lower extremity. CT demonstrated marked coarse diffuse honeycombing of the subcutaneous fat of the hip and thigh compatible with lymphedema. There was marked skin thickening compared to the normal left side. There was also diffuse enlargement of the underlying muscle groups, particularly in the medial compartment, with very minimal decreased attenuation in the enlarged adductor magnus muscle. A minimal amount of fluid was seen localized around the sartorius muscle. It was felt that these findings represented lymphedema with a mild myositis. This responded initially to antibiotics. However, she subsequently returned with upper extremity pain and swelling, and a triceps abscess.

Lymphedema creates more of a textured or reticulated subcutaneous pattern on CT, with tissue-attentuation septae running through the more normal subcutaneous fat attenuation (Figure 22.4). Lymphedema may be primary or secondary to a more proximal obstructive/destructive process. Either way, the edema and sluggish lymphatic fluids may encourage secondary or opportunistic infection. CT can be useful in characterizing lymphedema, and in searching for the more proximal mass or adenopathy which may be responsible for the extremity changes. Kaposi's sarcoma may cause more proximal lymphadenopathy and obstruction [4,5].

Muscle and soft-tissue infection

Myositis has been reported secondary to multiple bacterial agents [2,6]. Changes in muscle size, contour,

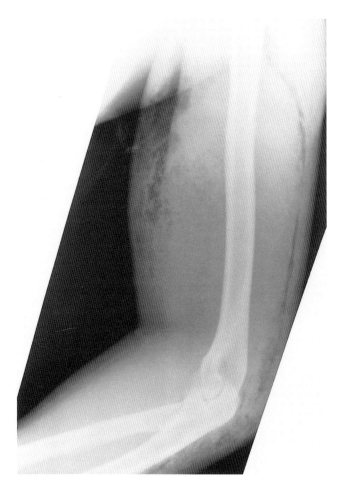

Figure 22.6. A 29-year-old HIV-positive IVDA female, presenting in septic shock. She had soft tissue crepitence of the upper extremity, shoulder and chest wall. A plain film of the upper arm demonstrated extensive gas, which appeared to follow fascial planes of the posterior upper arm but which were diffusely distributed over the anterior arm and the chest wall. She was admitted directly to the operating room in shock, and it was anticipated she would not survive. The upper extremity was partially degloved with stripping of the fascia; at the debridement, extensive necrotic fascia was resected, with far less involvement of underlying muscle than had been expected. Cultures were positive for hemolytic streptococcus, apparently confined to the fascia. There was extensive superficial venous thrombosis. The patient survived the procedure and subsequently underwent reconstruction and soft tissue grafts.

CT attenuation, or MRI signal may be seen in the absence of associated osteomyelitis or trauma. The overlying subcutaneous fat may remain normal, or may demonstrate lymphedema or cellulitis [6]. Although intact skeletal muscle ordinarily resists infection, the patient with HIV combines multifactorial immuno-suppression with potentially myotoxic medications [7] and, in some cases, intravenous drug abuse. Injections

may traumatize muscle, creating hematoma or com-promised tissue easily colonized either by direct inoculum or secondary to septicemia.

Myonecrosis may be produced under sterile con-ditions, or may be secondary to or complicated by infection. Non-clostridial infection appears to be com-mon at our institution, where the majority of HIV patients have a history of intravenous drug abuse. Tissue trauma under non-sterile circumstances, occa-sionally compounded by prolonged immobility, rapidly destructive and progressive infection. CT of involved muscle shows feathery intramuscular air in clostridial myonecrosis; but intramuscular gas may also occur secondary to inoculation, trauma, or intestinal perfo-ration. On CT, myonecrotic tissue has a lower attenuation than normal muscle, and is often swollen or distorted. Unlike abscess, this tissue is diffusely devascularized and will not enhance with contrast injection at CT or MRI.

Soft-tissue gas also may be seen with necrotizing fascitis (often streptococcal) or crepitant cellulitis (Figure 22.6). Conventional radiography may suggest a fascial plane distribution, although CT will provide a far more precise confirmation and characterization of gas distribution. At CT, fascitis is represented by extramuscular gas collections following fascial planes, with relatively normal underlying muscle attenuation and contour.

CT may be the next logical step in pursuing suspected, deep, soft-tissue infection or drainage, or re-section as deemed clinically appropriate. Diffuse homo-geneous changes in attenuation may be more difficult to appreciate than a focal finding such as abscess or calcification. Routine review of each study with narowed ('soft tissue or 'liver') window center and window width, and comparison to the contralateral (presumably normal) side, are helpful in enhancing appreciation of subtle attenuation changes. Where the contralateral side is not available, other muscle may provide an internal standard; myonecrosis may be multifocal but tends not to involve multiple compart-ments within an extremity. Intravenous contrast will increase the attenuation of normal muscle, widening the gap between normal and necrotic tissue, and can be used where the unenhanced study is borderline or equivocal.

MRI is even more sensitive than CT to changes in muscle or fascia. Primarily, intramuscular processes should be accompanied by only minimal, if any, changes in the signal characteristics of overlying

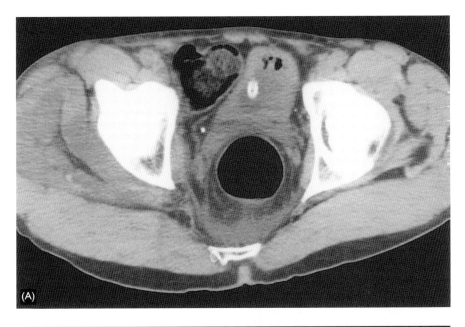

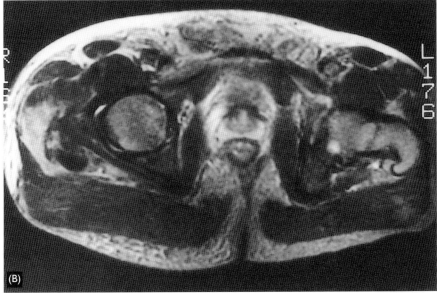

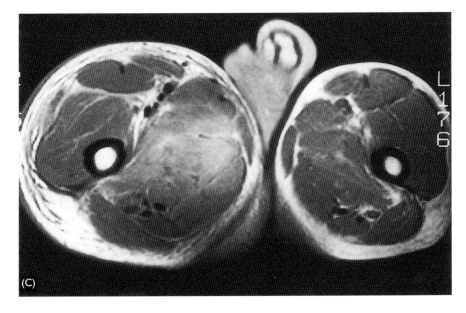

Figure 22.7. (A) A 41-year-old Black male, HIV-positive IVDA, who fell down a flight of steps during an episode of altered mental status. Transaxial CT scan through the hips shows marked enlargement and decreased attenuation of the right gluteus medius, with preservation of fascial planes and no focal fluid collections, compatible with myonecrosis. (B) this was confirmed on an MRI (1.5 T, TR 2500, TE 20), which also showed increased signal density and enlargement of the same muscle, with preservation of normal margins and interfaces. (C) MRI through the proximal thigh demonstrates diffuse enlargement and slightly heterogeneous increased signal attenuation of the right adductor muscle groups and diffuse enlargement of the entire thigh, primarily due to this compartment's enlargement. There is some right subcutaneous edema. The findings and clinical course were compatible with non-clostridial myonecrosis.

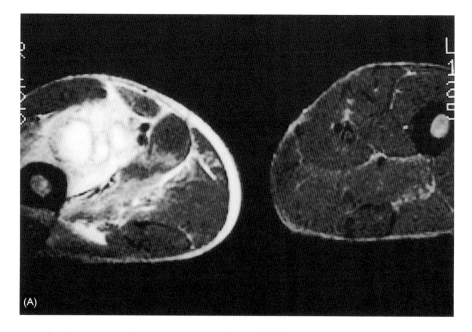

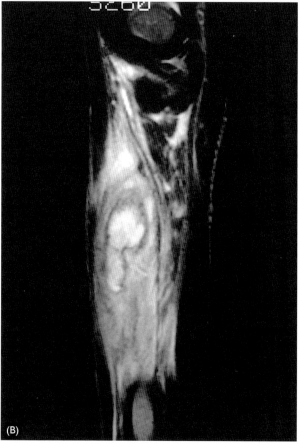

Figure 22.8. (A) Intramuscular abscess. A 34-year-old HIV-positive male with new onset seizures and one month of right knee and thigh pain. CT of the brain showed multiple lesions in the right frontal lobe suggesting toxoplasmosis, lymphoma, or metastasis. Transaxial MRI of the thigh (!.5 T, TR 2500, TE 80) demonstrated enlargement of the vastus intermedius and medialis with diffuse increased signal intensity. An 11 × 5 × 5 cm high signal intensity area of central fluid or necrosis was seen, which on T_1-weighted images had a suggestion of peripheral hemorrhage. (B) Coronal MRI (TR 2400, TE 80) confirmed the sharply demarcated fluid or abscess with the lower signal attenuation margin.

subcutaneous tissues. In myonecrosis, intravenous enhancement will be unable to perfuse the devascularized muscle, increasing the signal contrast between normal and affected muscle. As with CT, changes in signal, size, and contour may be readily noted when the contralateral side can serve as a control (Figure 22.7). Myonecrosis may be difficult to identify on T_1-weighted images but may be seen as high signal intensity on STIR or spin-density $>T_2$-weighted images [8]. MRI readily distinguished between fat and edema, increasing specificity.

It has been suggested that MRI may be useful in distinguishing superficial, non-necrotizing cellulitis from the clinically more urgent, necrotizing, soft-tissue infection. Necrotizing infections appear to be associated with a hyperintense signal from the deep fascia on T_2-weighted images, probably due to fluid from necrosis. Superficial processes do not affect the deeper tissue planes. It is also suggested that selective fat-saturated T_2-weighted images (for edema) or post-contrast fat-saturated T_1 images (for pathologic changes) may increase detection of subtle deep tissue changes [9].

Abscess

At either CT or MRI, a focal soft-tissue abscess may be defined as a focal abnormality with attenuation or signal characteristics suggesting a fluid content, with or without a distinct tissue rim (Figures 22.8 and 22.9). The relative hyperemia of the rim may produce ring

enhancement when intravenous is used in the CT study. CT can be used for identification, localization, percutaneous aspiration, or drainage, and to confirm resolution. Recent MRI reports have noted the presence of a hyperintense rim on T_1-weighted images, and speculate that paramagnetic material may be responsible for the peripheral drop in T_1 [2,8]. However, to date there have been insufficient cases studied and biopsied to allow firm conclusions to be drawn.

Osteomyelitis

The conventional radiographic features of osteomyelitis are well documented in the literature. Radiographs cannot detect very early osteomyelitis, although the HIV patient tends to present with more advanced disease than the non-immunocompromised population. Host factors both facilitate the progression of infection and mute its clinical expression, delaying diagnosis and treatment. Response to therapy may be slow or incomplete. Both the axial and appendicular skeleton are at risk. While the agents most common in the non-compromised population (*Staphylococcus aureus*, *Salmonella*) continue to predominate, they are joined by opportunistic agents such as *Nocardia asteroides*, *Cryptococcus neoformans*, or *Mycobacterium haemophilum* (or, more commonly, *Mycobacterium avium*). There is an increased risk of post-operative musculoskeletal infections in the postoperative orthopaedic patient, with or without implanted hardware (Figure 22.10).

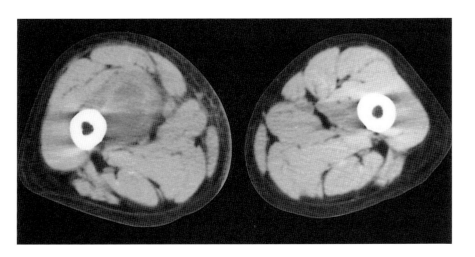

Figure 22.9. A 35-year-old female with a history of IVDA and HIV infection, with a drainage-proven abscess of the right vastus medialus. Non-contrast transaxial CT of the proximal thigh at tissue windows demonstrates enlargement and slight decrease in attenuation of the right vastus medialus, with a large, loculated, lower attenuation fluid collection centrally. The anterior and medial subcutaneous tissue demonstrates some streaky increased attenuation compatible with local cellulitis. Technetium-99m bone scan demonstrated increased blood flow and blood pooling without osteomyelitis. This 13 cm long collection was percutaneous drained, with adequate drainage of the locules confirmed by post-procedure CT.

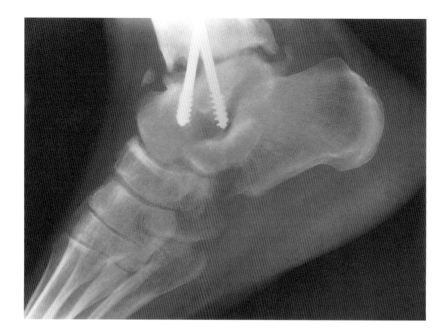

Figure 22.10. A 31-year-old HIV-positive male with a CD4 of 650 and infected non-union of the tibio-talar joint. Lateral film of the ankle shows sclerosis of the apposed tibio-talar remnants, without definite signs of osteomyelitis and without definite screw loosening. Surgically proven osteomyelitis.

As the HIV epidemic has progressed, a new form of multisystemic bacterial infection occasionally producing symptomatic osteolytic lesions and responding to antibiotics, bacillary angiomatosis, has been described [10]. The agent is believed to be a ricksettsial-type bacteria. Bone lesions, skin lesions, and systemic symptoms may be present, although synchronous; cutaneous presentation is the most common and may resemble Kaposi's sarcoma. Bacillary angiomatosis, however, responds rapidly to antibiotic treatment, even in the setting of immunocompromise.

In our institution, a number of HIV-positive patients with vague abdominal pain have been found at CT to have previously unsuspected thoracolumbar tuberculosis [4] (Figure 22.11). Tuberculosis is disproportionately present in the HIV-positive population; and can be expected to become more of a problem as increasingly drug-resistant strains continue to emerge. Unusual or fastidious strains of mycobacterial osteomyelitis (*Mycobacterium haemophilum*, *Mycobacterium avium intracellulare*) have also been reported [11]. Pyogenic vertebral infections may also be clinically modified in the HIV-positive population, presenting with a vaguer, more subdued clinical picture (Figure 22.12).

Avascular necrosis

There have been reports of avascular necrosis (AVN) in patients carrying the HIV [12,13], although causality is uncertain. Some, but not all, may be associated with previous steroid medication. Possible associated or contributing factors may include the autoimmune aspects of progressive HIV infection, vasculitis and subsequent vascular compromise, zidovudine therapy, or circulating antiphospholipid antibodies [12,13].

The HIV-positive patient with hip pain and radiographic AVN may pose a diagnostic dilemma. It may be impossible to distinguish between sterile and septic causes of new or increasing hip pain.

Anecdotally speaking, in our institution, where HIV most commonly is associated with IVDA, we have seen several patients with sufficient radiographic AVN (and insufficient clinical evidence of infection) to explain hip symptoms. However, diagnostic aspiration produced culture-proven acute infections in three such patients, only one of whom had any radiographic signs suggesting the coexistence of two disease processes (Figure 22.13). We have a low threshold to aspirate patients even with typical radiographic AVN, and move promptly in any patient with even minimal focal asymmetric osteopenia or trabecular loss, bone erosion, or permeative pattern superimposed on conventional radiographic AVN.

Rheumatic disease

There have been many, often conflicting, reports examining the possible association between non-septic, rheumatoid variant arthritides and HIV infection

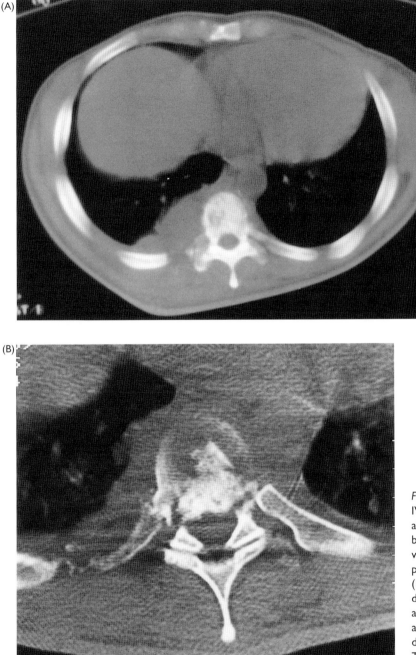

Figure 22.11. (A) A 39-year-old, male, HIV-positive IVDA seen elsewhere for fever and ill-defined abdominal pain. At transfer to our hospital, he brought an outside CT demonstrating lower thoracic vertebral body destruction, and marked paravertebral soft tissue mass or fluid collection. (B) A repeat CT zoomed to cone on the spine demonstrated extensive vertebral body destruction at T8, extending into the right transverse process and posterior rib, with a large, irregular, fluid density, soft-tissue mass in the paravertebral area. This turned out to be tuberculosis osteomyelitis.

[14–16]. Reiter's syndrome, psoriatic arthritis, polymyositis, Sjögren's syndrome, and undifferentiated seronegative spondyloarthropathies are among the possibly associated rheumatic or immune conditions. The relatively rare appearance of arthritis in AIDS associated with intravenous drug abuse, as opposed to AIDS associated with homosexuality, is a reminder of the complexity of the interacting risk factors. It will be difficult to separate the potential input of the pre-existing at-risk behaviors from the multifactorial input of systemic immunodepression, increased arthrotoxicity of the virus itself, or possible side effects of various therapies [17]. Reiter's syndrome was the first arthritis associated with HIV infections [18]. In such patients, Reiter's syndrome is believed to be otherwise identical to manifestations seen in non-infected patients; with asymmetric oligo-articular lower extremity involvement, enthesopathies, refractory erosive arthritis, and the usual non-musculoskeletal manifestations (Figure 22.14). The steroids or cytotoxic therapies to

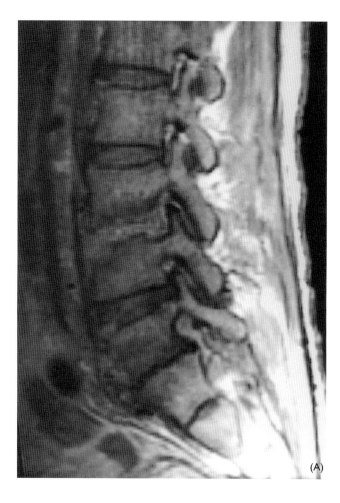

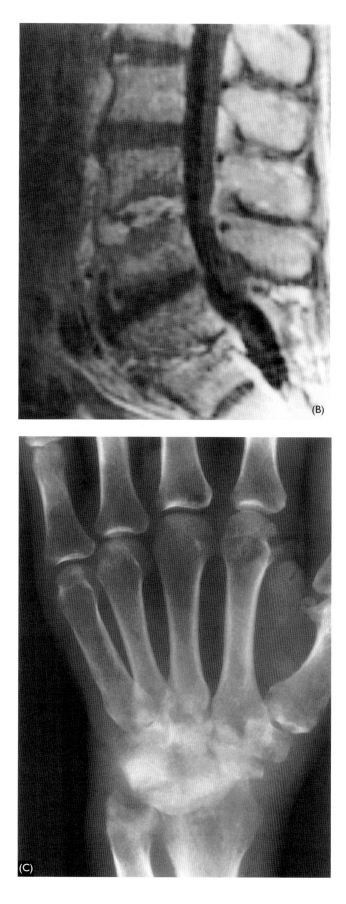

Figure 22.12. A 56-year-old HIV-positive man with increasing back pain, fevers, and polyarthritis. He also had S. Aureus subacute bacterial endocarditis. Lumbar spine MRI pre-(A) and post-(B) gadolinium injection demonstrates destruction of the inferior L3 and superior L4 end plates, preinjection (A, TR 3000, TE 28). Postinjection (B, TR 500, TRE 10) there is intense enhancement of the L3–4 disc, and mild enhancement at L5–1, with small fluid collection anterior to the L4 vertebral body which mildly enhances. The changes diagnosis was S. aureus discitis and osteomyelitis at L3–L4 extending through L5–S1, with probable abscess anterior to the L4 vertebral body. Plain films of multiple joints are obtained at the same time, demonstrating small needle fragments in the neck. (C) A plain film of the wrist showed marked osteopenia and destruction of the articular distal radius and ulna and proximal carpus, suggesting multifocal septic arthritis.

(A)

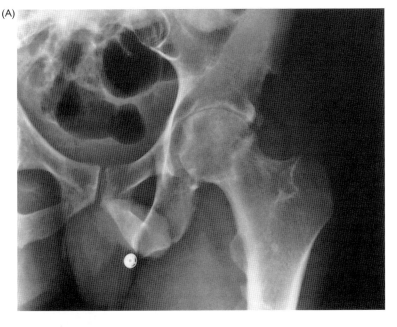

(B)

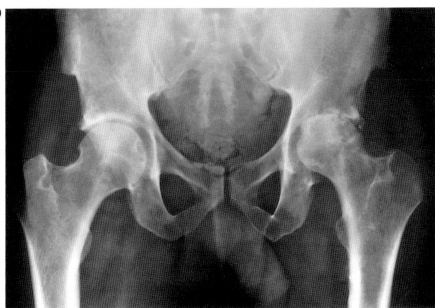

Figure 22.13. A 45-year-old, male, HIV-positive IVDA with a remote history of left thigh gunshot injury, and a history of psoas abscess 8 weeks prior to presenting with left hip pain. Initial plain film showed early collapse of the left femoral head superior pole from AVN, with superior joint space narrowing. There were no clinical or CT signs of infection at this time, and it was felt that the AVN explained his symptoms. However, he returned 6 weeks later complaining of increasing pain. (B) A radiograph at this time showed increase in femoral head sclerosis and deformity compatible with progression of AVN, but also showed increasing loss of definition of the trabeculae of the roof, suggesting possible superimposed infection. Aspiration was positive for *S. aureus* and he underwent resection arthroplasty. Postoperatively, he continued to spike fevers and was re-explored.

which non-infected patients may respond are contra-indicated in the presence of known HIV infection, compromising therapeutic response in this and other arthritic conditions.

While the causality remains in dispute, it is important for orthopaedists, rheumatologists, and musculo-skeletal radiologists to consider the possibilty of HIV infection when patients of known or suspected high risk present with Reiter's disease, cutaneous or skeletal psoriasis, seronegative spondyloarthropathy or entheso-pathy, or any unexplained oligoarthritis.

Neoplasms

If the immune system participates in life-long vigilance against neoplasm, then it follows that epidemic immunosuppression will allow a rise in the incidence of neoplasms. Kaposi's sarcoma was the first associated neoplasm; while involving mutiple organ systems, this tumor tends to spare the bone and bone marrow. One report described one patient with multifocal osteolytic leions of the axial skeleton, and a second patient with permeative local destruction [2]. Biopsy confirmation

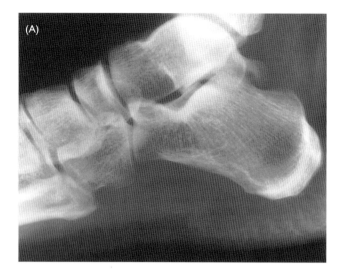

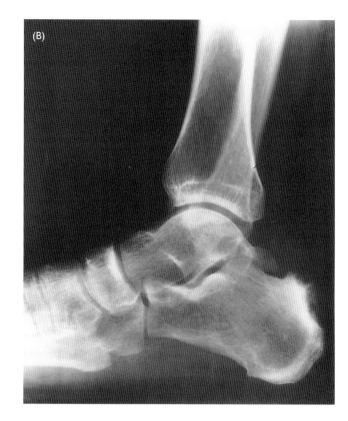

Figure 22.14. (A) A 39-year-old male with multiple risk factors for HIV infection, with radiographically documented rapid onset of changes compatible with Reiter's disease in the hind foot over a 23 month period. Initial radiograph demonstrated ill-defined focal soft tissue swelling posterior to the calcaneus, no significant bony abnormality. (B) Less than 2 years later, there are fluffy erosions and periostitis of the posterior superior calcaneus at the insertion of the gastrocnemius and a small plantar spur. There had also been one episode of urethritis.

may be necessary to direct therapy. It is of interest and importance to note that not all of the recognized sites in the first patient demonstrated technetium-99m MDP uptake; such a survey, if negative, is not conclusive. Radiographs detect such lytic lesions but are less sensitive than CT or MRI. However, both of the latter are usually reserved for targeted studies rather than skeletal surveys. CT will be of more use with primarily osseous findings, for Kaposi's sarcoma or other neoplasms. MRI may be more useful for muscle or marrow involvement.

Non-Hodgkin lymphoma may be as much as 60 times more common in AIDS patients than in the general population [19]. Both secondary and primary bone and bone marrow involvement have been described. HIV-associated lymphoma is aggressive and carries a poor prognosis.

Conclusion

We have not yet developed an effective vaccine or treatment for HIV infection. The progression and maturation of this epidemic has changed the practice of medicine. Musculoskeletal imaging, as other medical fields, is confronted with an increasingly complex array of associated infections, inflammatory, arthritic, and neoplastic conditions. A high level of suspicion and an awareness of the non-specificity of the clinical and radiographic manifestations of many of these conditions may help in recognizing and diagnosing these abnormalities.

References

1 Rivera J, Monteagudo I, Lopez-Longo J, Sanchez-Atrio A. Septic arthritis in acquired immunodeficiency syndrome, with human immordeficiency virus infection. *J Rheum* 1992; **19**: 12–14.

2 Steinbach LS, Tehranzadeh J, Fleckenstein JC, Vanarthos WJ. Human immunodeficiency virus infection: musculoskeletal manifestations. *Radiology* 1993; **186**: 833–838.

3 Sabbagh M, Meyer O, DeBandt M et al. Bone manifestations associated with AIDS. *Ann Med Interne* 1992; **143**: 50–56.

4 Magid D, Fishman EK. Musculoskeletal infections in patients with AIDS: CT findings. *AJR* 1992; **158**: 603–607.

5 Magid D, Fishman EK. Musculoskeletal infections. In: Kuhlman JE (ed) *CT of the Immunocompromised Host. Contemporary Issues in Computed Tomography*, Vol. 14. Edinburgh: Churchill-Livingstone, 1991: 155–137.

6 Fleckenstein JL, Burns DK, Murphy FK, Jayson HT, Bante FJ. Differential diagnosis of bacterial myositis in AIDS: evaluation with MR imaging. *Radiology* 1991; **179**: 653–658.

7 Bessen LJ, Greene JB, Louie E, Seitzman P, Weinberg H. Severe polymyositis-like syndrome associated with Zidovudine therapy of AIDS and ARC (letter). *N Engl J Med* 1988; **318**: 708–709.

8 Fleckenstein JL. Magnetic resonance imaging and computed tomography of skeletal muscle pathology. In: Bloehn JL, Sartois DJ (eds) *MR and CT of the Musculoskeletal System*. Baltimore: Williams & Wilkins, 1992: 172–188.

9 Rahmouni A, Chosidow O et al. MR imaging in acute infections cellulitis. *Radiology* 1994; **192**: 493–496.

10 Baron AL, Steinbach LS, LeBoit PE, Mills CM, Gee JH, Berger TG. Osteolytic lesions and bacillary angiomatosis in HIV infection: radiologic differentiation from AIDS-related Kaposi sarcoma. *Radiology* 1990; **177**: 77–81.

11 Gupta I, Kocher J, Miller AJ, Weishotz SV, Perz J, Scully M. Mycobacterium haemophilum osteomyelitis in an AIDS patient. *N Jersey Med* 1992; **89**: 201–202.

12 Belmonte MA, Garcia Portales R, Domenech I, Fernandez-Nebro A, Camps MT, Ramon ED. Avascular necrosis of bone in HIV infection and antiphospholipid antibodies. *J Rheum* 1993; **20**: 1425–1428.

13 Gerster JC, Camus JP, Chave JP, Koeger Ac, Rappoport G. Multiple site AVN in HIV infected patients. *J Rheum* 1991; **18**: 300–302.

14 Solinger AM, Hess EV. Rheumatic diseases and AIDS is the association real? *J Rheum* 1993; **20**: 678–683.

15 Espinoza LR, Jara LJ, Espinoza CG, Silverira LH, Martinez-Osuna P, Seleznick M. There is an association between HIV infection and spondyloarthropathies. *Rheum Clin North Am* 1992; **18**: 257–266.

16 Clark MR, Solinger AM, Hochberg MC. HIV infection is not associated with Reiter's syndrome. *Rheum Clin North Am* 1992; **18**: 267–276.

17 Monteagudo I, Rivera J, Lopez-Longo J, Cosin J, Garcia-Monforte A, Carreno L. AIDS and rheumatic manifestations in patients addicted to drugs: an analysis of 106 cases. *J Rheum* 1991; **18**: 1038–1041.

18 Winchester R, Berstein DH, Fischer HD et al. Co-occurrence of Reiter's syndrome and acquired immunodeficiency. *Ann Intern Med* 1987; **106**: 19–26.

19 Beral V, Peterman T, Berkelman R, Jaffe H. AIDS-associated non Hodgkin lymphoma. *Lancet* 1991; **337**: 805–809.

23 PEDIATRIC AIDS

Nancy B. Genieser
Keith Krasinski
Kevin J. Roche
Michael M. Ambrosino

Introduction

In slightly more than a decade, human immune deficiency virus type 1 (HIV-1) infection and acquired immune deficiency syndrome (AIDS) in children has evolved from a clinical syndrome meeting with skepticism as to its relationship to immunosuppressive disease in adults, to a well-characterized disease process, becoming the ninth leading cause of death in children and the seventh leading cause of death in adolescents in the USA [1]. The number of reported cases of AIDS among children in the USA now exceeds 7000 and it is estimated that there are five- to tenfold more children with HIV-1 infection. This epidemic is more explosive in developing areas of the world. Over the same period, there have been dramatic advances in our undertanding of human immunology and HIV-1, the causative agent of AIDS. New developments in radiologic techniques and additional experience with infected populations have advanced our understanding of the disease, enhanced diagnostic sensitivity and specificity, limited the need for invasive techniques, and improved our therapeutic approach to pediatric patients.

Epidemiology

In the USA, epidemiologic factors associated with HIV-1 infection in children are principally associated with infection in women of childbearing age [2–5]. They include intravenous drug abuse (50%), heterosexual contact with an HIV-1 infection person (40%), and having received blood or blood products before 15 April 1985, when screening of donated blood for HIV-1 became routine. Approximately 90–95% of infected children have acquired the infection from their mothers [6–8]. The other major transmission mechanism to children has been treatment with blood or blood products, principally in newborn nurseries or for coagulation defects [9–11]. Among the adolescent age group, experimentation with adult sexual and drug use behavior contributes to the risk of HIV-1 infection [12,13]. The proportion of adolescents with sexual contact or drug use increases steadily from 9% among 13–14-year-olds, to 24% among 15–16-year-olds, to 69% among 17–19-year-olds [3]. The largest contribution derives from sexual contact between males, accounting for 36% of adolescent cases. A small proportion (1–2%) of cases in the USA result from sexual abuse of children and sexual exploitation of adolescents.

In developing countries, contaminated blood or blood products, and use of contaminated needles continues to be associated with spread of disease. Breast milk has an incremental transmission risk of 15% over and above the risk of perinatal transmission [14,15]. Although the risk appears highest during primary infection of the mother, with colostrum and early breast milk, there is an accrual of risk for the duration of breast feeding. In the USA breast feeding by HIV-1-infected women is contraindicated. In the developing world, safe and affordable milk substitutes are unavailable, and there is substantial morbidity and mortality from diarrheal diseases of childhood. Since breast milk is known to reduce the problem, breast feeding is recommended. This recommendation is being reviewed by the World Health Organization (WHO).

Perinatal transmission

Only 10–30% of infants delivering to HIV-1-infected women will ultimately prove to have HIV-1 infection. The maternal use of drugs, resulting in placental infarction, or the presence of infections, such as syphilis or toxoplasmosis that cause placental inflammation and consequent breakdown of the barrier, may be cofactors of transmission and gestational HIV-1 infection. Infants who escape infection prior to delivery are at risk from invasive monitoring intrapartum, and direct cutaneous and mucosal exposure to HIV in mother's blood, and cervical and vaginal secretions. Prenatal, intrapartum and newborn prophylaxis with zidovudene can reduce transmission to 4–8%.

Using viral culture and the polymerase chain reaction (PCR), *vide infra*, as many as 50% of those infants delivering to HIV-1-infected women, who ultimately prove to be HIV-1 infected can be diagnosed in the newborn period [16]. This suggests that in half of infected children, infection was transmitted at some time prior to delivery, resulting in sufficient viral replication to allow for detection. Fetal infection can occur as early as the 12th week of gestation [17,18]. However, the early detection of virus could also result from a large inoculum size at the time of delivery.

Clinical diagnosis

In the past, the clinical diagnosis of HIV-1 infection had been based on meeting the case definition for AIDS. Before the etiologic agent was known, patients with illnesses that were moderately predictive of severe immunosuppression, in the absence of other recognized immunosuppressive illnesses or therapy, were identified as having AIDS. Indicator diseases associated with this degree of immunosuppression are shown in Table 23.1. The discovery of HIV-1, the ability to detect the virus and its immunological consequences allowed for the creation of the revised Centers for Disease Control and Prevention (CDC) classification for HIV infection in children [19] (Table 23.2). This takes cognisance of the fact that antibody-positive infants may have transplacental passively acquired maternal antibody and remain uninfected. It also allows the association of laboratory markers of immune function with clinical syndromes, and recognition of symptomatology.

Table 23.1.   Diseases indicative of immuno-compromise.

Bacterial
Recurrent severe bacterial infections
Environmental mycobacterial infections
Disseminated or extrapulmonary *Mycobacterium tuberculosis*

Fungal
Candidiasis of the trachea, bronchi, lungs, or esophagus
Extrapulmonary or disseminated coccidioidomycosis
Extrapulmonary crytococcosis
Disseminated or extrapulmonary histoplasmosis

Viral
Cytomegalovirus disease of any organ system, beyond the newborn period
Herpes simplex, chronic mucosal ulceration, esophagitis, or pneumonitis
HIV encephalopathy
Progressive multifocal leukoencephaly

Parasitic
Cryptosporidiosis
Isporiasis
Pneumocystis carinii pneumonia (classified by some as fungal)
Toxoplasmosis beyond the newborn period

Neoplastic
Kaposi's sarcoma

Other/unclassified
Lymphocytic interstitial pneumonitis (LIP)
Wasting syndrome

Laboratory diagnosis

Early diagnosis is now requisite for proper management. The development of diagnostic tests first allowed serodetection of antibodies to HIV-1, subsequently detection of viral antigens, recovery of virus in culture from a clinical specimen, and, more recently, the ability to detect small amounts of viral nucleic acids using gene amplification with the PCR. Cell-mediated host responses that are specific to viral antigens can also be detected. Laboratory tests for HIV-1 are indicated in Table 23.3 [20]. Children beyond 15–18 months of age with detectable anti-HIV-1 are regarded as infected. Occasionally, HIV-infected children are antibody negative. However, this does not result in a diagnostic dilemma because these children tend to have advanced immunosuppression associated with hypogammaglobulinemia, and are easily recognized clinically. Similarly, beyond the newborn period,

Table 23.2.   Definition of HIV infection in children[1]

1. HIV-infected
   - Child <18 months known to be HIV+ or born to HIV+ mother
     and
     has positive results on 2 separate determinations from one or more HIV culture, HIV PCR, HIV p24 antigen.
   - Child ≥ 18 months born to HIV+ mother or infected by blood products, sexual contact who is HIV antibody+
     by ELISA and Western blot or +HIV culture, PCR or p24 antigen.
2. Perinatally Exposed (E): A child who does not meet criteria above but
   - is HIV seropositive and <18 months of age
   - unknown antibody status but born to HIV+ mother
3. Seroreverter:
   - (CDC definition): A child born to HIV+ mother: Documented HIV negative (2 or more neg. EIA at 6–18 months,
     or 1 neg. EIA at >18 months) and no other lab evidence of infection and not had an AIDS-defining condition
4. Viral reversion:
   - (Pediatric AIDS Foundation): +PCR assay or viral cultures on blood samples (not cord blood) on 2 occasions, no
     HIV infection evident, no HIV antibody on 2 tests at age >18 months, + genetic relatedness of viruses in mother
     and infant. Those not meeting these criteria classed as "ambiguous" (*NEJM* **334**:801, 1996).

1994 CDC pediatric HIV classification[1]

Immunologic categories	Clinical categories			
	N: No signs/ symptoms	A: Mild signs/ symptoms	B: Moderate signs/symptoms	C: Severe signs/ symptoms
1: No evidence of suppression	N1	A1	B1	C1
2: Evidence of moderate suppression	N2	A2	B2	C2
3: Severe suppression	N3	A3	B3	C3

Immunologic categories					
Age of child					
	<12 months		1–5 years		6–12 years
Immunologic category	CD4 μL	(%)	CD4 μL	(%)	CD4 μL	(%)
1: No evidence of suppression	≥1,500	(≥25)	≥1,000	(≥25)	≥500	(≥25)
2: Evidence of moderate suppression	750–1,499	(15–24)	500–999	(15–24)	200–499	(15–24)
3: Severe suppression	<750	(<15)	<500	(<15)	<200	(<15)

[1]1994 revised classification system for HIV infection in children less than 13 years of age [*MMWR* **42**(RR-12):1–10, 1994]

Clinical Categories for Children With Human Immunodeficiency Virus (HIV) Infection

CATEGORY N: NOT SYMPTOMATIC
Children who have no signs or symptoms considered to be the result of HIV infection or who have only one of the conditions listed in Category A.

CATEGORY A: MILDLY SYMPTOMATIC
Children with two or more of the conditions listed below but none of the conditions listed in Categories B and C.
- Lymphadenopathy (≥0.5 cm at more than two sites; bilateral = one site)
- Hepatomegaly
- Splenomegaly
- Dermatitis
- Parotitis
- Recurrent or persistent upper respiratory infection, sinusitis, or otitis media

Table 23.2. Continued

CATEGORY B: MODERATELY SYMPTOMATIC
Children who have symptomatic conditions other than those listed for Category A or C that are attributed to HIV infection. Examples include but are not limited to:
- Anemia (<8 gm/dL), neutropenia (<1,000/mm^3), or thrombocytopenia (<100,000/mm^3) persisting ≥30 days
- Bacterial meningitis, pneumonia, or sepsis (single episode)
- Candidiasis, oropharyngeal (thrush), persisting (>2 months), in children >6 months of age
- Cardiomyopathy
- Cytomegalovirus infection, with onset before 1 month of age
- Diarrhea, current or chronic
- Hepatitis
- Herpes simplex virus (HSV) stomatitis, recurrent (more than 2 episodes within 1 year)
- HSV bronchitis, pneumonitis, or esophagitis with onset before 1 month of age
- Herpes zoster (shingles) involving at least 2 distinct episodes or more than 1 dermatome
- Leiomyosarcoma associated with EBV (*NEJM* **332**:12, 1995)
- Lymphoid interstitial pneumonia (LIP) or pulmonary hyperplasia complex
- Nephropathy
- Nocardiosis
- Persistent fever (lasting >1 month)
- Toxoplasmosis, onset before 1 month of age
- Varicella, disseminated (complicated chickenpox)

CATEGORY C: SEVERELY SYMPTOMATIC
- Serious bacterial infections, multiple or recurrent (i.e., any combination of at least 2 culture-confirmed infections within a 2-year period), of the following types: septicemia, pneumonia, meningitis, bone or joint infection, or abscess of an internal organ or body cavity (excluding otitis media, superficial skin or mucosal abscesses, and indwelling catheter-related infections)
- Candidiasis, esophageal or pulmonary (bronchi, trachea, lungs)
- Coccidiodomycosis, disseminated (at site other than or in addition to lungs or cervical or hilar lymph nodes)
- Cryptococcosis, extrapulmonary
- Cryptosporidiosis or isosporiasis with diarrhea persisting >1 month
- Cytomegalovirus disease with onset of symptoms of age >1 month (at a site other than liver, spleen, or lymph nodes)
- Encephalopathy (at least one of the following progressive findings present for at least 2 months in the absence of a concurrent illness: (a) failure to attain or loss of development milestones or loss of intellectual ability, (b) impaired brain growth or acquired microcephaly demonstrated by head circumference measurements or brain atrophy demonstrated by CT or MRI, (c) acquired symmetric motor deficit manifested by ≥2 of the following: paresis, pathologic, reflexes, ataxia, or gait disturbance
- Herpes simplex virus infection causing a mucocutaneous ulcer that persists for >1 month; or bronchitis, pneumonitis, or esophagitis for any duration affecting a child >1 month of age
- Histoplasmosis, disseminated (at a site other than or in addition to lungs or cervical or hilar lymph nodes)
- Kaposi's sarcoma
- Lymphoma, primary, in brain
- Lymphoma, small, noncleaved cell (Burkitt's), or immunoblastic or large cell lymphoma of B-cell or unknown immunologic phenotype
- Mycobacterium tuberculosis, disseminated or extrapulmonary
- Mycobacterium, other species or unidentified species, disseminated (at a site other than or in addition to lungs, skin, or cervical or hilar lymph nodes)
- Mycobacterium avium complex or Mycobacterium kansasili, disseminated (at site other than or in addition to lungs, skin, or cervical or hilar lymph nodes)
- Pneumocystis carinii pneumonia
- Progressive multifocal leukoencephalopathy
- Salmonella (non-typhoid) septicemia, recurrent
- Toxoplasmosis of the brain with onset at >1 month of age
- Wasting syndrome: (a) persistent weight loss >10% of baseline OR (b) downward crossing of at least 2 of the following percentile lines on the weight-for-age chart (e.g., 95th, 75th, 50th, 25th, 5th) in a child ≥1 year of age OR (c) <5th percentile on weight-for-height chart on 2 consecutive measurements, ≥30 days apart PLUS (a) chronic diarrhea (i.e., at least 2 loose stools per day for ≥30 days) OR (b) documented fever (for ≥30 days, intermittent or constant)

Table 23.3. Laboratory diagnosis of HIV-I infection.

Serologic diagnosis
Screening test: enzyme linked immunosorbent assay (ELISA), latex agglutination, dot-blot ELISA
Confirmatory tests: Western blot analysis (WB), immunofluorescence (IF), radioimmune precipitation (RIPA)

Viral antigen detection
Enzyme immunoassays (p24)
Immune complex dissociated p24 antigen detection (ICD p24)

Viral culture
Molecular detection of HIV-I nucleic acids
Gene amplication using the polymerase chain reaction

Research-based detection of host response to virus
Neutralizing anti-HIV-I antibody, isotypic anti-HIV-I response, specific IgM, specific IgA, *in vitro* production of antibody
   (IVAP), *in vitro* detection of antibody producing cells, lymphocyte proliferative responses to HIV-I antigen

reproducible detection of virus, viral genome, or viral antigens are diagnostic of infection (Table 23.3). The detection of a host response, with generation of anti-HIV-1-specific IgG, IgA, or IgM antibodies, or the detection of anti-HIV-1-specific cell-mediated immunity, suggests infection. However, these should not replace detection of virus as a diagnostic tool.

Prognosis

Before the etiology of AIDS was known, and diagnostic laboratory tests were available, there was substantial ascertainment bias towards severe disease [21]. Ultimately, this was codified in the CDC's 1987 case definition (Table 23.3) [19,22]. Reports from 1989 indicate an 83% 12-month survival from time of diagnosis [23]. There appears to be an effect of era associated with improved survival, which may be partially caused by improved ability to establish the diagnosis of infection at younger ages without advanced disease, and partially by prophylactic and therapeutic interventions.

Differences in survival among various clinical syndromes that clinically define AIDS among children confound any understanding of prognosis. Those syndromes associated with the worst prognosis, defined as limited survival include: PCP, progressive neurological disease, and infection due to *Mycobacterium avium-intracellulare*. AIDS-defining illnesses with an intermediate prognosis include lymphoid interstital proliferation (LIP) and recurrent severe bacterial infections. HIV-1-associated diseases with relatively good short-term prognosis include: hepatosplenomegaly,

lymphadenopathy syndrome, parotitis, and respiratory infections [22,24].

Reasons for prolonged periods of apparent good health in children who have perinatally acquired disease are not understood, but may include timing of infection, transplacental versus neonatal, inoculum effects, viral phenotype and possibly genetic determined host responses [25,26]. Children presenting at young ages tend to have shorter survival from presentation than older children with the same clinical syndromes [22]. Similarly, children acquiring HIV infection beyond the neonatal period have a better prognosis [23].

Radiologic manifestations

Pulmonary

Pneumocystis carinii pneumonia

Pneumocystis carinii pneumonia (PCP) is the disease entity with the single worst prognosis in children with AIDS. The disease is preventable, and when properly treated with trimethoprim-sulfamethoxazole, steroids and supportive care, more than 50% of children currently survive an episode of PCP. They have a post-PCP mean and median survival of approximately 19 additional months, with some surviving over 5 years. Clinical resolution usually requires 3–6 weeks but may continue for months. Steroid therapy early in the disease often shortens recovery time. Nation-wide, approximately 70% of PCP occurs in children who have not had prophylaxis. One half of these children have not been previously diagnosed as HIV-1-infected. Others developed PCP despite having CD4 counts above the suggested level for prophylaxis.

PCP can present at any age. It occurs in approximately 39% of children with AIDS. In infants, the infection is often insidious, with cough, low-grade fever, and tachypnea that worsens over a period of 1–4 weeks. Death can occur in a matter of days. Rales may be few or absent. In older children the onset is often abrupt. No rales are heard. There is often striking contrast between severe clinical distress and lack of pulmonary findings.

Early chest radiographs are frequently normal. There is no specific radiographic pattern for PCP. Cytomegalovirus (CMV) often duplicates the same clinical and radiographic findings. The lungs can show progressive air-space changes with bronchograms. Infants who respond poorly to therapy and require intubation often exhibit air block with interstitial air, complicated by pneumothorax and pneumomediastinum. The stiff lungs partially collapse with pneumothrax. High-resolution computed tomography (HRCT) performed on infants showed diffuse, segmental, ground-glass opacification with bronchial wall thickening (Figure 23.1). Pleural effusions are usually absent. Hilar adenopathy may be present. Older children, recovering from PCP, can develop bullae and cysts Figure 23.2) [27–29]. Atypical patterns, including focal parenchymal lesions and nodules, have been described [30].

Lymphocytic interstitial pneumonitis

Approximately 30–40% of HIV-1-symptomatic children over the age of 1 year have pulmonary parenchymal and airway infiltrations of lymphocytes [31–34]. The etiology of LIP has been linked to a local response to antigenic stimulation [35], a direct result of lung infection by the HIV-1 virus [36, 37], Epstein–Barr virus (EBV) or other organisms. These patients frequently have positive serologic testing for EBV infection [34]. Histologically, lymphocytes, plasma cells, and immunoblasts diffusely infiltrate the alveolar septa and peribronchiolar areas. Lymphoid nodules with and without germinal centers, and granuloma-like collections of mononuclear and multi-nucleated giant cells may be present [31]. In the proper setting, LIP is a clinical and radiologic diagnosis, and lung biopsy is usually not required. Other lymphocytic interstitial lung disease that can resemble LIP radiographically include: polyclonal B-cell lymphoproliferative disease (PBLD), miliary tuberculosis,

chronic interstitial pneumonitis (CIP), follicular bronchiolitis, immunoblastic sarcoma, bronchiolar-associated lymphoid tissue (BALT) and desquamative interstitial pneumonitis (DIP) [38].

LIP has an intermediate prognosis in the limited survival of children with AIDS. The course is chronic with superimposed infections. Clinically, children present with cough, wheezing, tachypnea, and occasionally clubbing. As lymphocyte proliferation and infiltration of interalveolar septa and peribronchial spaces increases, there is impairment of gas flow and reduced lung compliance with normal expiratory flow [32]. Patients are usually treated symptomatically with oxygen, bronchodilators and later cortical steroids to suppress the lymphocytic proliferation.

Radiographs are often more impressive than clinical signs (Figure 23.3). Patients with symptoms compatible with LIP may only show hyperinflation on chest radiograph. Lymphocytes and plasma cells in the alveolar and interlobar septa probably account for the reticular radiographic pattern while nodules of lymphocytes, plasma cells, immunoblasts and plasma-cytoid lymphocytes in a peribronchiolar pattern are most likely responsible for the nodular pattern. The two findings are often lumped together as PLH/LIP (PLH: pulmonary lymphocytic hyperplasia) or LIP. In our patients, we have observed the three types of LIP defined by Oldham on chest X-rays in adults (Figure 23.4):

- Type 1, reticular or finely reticulonodular infiltrates;
- Type 2, coarse reticulonodular interstitial infiltrates;
- Type 3, the findings of types 1 or 2 with superimposed areas of patchy alveolar infiltrate [39].

The lung nodules usually enlarge as the disease progresses, although this is not always the case [40]. The nodules can disappear totally, remain stable, or come and go [32]. Nodules have been reported to appear suddenly on chest radiography following a positive PLH/LIP biopsy when no nodules were present on the prebiopsy chest film [32]. The early reticulonodular infiltrates are best seen on chest X-ray at the lung periphery or bases [41,42]. HRCT can show interstitial thickening and nodularity when the chest radiograph is negative. During hypoxic (P_aO_2 <65 mmHg) LIP 'flares', there is coarsening of the reticulonodular changes. They usually return to baseline as a child responds to steroid therapy.

(A)

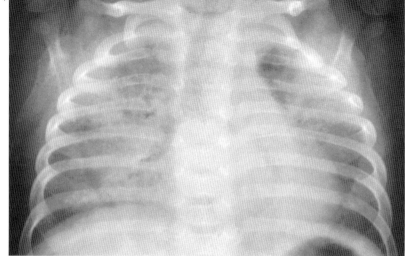

(B)

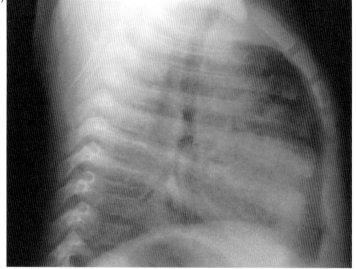

(C)

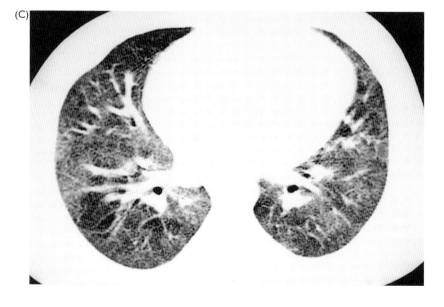

Figure 23.1. A 4-month-old male with PCP by bronchoscopy born to a drug-abusing HIV-1-positive mother. (A,B) Posterior-Anterior and lateral views of the chest show diffuse haziness throughout both lung fields with air bronchograms. (C) HRCT through the lower lobes show a ground-glass appearance with airspace disease.

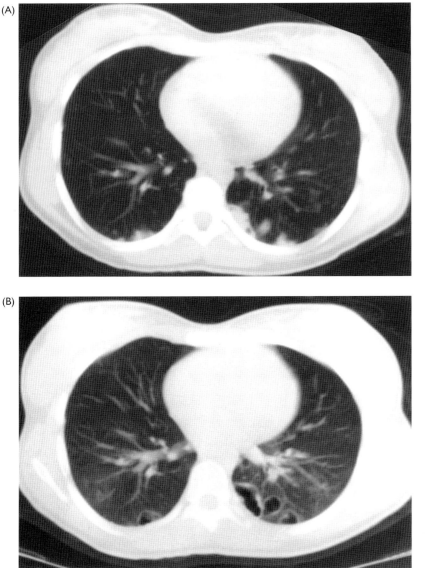

Figure 23.2. A 13-year-old sexually abused child who is HIV-1-positive with PCP. (A) A CT scan shows bilateral basilar alveolar infiltrates. (B) Four weeks later, the infiltrates show cavitation.

Children with LIP are living longer and developing more chronic lung changes. Imaging studies show increasing lower-lobe disease with volume loss, bronchiectasis, and cystic changes [43]. The cystic findings usually consist of small blebs, although cysts similar to those seen in histiocytosis-X have been described [44]. The blebs can rupture with resultant pneumothorax. Cor pulmonale is frequently observed.

At our institution, all children with LIP had significant hilar adenopathy. The adenopathy increased in size during pulmonary superinfection but the reculonodular pattern often remained unchanged. Mild adenopathy was seen when CD4 levels were close to 10%. However, no adenopathy was seen when CD4 fell below 7%. This has not been the experience of others where the presence of hilar adenopathy was inconsistent [31,32,45,46].

Cytomegalovirus pneumonia

CMV infection occurs in approximately 45% of children with symptomatic HIV infection and in 10% of those under 18 months of age with an indeterminate infection status. Immunocompetent infants and HIV-infected infants can both present with similar clinical findings. Therefore, CMV cannot be used as a diagnostic indicator for AIDS in this age group. Beyond the newborn period, symptomatic CMV infection is unusual, occurring in approximately 5% of HIV-

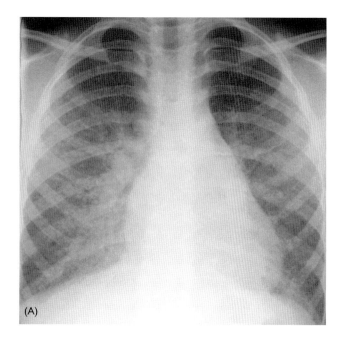

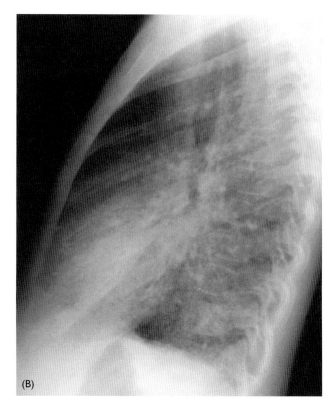

Figure 23.3. A 6-year-old male with LIP who is asymptomatic. (A,B) PA and lateral chest show type III LIP.

infected children [47]. Disseminated disease, which carries a poor prognosis, tends to occur below 6 months of age in HIV-1 CMV coinfected children. Disseminated disease, which carries a poor prognosis, tends to occur below 6 months of age in HIV-1 CMV coinfected children. CMV is often superimposed on LIP or PCP [48]. It can begin insidiously or with acute respiratory failure. Infants can present with hepatosplenomegaly, lymphadenopathy, and microencephaly. The radiographic pattern correlates with the clinical course. Those patients with insidious onset show a reticulonodular pattern, while a miliary pattern predominates in the more acutely ill patients [44,49]. The findings are non-specific, and open lung biopsy or bronchial washings are required for definitive diagnosis [48].

Mycobacterial infections

Tuberculosis accounts for approximately 1% of AIDS-defining illnesses among our pediatric population. It is usually primary disease acquired from a family member. There is little to suggest that the pathophysiology of the tuberculosis is different in this group.

However, as might be expected among children with impaired cellular immunity, disease progression and dissemination is more common. Because of impaired delayed typed hypersensitivity, children with HIV and tuberculosis often have negative tuberculin skin tests. HIV-infected children with tuberculosis typically present with prolonged fever, and respiratory signs and symptoms. Extrapulmonary manifestations, including scrofula, meningitis, and osteomyelitis, have occurred. On chest X-ray there is frequently adenopathy with atelectasis [44]. Pulmonary disease may progress to cavitation, which is rare in non-immunocompromised children (Figure 23.5). Radiographically, it is difficult to distinguish with certainty the miliary pattern of tuberculosis from LIP [38,41].

Mycobacterium avium-intracellulare

Mycobacterium avium-intracellulare (MAI) is detected in a greater proportion of HIV-1-infected children than adults. It is one of the infections in AIDS children that carries the worst prognosis for long-term survival [50]. The median survival following diagnosis is

(A)

(B)

(C)

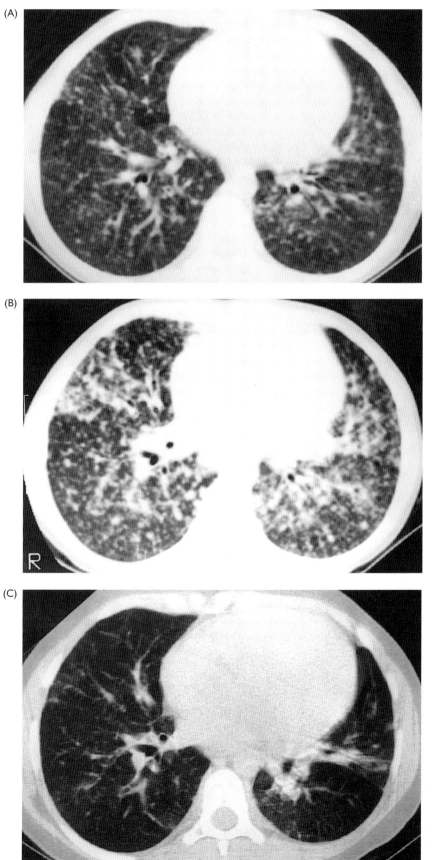

Figure 23.4. A 7-year-old male with LIP. CT of the lower lobes shows the changing LIP pattern. (A) Type II LIP. (B) Two weeks later there is coarsening of the reticular nodular pattern with airspace disease, type III. (C) The patient is treated with steroids and converts to type I. Note left lower lobe infiltrate.

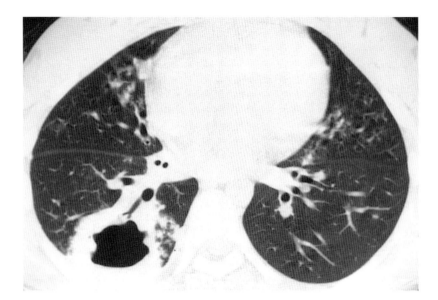

Figure 23.5. A 15-year-old female with tuberculosis who is HIV-1-positive and sexually active. A CT scan shows a thick-walled cavity in the right lower lobe.

approximately 4 months. The incidence of infection varies between 4% and 15%. The age of onset is variable, often occurring in the first year of life, but may also be found among adolescents. There is a variable interval from symptom onset to culture positivity from 0 to 19 months. At least 90% of children diagnosed as having MAI have another preexisting AIDS defining illness.

Clinical signs and symptoms include: persistent failure to gain weight, anorexia, abdominal pain and tenderness, persistent or recurrent fever, transfusion-dependent anemia, intermittent or persistent diarrhea, night sweats and joint pain.

The radiographic findings of alveolar or nodular infiltrates accompanied by adenopathy are non-specific. Areas of collapse may be present. HRCT scans show non-specific changes (Figure 23.6). Biopsy, bronchoscopic washings or sputum are required for diagnosis. A positive culture may be obtained from the lung, even if the chest radiograph is negative; in such a case, the disease is assumed to be disseminated [51]. Therapy may effect reductions in the circulating load of mycobacteria. However, the infection is usually not eradicated.

Varicella zoster virus

Children who are HIV-1-infected, but still have intact immune function, who contact *Varicella* show the usual course of chickenpox [52]. Those children who are immunosuppressed have a prolonged illness and are at risk for *Varicella* pneumonia, encephalitis, pancreatitis, and hepatitis [52]. Superinfection by bacteria or fungi is common with secondary osteomyelitis, bacterial/

fungal pneumonia. Fifty per cent of HIV-infected children will have chronic *Varicella* infections, 15% will succumb, and 35% will recover completely [52].

The diagnosis of *Varicella* is usually made clinically. In the absence of an exposure history, viral culture is sometimes requested to differentiate disseminated

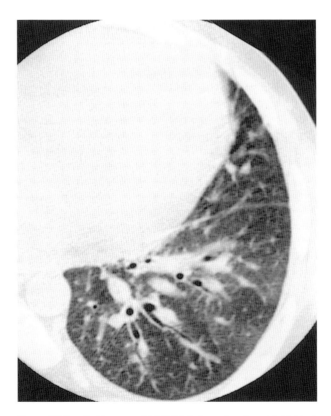

Figure 23.6. A 10-year-old HIV-1-infected male with MAI. A CT scan of the left lower lobe shows non-specific peribronchial thickening.

Herpes simplex infection. Persistent and or progressive *Zoster* occurs in these immunodeficient hosts between 8 months to 3 years following the initial insult [53].

Chest radiographs demonstrate diffuse nodular densities that often coalesce into areas of focal consolidation. The latter is usually a sign of acute superimposed bacterial pneumonia [48].

Measles

Measles pneumonia can occur in children with HIV-1 who have not been vaccinated or in whom there has been a vaccination or immune system failure [54]. The disease can be similar to the immunocompetent child or can result in a severe giant-cell pneumonia which occurs without the typical measles rash. Chest radiographs are non-specific. The diagnosis is made by specific IgM and IgG measles serology or by recovery of virus [48].

Additional pulmonary infections

In our series, 'common' bacterial infections have occurred in approximately 18% of HIV-1-infected children. The most common pathogens causing bacteria pneumonias include *Streptococcus pneumoniae* and *Haemophilus influenzae*. *Staphylococcus aureus*, and *Salmonella* spp. have also occurred. *Acinetobacter, Pseudomonas*, and enterococcal pneumonias, *Aerobacter, Campylobacter* spp., *Serratia* spp., *Morganella, Branhamella, Acinetobacter, Klebsiella* spp., *Proteus mirabilis, Enterobacter* spp., *Pseudomonas, Escherichia coli, Staphylococcus aureus, Streptococcus viridans*, and *Staphylococcus epidermidis*, have also been associated with lower respiratory infections in HIV-1-infected children.

Adenovirus and respiratory syncytial virus can produce severe pulmonary disease, especially in infants and young children. Pulmonary candidiasis is seen in those patients with central intravenous lines or on intensive antibiotic therapy (Figure 23.7). The infection is usually superimposed upon a preexisting condition. Aspergillosis of the lung has been described [55]. Acute onset of disease associated with fever and tachypnea is often properly interpreted as suggesting pneumonia.

Chest radiographs are non-specific. HRCT often shows multiple subsegmental pulmonary consolidations with poorly defined margins [56]. These consolidations frequently fail to clear completely with treatment and a subclinical infection persists. They often recur

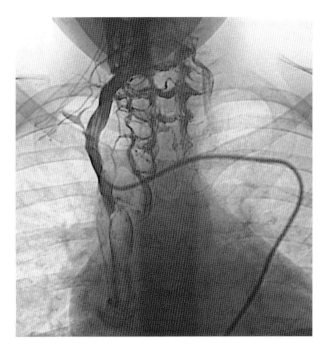

Figure 23.7. A 13-year-old HIV-1-positive female with *Candida* sepsis. A venous angiogram through a Broviac catheter shows a large thrombus of the superior vena cava extending into the right atrium.

in the same areas when the patient becomes clinically compromised. The pathogens are mainly encapsulated bacteria, although more than one organism is often identified.

Cardiac disease

The reported incidence of cardiac disease in HIV-1-infected children varies from 27% to 72% [57,58]. Cardiomyopathy is the most characteristic manifestation, although conduction abnormalities, especially sinus arrhythmia with wandering atrial pacemaker, can be present [59,60]. The etiology of these cardiac abnormalities remains unclear, but may sometimes be due to HIV infection of the heart [57]. CMV is also known to cause myocarditis. Most infected children with cardiac symptoms are over 1 year old, although congestive heart failure (CHF) has been seen in a 2-month-old infant [57]. Many of the cardiac problems are related to lung disease which causes pulmonary hypertension and hypoxemia. Cor pulmonale is associated with LIP. AIDS deaths in children are not usually due to cardiac causes.

Congestive heart failure and cardiomegaly are the commonest cardiac abnormalities observed on chest

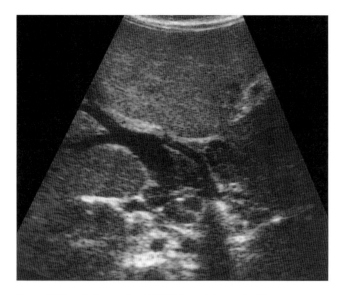

Figure 23.8. A 7-month-old HIV-1-positive male. Transverse ultrasound shows multiple hypoechoic nodes in the region of the porta hepatis.

radiographs. Enlargement of cardiac size on serial films should suggest myocardial involvement [42]. Occasionally a pericardial effusion is detected [60].

At postmortem, the heart is enlarged with marked left or biventricular dilatation. The myocardial fibers are hypertrophied with necrosis and sparse focal myocarditis. Bacterial endocarditis, valcular and chordae thickening, myocardial infarction and coronary thrombosis, and aneurysms have all been described [60,61].

HIV-related ateriopathy consisting of endothelialitis and fragmentation of elastic lamina and mineralization of the vessel walls can involve many organs. The small and medium-sized cardiac vessels are affected [62].

Lymph nodes

Lymph node involvement with HIV-1 is an integral part of the disease process. The body burden of HIV-1 may be largely sequestered in lymph nodes. From biopsy material correlated with clinical and virologic laboratory parameters, it appears that lymph node involvement precedes viremia associated with progressive disease, with the viremia resulting from the inability of stationary lymphocytes to continue to restrict HIV. MAI may also be responsible for lymph node enlargement.

Histologic examination of the nodes may show follicular hyperplasia with normocellular or depleted paracortical zone, or follicular atrophy with absence of germinal centers and lymphocytic depletion of the paracortical zone [63,64]. In MAI patients, microscopic examination can demonstrate poorly formed granulomas or sheets of histocytes packed with mycobacteria.

The paucity of retroperitoneal fat in children makes ultrasound an excellent method for assessing lymph node enlargement (Figure 23.8). Computed tomography (CT) frequently provides additional information. Involved nodes are usually found in the paraaortic, caval, mesenteric, and porta hepatis regions.

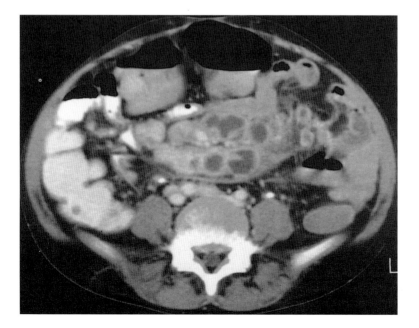

Figure 23.9. A 10-year-old male who is HIV-1-positive with MAI. A CT scan of the abdomen shows multiple mesenteric nodes of low attenuation.

Nodes can be hyperechoic or hypoechoic [40], depending on the histological or infectious composition (Figure 23.9).

Parotid gland infections

Parotid glands become enlarged (40%) with cystic sialectasis or diffuse infiltrates from CD8 lymphocytes [42,65] (Figure 23.10). There is often accompanying cervical adenopathy [42,65,66]. In children aged 9–12 years, Sjogren's syndrome has been seen at the initial presentation of HIV infection [67].

Hepatic disease

Although a significant number of HIV-1-infected children develop hepatosplenomegaly with abnormal liver enzymes, symptomatic liver disease is rare in older children [57]. Occasionally, patients may present with a clinical syndrome of cholestasis and hepatitis as the first manifestation of HIV infection [68]. Cholestatic hepatitis may be the presenting finding of HIV-1 infection in infancy. Chronic liver inflammation has been reported in 10% of pediatric AIDS patients. Hepatitis B infection is almost always caused by perinatal transmission. In addition, systemic viral illness, including EBV, CMV hepatitis A, and hepatitis C can all cause hepatitis. The most common intrahepatic opportunistic infection is MAI. It is usually disseminated when the diagnosis is made. MAI infection can mimic tumor nodules when present as the histoid or pseudosarcomatous variant. Chronic hepatic inflammation can lead to progressive liver failure resulting in bleeding abnormalities.

To date, sonography and computed tomography have not been helpful in differentiating causes of diffuse hepatic disease. Ultrasound can be used to guide liver biopsies, which can sometimes be helpful by showing CMV inclusions, Kaposi's sarcoma, central vein necrosis, giant cell hepatitis, portal inflammation, steatosis, cholestasis and granulomatous hepatitis [69].

Gastrointestinal disease

HIV-1-infected children with esophageal lesions present with dysphagia and odynophagia. The common organism is *Candida albicans*, followed by CMV and *Herpes simplex* virus. These viral infections can produce esophagitis, but more commonly cause oral mucosal ulcerations [57]. Rarely, similar findings are seen with disseminated histoplasmosis and cryptococcus. Barium esophogram demonstrates mucosal edema, plaques, and ulcerations, resulting in a cobblestone or shaggy appearance. Pseudodiverticulum can develop. CMV causes a vasculitis leading to ischemia with necrosis and ulceration. These findings are nonspecific and can resemble candidiasis [70].

Children with HIV infection can have either typical bacterial gastrointestinal pathogens of childhood or opportunistic infections [71,72]. *Cryptosporidium*, best diagnosed by stool analysis or duodenal aspirate, is felt to account for a significant number of cases of diarrhea in children [73]. It commonly involves the small bowel but can be seen throughout the entire gastrointestinal tract [74] (Figure 23.11). The proximal small bowel shows thickened folds, spasm, dilatation, and fragmentation of barium. In severe cases, there is

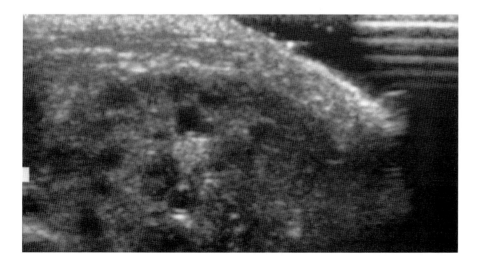

Figure 23.10. A 2-year-old male with AIDS born to a drug-abusing mother. Longitudinal ultrasound of the parotid shows an enlarged gland with hypo- and hyperechoic areas.

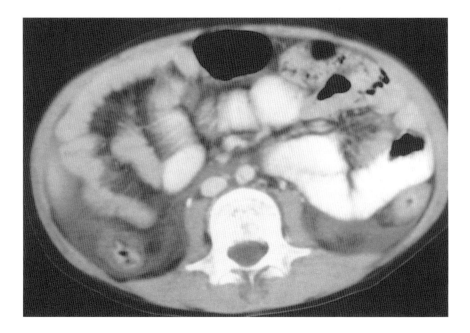

Figure 23.11. A CT scan of an 8-year-old male with cryptosporidium of the gastrointestinal tract and AIDS contracted from blood products during surgery for congenital heart disease. A CT scan shows non-specific dilatation of small bowel with some thickening of the folds.

a smooth featureless mucosa with loss of the normal folds [42]. Thickened gastric folds on UGI (upper gastrointestinal) series can be secondary to cryptosporidiosis, *Helicobacter*, or lymphoproliferative disorder (gut-associated lymphoid tissue). CMV can produce thickening of the pylorus and proximal duodenum resembling pyloric stenosis [75].

MAI produces a pseudo-Whipple pattern with fine nodularity and thickening of proximal jejunal folds on UGI or CT scan [76]. It is associated with enlarged, often necrotic, mesenteric and retroperitoneal lymph nodes [77]. The colon is commonly affected by CMV [78]. Radiographic findings include stricture, perforation, typhlitis, pneumatosis, and pseudomembranous colitis. Diagnosis in all cases requires biopsy or culture. Loss of mucosal integrity is common. This loss, coupled with deficient coagulation parameters, is probably responsible for upper and lower gastrointestinal hemorrhages. One infant, who presented with gastrointestinal hemorrhage, showed multiple chronic small bowel ulcers, which on electron microscopic studies of intestinal epithelial cells showed virus-like particles [19] suggesting HIV [79].

Renal disease

HIV-1-associated renal nephropathy is frequently encountered. It consists of proteinuria and mild hypertension, and can lead to nephrotic syndrome with hypoalbuminemia and edema [73,80]. It can be seen in all stages of HIV-1 infections and has presented as the first manifestation of AIDS [81]. Hematuria with or without pyelonephritis has been observed. The pathogenesis of renal disease in HIV-1 children is not known but may be related to circulating immune complexes [73,82]. Focal segmental glomerulosclerosis [83] and mesangial proliferative glomerulonephritis [8] have been demonstrated [73,84]. On ultrasound, the kidneys can be enlarged and hyperechoic, often with loss of corticomedullary definition (Figure 23.12).

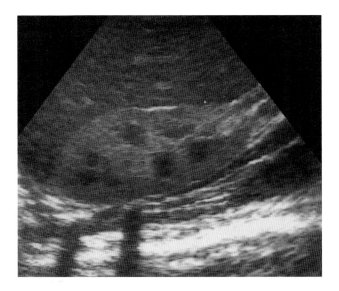

Figure 23.12. A 1-year-old female who is HIV-1-positive. Renal ultrasound shows loss of the normal cortical medullary junction and increased echogenicity.

(A)

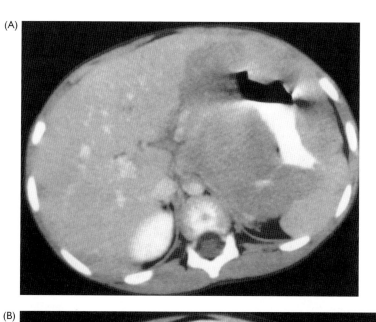

(B)

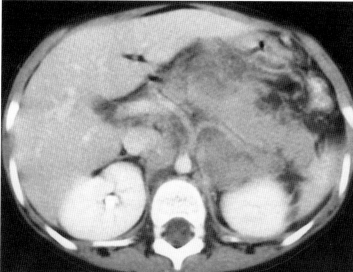

(C)

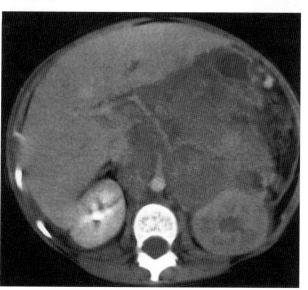

Figure 23.13. A 6-year-old male who is HIV-1 positive with Burkitt's lymphoma. (A) A CT scan shows thickening of the wall of the stomach with ulceration. (B) A CT scan at the level of the celiac axis shows the celiac axis to be stretched with extensive adenopathy and delayed perfusion of left kidney. (C) A scan performed 2 weeks later shows the rapid doubling time of the tumor.

Glomerulomegaly, tubular dilatation and infiltrates may help explain the enlarged kidneys.

Recurrent infections

Over 60% of our children with symptomatic HIV infection suffer from recurring and/or chronic infections. Bacterial diseases can present as sepsis, pneumonia, urinary tract infection, and meningitis, bone and joint infection, parotiditis, sinusitis and otitis media. Organisms causing disease are commonly pneumococcus, *Haemophilus influenzae* type b, enterococcus, both typical and atypical mycobacterial species, and Gram-negative enteric bacilli, i.e. *E. coli*, *Klebsiella* and *Salmonella* species. *Pseudomonas aeuroginosa* has complicated the terminal stages of illess in some of our patients. Nearly all our patients have otitis media and a large number have clinically significant sinusitis. In our experience, CT has been helpful in assessment of chronic sinusitis and otitis in young infants.

Malignancy

The incidence of neoplastic disease in pediatric AIDS has been reported to be 7% [73]. The characteristic malignancy is B-cell lymphoma, often Burkitt's [85,86]. The usual presentation is intestinal involvement with extensive mesenteric adenopathy, although other primary sites have been reported [87]. Burkitt's tumor tends to be extremely aggressive with an initial response to chemotherapy, followed by a rapid down-

hill course (Figure 23.13). Hodgkin's lymphoma, although one of the currently accepted malignancies for making the diagnosis of AIDS, may not occur more frequently in HIV-1 children than in the general population [57]. Hodgkin's disease is usually seen in children over 10, but has been reported in a 4-year-old HIV-1-positive male [88]. Two cases of polyclonal polymorphic B-cell lympoproliferative disorder have been described [89].

It is felt that soft-tissue tumors are disproportionately represented among children with AIDS. Kaposi's sarcoma has been described in childhood [90] and, in two infants, involving lymph nodes, spleen and thymus [91]. Rhabdomyosarcoma has been reported with one case involving the gallbladder [92]. Fibrosarcoma of the liver was identified in one African HIV-infected child [93]. Three children, infected with HIV-1 as infants, developed gastrointestinal tract and lung tumors by age 8 [94,95]. One of our HIV hemophiliac patients had soft-tissue sarcoma of the thigh with metastatic disease to the thorax, liver, and adrenals (Figure 23.14).

Central nervous system abnormalities

In children with AIDS, central nervous system disease is often protracted and related to direct invasion of neural tissue by HIV [96–98] resulting in progressive encephalopathy. These clinical findings may be superimposed on static neurologic problems associated with maternal drug use, congenital infection, and birth

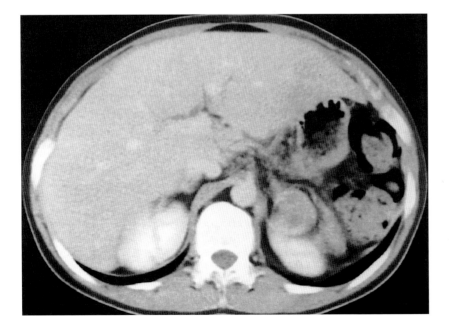

Figure 23.14. A 16-year-old hemophiliac with AIDS from acquired blood product. A CT scan shows metastatic sarcoma to the left adrenal (arrows).

asphyxia. The virus appears to infect predominantly cells of the monocyte–macrophage lineage and has been identified in microglial mononuclear cells and multinucleated giant cells [64]. The clinical signs and symptoms include: loss of devleopmental milestone lag, apathy, weakness, spastic paresis, secondary microencephalopathy, and generalized seizures.

Routine CSF examination is often normal or has a slight protein elevation. Cytomegalovirus affecting the brain *in utero* can become reactivated after birth when immunodeficiency develops. This has been described in an infant with AIDS and typical periventricular enhancing mass lesions on CT [99]. Toxoplasma encephalitis has also been seen in infants with AIDS, although it was unclear whether this was intrauterine infection or postnatally acquired disease [100]. Progressive multifocal leukoencephalopathy is caused by a member of the papovavirus family. This causes a slow, subacute, demyelinating disease. CT scans can show calcifications in the basal ganglia or cortical atrophy [101]. Magnetic resonance imaging (MRI) may identify alterations in basal ganglia relaxation parameters before calcification occurs. Head ultrasound has demonstrated hyperechoic foci in the basal ganglia and periventricular white matter [102]. Although primary lymphomas of the central nervous system are uncommon in children [103], we have observed several children with this entity (Figure 23.15). They are frequently multicentric lesions that enhance with contrast on CT [42]. The children have progressive focal neurologic deficits. In the spinal cord, vacuolar myelopathy secondary to swelling of myelin sheaths, with vacuolar degeneration affecting the lateral and posterior columns of the thoracic spinal cord has been seen. The pathogenesis is unclear [73].

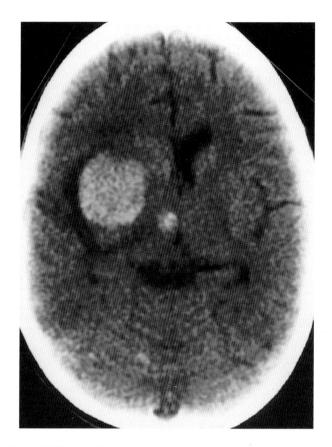

Figure 23.15. A CNS lymphoma in a 6-year-old child with AIDS. A contrast-enhanced CT scan at the level of the quadrigeminal plate cistern shows lymphoma enhancing lesion with parenchymal edema.

References

1 NCHS. *Annual Summary of Births, Marriages, Divorces and Deaths: United States 1992.* US Department of Health and Human Services, 1993.

2 Gwinn M, Pappaioanou M, George JR et al. Prevalence of HIV infection in childbearing women in the United States. *JAMA* 1991; **265**: 1704–1708.

3 Kanki P, Coutinho R. Epidemiology. *VIII International Conference on AIDS/III STD World Congress.* Amsterdam: Harnard AIDS Institute, 1992: 22–32.

4 World Health Organization. *AIDS Surveillance in Europe.* Paris WHO Collaborating Centre on AIDS. Paris: WHO, 1989.

5 Anderson VM, Kahn E, Greco MA. Pediatric AIDS pathology. In: Weinstein, RS (ed) *Advances in Pathology and Laboratory Medicine.* St Louis: Mosby-Year Book, Inc., 1993.

6 Caldwel MB, Rogers MF. Epidemiology of pediatric HIV infection. *Pediat Clin North Am* 1991; **38**: 1–16.

7 Goedert J, Duliege, Amos CI et al. High risk of HIV-1 infection for first born twins. *Lancet* 1991; **338**: 1471–1475.

8 Children born to women with HIV-1 infection: natural history and risk of transmission. European Collaborative Study. *Lancet* 1991; **337**: 253–260.

9 Hilgarther M. AIDS in the transfusion recipient. *Pediat Clin North Am* 1991; **38**: 1.

10 Lawrence DN, Lui K, Peterman TA et al. Characteristics of incubation periods (IP) in pediatric cases of transfusion-associated acquired immune deficiency syndrome (TA-AIDS). *Second International Conference on AIDS*, Paris 1986, Vol. 20; p. 33.

11 Shannon KM, Ammann A. Acquired immune deficiency syndrome in childhood. 1985; *J. Paediat* **106**: 332–341.

12 Kingson RW, Strohim C, Berlin B. Acquired immuno-deficiency syndrome transission changes in knowledge and behavior among teenagers. Massachusetts Statewide Surveys 1986–1988. *Pediatrics* 1990; **85**: 24–29.

13 Rubinstein A. Pediatric AIDS. *Curr Prob Pediat* 1986; **7**: 361–409.

14 Palasanthrim JB, Ziegler GL. Breast feeding during primary maternal human immunodeficiency virus infection and risk of transmission from mother to infant. *J Infant Dis* 1993; **167**: 441–444.

15 Dunn DT, Newell M, Ades E. Risk of human immuno-deficiency virus type 1 transmission. *Lancet* 1992; **340**: 585–588.

16 Borkowsky W, Krasinski K, Pollack H et al. Early diagnosis of human immunodeficiency virus infection in children <6 months of age: coparison of polymerase chain reaction, culture and plasma antigen captive techniques. *J Infect Dis* 1992; **166**: 616–619.

17 DiMaria H, Courpotin C, Rouzioux C. Transplacental trans-mission of human immunodeficiency virus. *Lancet* 1986; **2**: 215–216.

18 Sprecher S, Soumenkoff G, Puissant F. Vertical transmission of HIV in a 15 week fetus. *Lancet* 1986; **2**: 288–289.

19 Centers for Disease Control. Revision of the CDC surveil-lance case definition for acquired immunodeficiency syn-drome. *MMWR* 1994; **43** (RR–IZ): 1–10.

20 Krasinski K, Borkowsky W. Laboratory diagnosis of HIV infection. *Pediat Clin North Am* 1991; **38**: 17–35.

21 Scott G, Buck B, Leterman J. Acquired immunodeficiency syndrome in infants. *N Engl J Med* 1984; **310**: 76–81.

22 Turner B, Denison M, Eppes S. Survival experience of 789 children with the acquired immunodeficiency syndrome. *Pediat Infect Dis J* 1993; **12**: 310–320.

23 Krasinski K, Borkowsky W, Holzman R. Prognosis of human immunodeficiency virus infection in children and adolescents. *Pediat Infect Dis J* 1989; **8**: 216–220.

24 Tovo PA, DeMartino M, Gabiano C et al. Prognostic factors and survival in children with perinatal HIV-1 infection. *Lancet* 1992; **339**: 1249–1253.

25 Persaud D, Chandwani S, Rigaud M. Delayed recognition of human immunodeficiency virus infection in pre-adolescent children. *Pediatrics* 1992; **90**: 688–691.

26 Itescu S, Brancat L, Winchester R. A sicca syndrome in HIV infection associated with HLA-DR5 and CD8 lymphocyto-sis. *Lancet* 1989; **334**: 466–468.

27 Naidich D, McGuinness G. Pulmonary manifestations of AIDS: CT and radiographic correlations. *Radiol Clinics North Am* 1991; **29**: 999–1017.

28 Sandhu JS, Goodman PC. Pulmonary cysts associated with penumocystis carinii pneumonia in patients with AIDS. *Prog Surg Pathol* 1989; **12**: 181–215.

29 Ledesma-Medina J, Green M, Newman B. Transplantation and the pediatric chest. *Radiol Clinics North Am* 1993; **31**: 465–477.

30 Kuhn J. High resolution computed tomography of pediatric pulmonary parenchymal disorders. *Radiol Clinics North Am* 1993; **31**: 51–53.

31 Heitzman RE. Pulmonary neoplastic and lymphoproliferative disease in AIDS: a review. *Radiology* 1990; **177**: 347–351.

32 Marquis JR, Berman C, DiCarol F et al. Radiographic patterns of PHL/LP in HIV positive children. *Pediatr Radiol* 1993; **23**: 328–330.

33 Connor EM, Marquis J, Oleske IM. Lymphoid interstitial pneumonitis. In: Pizzo PA, Wilfert C (eds) *Pediatric AIDS*. Baltimore: Williams and Wilkins, 1991: 343.

34 Pitt J. Lymphocytic interstitial pneumonia. *Pediat Clinics North Am* 1991; **38**: 89–95.

35 Iescu S, Brancato L, Busbaum J et al. A diffuse infiltrative CD8 lymphocytosis syndrome in human immunodeficiency virus (HIV) infection: a host immune response associated with HLA-DR5. *Ann Intern Med* 1990; **112**: 3–10.

36 Ho D, Pomerantz R, Kaplan J. Pathogenesis of infection with immunodeficiency virus. *N Engl J Med* 1987; **317**: 278–286.

37 Plata F, Autran B, Martins L. AIDS virus-specific cytoxic T lymphocytes in lung disorders. *Nature* 1987; **328**: 348–351.

38 Zimmerman BL, Haller J, Price AP et al. Children with AIDS – is pathologic diagnosis possible based on chest radiographs? *Pediat Radiol* 1987; **17**: 303.

39 Oldham S, Castillo M, Jacobson F et al. HIV-associated lym-phocytic interstitial pneumonia: radiological manifestations and pathologic correlation. *Radiology* 1989; **170**: 83–87.

40 Amodio J, Abramson S, Berdon W. Pediatric AIDS. *Semin Roentgenol* 1987; **22**: 66–76.

41 Bradford BF, Abedenour GE Jr, Frank JL et al. Usual and unusual radiologic manifestations of acquired immuno-deficiency syndrome (AIDS) and human immunodeficiency virus (HIV) in children. *Radiol Clinics North Am* 1988; **26**: 341–353.

42 Haney PH, Yale-Loehr A, Nussbaum NA et al. Imaging of infants and children with AIDS. *AJR* 1989; **152**: 1033–1041.

43 Amorosa JK, Miller R, Laraya-Cuasay L et al. Bronchiectasis in children with LIP and AIDS. *Pediatr Radiol* 1992; **22**: 603–507.

44 Berdon WE, Mellins R, Abramson SJ et al. Pediatric HIV infection in its second decade – the changing pattern of lung involvement. *Radiol Clinics North Am* 1993: **31**: 453–463.

45 Morris J, Rosen M, Marchevsky A et al. Lymphocytic inter-stitial pneumonia in patients at risk for the acquired immune deficiency syndrome. *Chest* 1987; **91**: 63–67.

46 Goodman PC. Pulmonary disease in children with AIDS. *J Thorac Imag* 1991; **6**: 60–64.

47 Krasinski K, Borkowsky W, Holzman R et al. Prognosis of human immunodeficiency virus infection in infants and chil-dren. *Pediat Infect Dis J* 1989; **8**: 216.

48 Ambrosino MA, Genieser N, Kransinski K et al. Oppor-tunistic infections and tumors in immunocompromised chil-dren. *Radiol Clinics North Am* 1992; **30**: 639–658.

49 Beschorner W, Hutchins G, Burns W et al. Cytomegalovirus pneumonia in bone marrow transplant recipients: miliary and diffuse patterns. *Am Rev Respir Dis* 1980; **122**: 107–114.

50 Hoyt L, Oleske J, Holland B. Non tuberculosis mycobacteria in children with acquired immunodeficiency syndrome. *Pediat Infect Dis J* 1992; **11**: 354–360.

51 Marinelli D, Albeda S, Williams T et al. Nontuberculous mycobacterial infection in AIDS: clinical, pathologic, and radiographic features. *Radiology* 1986; **160**: 77–82.

52 Jura E, Chadwick E, Joseph S. Varicella-zoster virus infections in children with acquired immunodeficiency virus. *Pediat Infect Dis* 1989; **8**: 586–590.

53 Prose NS, Mendez H, Menikoff H et al. Pediatric human immunodeficiency virus infection and its cutaneous manifestations. *Pediat Derm* 1987; **4**: 67–74.

54 Krasinski K, Borkowsky W. Measles and measles immunity in children infected with human immunodeficiency virus. *JAMA* 1989; **26**: 2512–2516.

55 Wright M, Fikrig S, Haller JO. Aspergillosis in children with acquired immune deficiency. *Pediat Radiol* 1993; **23**: 492–494.

56 Ambrosino MM, Genieser N, Roche KJ et al. Feasibility of high resolution, low dose chest CT in evaluating the pediatric chest. *Pediat Radiol* 1994; **24**: 6–10.

57 Burroughs MH, Edelson PJ. Medical Care of the HIV-infected child. *Pediat Clinics North Am* 1991; **38**: 45–67.

58 Lipschultz SE, Chanock Sanders SP. Cardiovascular manifestations of human immunodeficiency virus infection in infants and children. *Am J Cardiol* 1989; **63**: 1489.

59 Bharati S, Joshi VV, Connor Em. Conduction system in children with acquired immunodeficiency syndrome. *Chest* 1989; **96**: 406.

60 Joshi VV, Kaufman S, Oleske JM et al. Dilated cardiomyopathy in children with acquired immunodeficiency syndrome: a pathologic study of five cases. *Human Pathol* 1988; **19**: 69.

61 Steinherz LJ, Brochstein J, Robin J. Cardiac involvement in congenital acquired immunodeficiency syndrome. *Am J Dis Child* 1988; **140**: 1241.

62 Joshi VV, Pawal B, Connor E et al. Arteriopathy in children with acquired immune deficiency syndrome. *Pediat Pathol* 1987; **7**: 261.

63 Joshi VV, Oleski J, Minnefor AB et al. Pathology of suspected acquired immune deficiency syndrome in children: a study of eight cases. *Pediat Pathol* 1984; **2**: 71.

64 Kostianovsky M, Orenstein J, Schaff AZ et al. Cytomembranous inclusions observed in acquired immune deficiency syndrome. *Arch Pathol Lab Med* 1987; **111**: 218–223.

65 Williams M. Head and neck findings in pediatric acquired immune deficiency syndrome. *Laryngoscope* 1987; **97**: 713.

66 Chanock S, McIntosh K. Pediatric infection with the human immunodeficiency virus. *Otolaryngol Clinics North Am* 1989; **22**: 637.

67 Itescu S. Diffuse infiltrative lymphocytosis syndrome in human immunodeficiency virus infection – a Sjogren's like disease. *Rheum Dis Clinics North Am* 1991; **17**: 99–115.

68 Persaud D, Bangaru B, Grieco A. Cholestatic hepatitis: a presenting manifestation of HIV infection in infancy. *Pediat Infect Dis* 1993; **12**: 492–498.

69 Jonas MM, Roldan EO, Lyons HJ et al. Histopathologic features of the liver in pediatric acquired immune deficiency syndrome. *J Pediat Gastroenterol Nutr* 1989; **9**: 73.

70 Haller JO, Cohen HL. Gastrointestinal manifestations of AIDS in children. *AJR* 1993; **162**: 387–393.

71 Berkowitz CD, Seidell J. Spontaneous resolution of cryptosporidiosis in children with acquired immune deficiency syndrome. *Am J Dis Child* 1985; **13**: 967–969.

72 Bursztyn E, Lee B, Bauman J. CT of acquired immune deficiency syndrome. *Am J Neuroradiol* 1984; **5**: 711–714.

73 Joshi VV. Pathology of childhood AIDS. *Pediatr Clinics North Am* 1991; **38**: 97–120.

74 Soave R, Johnson W. Cryptosporidium and Isospora belli infections. *J Infect Dis* 1988; **157**: 225.

75 Victoria MS, Nangia B, Jindrak K. Cytomegalovirus pyloric obstruction in a child with acquired immunodeficiency syndrome. *Pediat Infect Dis* 1985; **4**: 550–552.

76 Roth RI, Owen R, Keren DF. AIDS with mycobacterium avium – intracellulare lesions resembling those of Whipple's disease. *N Engl J Med* 1983; **309**: 1324.

77 Radin DR. Intra-abdominal mycobacterium tuberculosis vs mycobacterium avium-intracellulare infections in patients with AIDS: distinction based on CT findings. *AJR* 1991; **156**: 487–491.

78 Joshi VV, Oleske J, Saad S et al. Pathology of opportunistic infections in chldren with acquired immune deficiency syndrome. *Pediat Pathol* 1986; **6**: 145.

79 Chandler FW, White E, Callaway CS et al. Unidentified virus-like particles in the intestine of patients with the acquired immune deficiency sydrome. *Ann Intern Med* 1984; **100**: 851–853.

80 Rao TKS, Freidman E, Nicastri AD. The types of renal disease in the acquired immune deficiency syndrome. *N Engl J Med* 1987; **316**: 1062.

81 Connor E, Gupta S, Joshi V et al. Acquired immunodeficiency syndrome-associated renal disease in children. *J Pediat* 1988; **113**: 39.

82 Calvelli TA, Rubenstein A. Intravenous gamma-globulin in infant acquired immunodeficiency syndrome. *Pediat Infect Dis* 1986; **5**: 8207.

83 Cohen AH, Nast CC. HIV-associated nephropathy: a unique combined glomerular tubular and interstitial lesion. *Mod Pathol* 1988; **1**: 87.

84 Strauss J, Abitbol C, Zilleruelo G et al. Renal disease in children with the acquired immunodeficiency virus infection. *N Engl J Med* 1989; **321**: 625.

85 Fahey JL, Oho-Amaize AE. Acquired immunodeficiency syndrome (AIDS) and neoplasia. *Am J Pediat Hematol Oncol* 1987; **9**: 193.

86 Kamani N, Kennedy J, Brandsma J. Burkitt's lymphoma in a child with human immunodeficiency virus infection. *J Pediat* 1988; **112**: 241.

87 Mukerji PK, Hilfer C. Burkitt's lymphoma with mandible, intra-abdominal and renal involvement – initial presentation of HIV infection in a 4 year old child. *Pediat Radiol* 1993; **23**: 76–77.

88 Montalvo FW, Casanova R, Clavell LA. Treatment outcome in children with malignancies associated with human immunodeficiency virus infection. *J Pediat* 1990; **116**: 735–738.

89 Joshi VV, Kaufman S, Oleske M et al. Polyclonal polymorphic B-cell lymphoproliferative disorder with prominent pulmonary involvement in children with acquired immune deficiency syndrome. *Cancer* 1987; **59**: 1455.

90 Connor E, Boccon-Gibod L, Joshi V et al. Cutaneous acquired immunodeficiency syndrome-associated Kaposi's sarcoma in pediatric patients. *Arch Dermatol* 1990; **126**: 791.

91 Buck BE, Scott GB et al. KS in two infants with acquired immune deficiency syndrome. *J Pediat* 1983; **103**: 911–913.

92 Case records of the Massachusetts General Hospital C9. A 40-month-old girl with the acquired immune deficiency syndrom and spinal cord compression. *N Engl J Med* 1986; **314**: 629.

93 Ninane J, Moulin D, Latinne D et al. AIDS in two African children – one with fibrosarcoma of the liver. *Eur J Pediat* 1985; **144**: 385.

94 Chadwick EG, Connor E, Hanson CG et al. Tumors of smooth-muscle origin in HIV-infected children. *JAMA* 1990; **263**: 3182–3184.

95 McLoughlin LC, Nord K, Joshi VV et al. Disseminated leiomyosarcoma in a child with acquired immune deficiency syndrome. *Cancer* 1991; **67**: 2618–2621.

96 Whelan M, Kricheff II, Handler M et al. Acquired immunodeficiency syndrome: computed tomographic manifestations. *Radiology* 1983; **149**: 477–484.

97 Curran JW, Lawrence DN, Jaffee H et al. Acquired immune deficiency syndrome (AIDS) associated with transfusions. *N Engl J Med* 1984; **310**: 69–75.

98 Elkin CM, Leon E, Grenell SL et al. Intracranial lesions in the acquired immune deficiency syndrome. *JAMA* 1985; **253**: 393–396.

99 Post MD, Curless R, Gregorios JB et al. Reactivation of congenital cytomegalic inclusion disease in an infant with HTLV III associated immunodeficiency: a CT-pathologic correlation. *J Comput Assist Tomog* 1986; **10**: 533–536.

100 Shanks GD, Refield R, Rischer GW. Toxoplasma encephalitis in an infant with acquired immunodeficiency syndrome. *Pediat Infect Dis* 1987; **6**: 70–71.

101 Epstein LG, Sharer L, Joshi VV et al. Progressive encephalopathy in children with acquired immune deficiency syndrome. *Ann Neurol* 1985; **17**: 488.

102 Sica GT, Norton K. Intracranial human immunodeficiency virus infection in an infant: sonographic findings. *Pediat Radiol* 1990; **20**: 64–65.

103 Epstein LG, DiCarlo FJ, Joshi VV et al. Primary lymphoma of the central nervous system in children with acquired immune deficiency syndrome. *Pediatrics* 1988; **82**: 355.

24 | WOMEN AND AIDS

Kees Boer
Mieke H. Godfried

Introduction

Women infected with the human immune deficiency virus (HIV) constitute half of the HIV-infected population in the world. Many aspects of HIV disease in men manifest themselves also in women, but some aspects are particular to women, related to the female genital tract. The most distinct of these is transmission from mother to child *in utero*, at birth, or during lactation.

Epidemiology

It is estimated that by 1 December 1996, 22.6 million people are living with HIV infection or AIDS [1]. Most of these are adults (21.8 million), some are children (830 000). Women constitute approximately 42% of the adult HIV-infected population, and their proportion is still growing. In industrialized countries, men still outnumber women, but the male to female ratio has begun to equalize. In the USA, the incidence of AIDS among women has increased from 8% of cases between 1981 and 1987 to 18% reported during 1993 to October 1995 [2]. In 1994, the median age of women with AIDS in the USA was 35 years, with women aged 15–44 years constituting 85% of cases[3]. Hispanic and Black women were disproportionally affected (77% of cases).

Women acquire HIV infection primarily through three modes of transmission: sexual, intravenous drug use with sharing of needles, and via blood transfusions or blood products. Globally, heterosexual contact with an HIV-infected partner probably is the main mode of transmission[4,5]. In Europe and the USA, injection drug users (IDU) still account for over half of all AIDS cases, but the proportion of cases associated with heterosexual transmission is increasing [3–6]. As AIDS reflects the incidence of HIV infection several years ago, it may be assumed, however, that the number of women infected heterosexually at present accounts for the majority of cases also in Europe and the USA. In non-industrialized countries, where screening for HIV infection is not routine, exposure to infected blood or blood products remains a real risk.

Natural history

Most information on the natural course of HIV infection and influences on or predictors of disease progression is derived from studies on male homosexual or male hemophiliac cohorts in the Western world. The manifestations of HIV disease specific to women are less well documented. Most of what is currently known is derived from studies in Europe and the USA, where injection drug use is the main risk factor [3–17].

We will first discuss how AIDS differs in general terms between men and women, and will then describe disease processes specific to women, including genital tract infections, neoplasms, and pregnancy.

Several studies have addressed the issue of possible gender differences with respect to the manifestations of HIV infection [4–17]. Earlier studies pointed to faster disease progression and shorter survival after AIDS diagnosis in women than in men [4–7]. However, after controlling for confounding factors, such as CD4+ cell count, socioeconomic status, access to medical care, and treatment variables, the available data provide little evidence for major differences[4–6]. In a study of 468 newly HIV-seroconverted IDU, 27% of whom were women, disease progression was similar for men and women [8]. Likewise, no differences in the rates of disease progression were found in a cohort of 1443 patients (111 women) with both early- and late-stage HIV disease [9]. However, rapid disease progression was reported in 160 female African sex workers with an estimated median duration from asymptomatic HIV infection to disease of 4.4 years [10]. This is considerably shorter than the estimates of 8–11 years that have been reported for male Western populations [19]. Several factors could explain the rapid disease progression in this population, among them genetic and environmental differences, high rates of other sexually transmitted diseases (STD) with resulting immunologic stimulation, and the possibility of simultaneous and repetitive infection with different HIV strains [10].

Data from studies on possible survival differences are conflicting. In New York City, survival was shorter for 552 women with AIDS than for 5281 men [7]. After 1 year, 59.8% of women had died versus 50.3% of men. A European study, that retrospectively examined the data of 2554 patients, including 566 women, found similar average survival times from AIDS diagnosis in men (median, 18 months) and women (median, 16 months) [11]. In contrast, in a large prospective study of 768 women and 3779 men, HIV-infected women had a poorer survival rate than men, even though rates of disease progression did not differ [12]. The adjusted relative risk (RR) for death in women was 1.33 [95% confidence interval (CI) 1.06–1.67]. The increased risk of death for women was primarily found among women with (a history of) injection drug use (RR: 1.68, 95% CI 1.20–2.35). No data on survival after AIDS diagnosis were given, however, which complicates comparison with other studies. In a cohort of 82 women, followed for a median of 13 months (range 3–61 months), median survival time following AIDS diagnosis was 27 months, which is much longer than survival in the above mentioned European study [11,13]. Unfortunately, no male control group was included in this study and the number of women followed was small, which may have influenced the outcome [13]. Interestingly, women who participated in antiretroviral therapy clinical trials had a significantly longer duration of survival.

Although minor gender differences have been reported, most studies report striking similarities in the occurrence of most HIV-related symptoms and of most of the AIDS-defining diseases. The retrospective multicentre 'AIDS in Europe' study included 2554 AIDS cases, 566 of whom were women. Only toxoplasmosis and *Herpes simplex* virus (HSV) ulceration occurred significantly more frequently in women. Kaposi's sarcoma (KS) occurred less frequently in

women than in men [11]. All other AIDS-defining diagnoses were found in equal rates in men and women. On the other hand Melnick et al. found an increased risk for bacterial pneumonia in women (RR: 1.38, 95% CI: 1.05–1.92) and a reduced risk for the development of KS and oral hairy leukoplakia, but no differences in the occurrence rate of toxoplasmosis or infections with HSV [12]. Their study was prospective, included more patients and corrected for possible confounding variables, like CD4+ cell count, age, race, history of injecting drug use, etc. An analysis of adult AIDS cases diagnosed in the USA between January 1988 and June 1991, and reported to the Centers for Disease Control and Prevention (CDC) also showed similar prevalences for men and women, when differences in race/ethnicity and mode of transmission were accounted for [14]. Subgroup analysis showed, however, that esophageal candidiasis, HSV disease and cytomegalovirus disease were reported more frequently among female IDU. In a cross-sectional analysis of 444 male and 118 HIV-infected IDU patients with early HIV disease a recent history of genital HSV was found more often in women than in men, but this difference could not be confirmed on physical examination [15]. The overall frequency of oral candidiasis and constitutional symptoms did not differ [15]. Although in most studies KS appears to be a rare complication of HIV infection in women, occurring in 1% or less of American women with AIDS, a recent retrospective study documented a much higher prevalence of 3.6%, especially among women born outside the USA [5,16].

Data on markers of disease progression among women are scarce and little comparative data concerning gender-related differences or similarities are available. It seems likely, however, that measures of immune deficiency and virologic parameters, such as the CD4+ cell count and viral load, predict progression to AIDS in women as they do in men [17,19,20]. Although in one study lower plasma HIV-RNA concentrations in women were reported, no gender differences in viral load were observed in a group of patients who were naive to antiretroviral therapy, and matched for age and CD4+ cell count [19,20].

In conclusion, hitherto no major differences in the natural history of HIV infection have been found between men and women. The fact that several studies have shown a worse prognosis for women due to differential access to medical care and socioeconomic differences remains of special concern.

Heterosexual transmission

World-wide the most important mode of HIV infection is through heterosexual transmission. Direct evidence that HIV infection of women can be transmitted via the genital tract came from the first report in 1985 that artificial insemination with semen from one HIV-infected donor caused HIV infection in four Australian women [21]. In a study from the USA seven (3.52%; 95% CI: 1.55–7.41%) out of 199 women inseminated with semen from any of five HIV-infected donors appeared to be infected [22].

Although heterosexual transmission is the most important mode of infection for both sexes, the effectiveness of infection does not appear to be the same. Two study groups on heterosexual transmission of HIV found that the efficiency of male to female transmission was 1.9 (95% CI: 1.1–3.3) and 2.3 (95% CI: 1.1–4.8) times greater than that of female to male transmission [24,25]. In the stable couples studied, consistent condom use appeared to protect against infection. Next to gender, having another sexual transmitted disease, peno-anal intercourse, frequent intercourse (≥twice weekly) and a partner with AIDS or with <400 CD4+ cells all more than doubled the risk of infection [24]. Similar risk factors and complete protection by condom use were found by the European study group [25]. In the last study, the seroconversion rate in 121 couples using condoms inconsistently or not appeared to be 4.8 per 100 persons-years (95% CI: 2.5–8.4). However, the cumulative index of seroconversion in the uninfected partner was as high as 48.7% when the partner had AIDS or <200 CD4+ cells as opposed to 7.8% when he or she did not.

Disruptions of mucosa of the lower genital tract, as evidenced by postcoital bleeding, were shown to increase male to female transmission 3–7-fold [26,27]. Interestingly, not only HIV infection, but also dyspareunia and heavy smoking were independent risk factors for postcoital bleeding, which suggests that (heavy) smoking increases susceptibility for HIV infection [28], as reported before in Haitian women [29]. However, the epithelium probably does not have to be disrupted for infection. In rhesus monkey, intact vaginal epithelium appeared to be crossed by simian immune deficiency virus, the analog of HIV in monkeys [30,31].

From the aforementioned studies on heterosexual transmission in Europe [23–25], it might be concluded that the risk of infection per coitus is below 1% and thus lower than the observed infection rate after insemination [22]. The risk of female to male transmission was even estimated to be as low as 0.1% per coitus [32]. A study from Thailand on 77 HIV-infected 21-year-old male military conscripts estimated the risk per sexual contact with an HIV-infected prostitute at 5.6% (95% CI: 4.1–7.5%)[33], whereas female to male transmission is less effective than the reverse. This relatively high transmission rate might explain the epidemic spread of HIV in South-East Asia. In a similar group of Thai military men, the annual incidence rate of infection during 2 years of military service was 2.43 per 100 person-years [34]. The most prominent mode of infection was sex with a female commercial sex worker.

HIV and gynecology

HIV infection and other sexually transmitted diseases in women

As sexual intercourse has been the route of HIV transmission in most HIV-infected women [35], it is not surprising that HIV-infected women are also at risk for other sexually transmittable diseases. First, it is possible to obtain multiple infections from the same partner. Second, if an ulcerative STD is present, the susceptibility for an HIV infection is increased, as is the infectiousness of an HIV-infected woman for her partner by increased shedding of HIV [36,37]. Some of these STDs, such as gonorrhea, are readily diagnosed and treated, but others are carried on because they do not cause clinical symptoms within many years, such as infections with human papilloma virus (HPV), or they cannot be eradicated, as in the case of HSV. HIV-infected women are not only at increased risk of infection with STD's, immune deficiency itself may contribute to the susceptibility for STDs and their manifestation or progress [38,39]. In this way, immune deficiency results in a concomitant increased prevalence of some gynecological diseases [40]. For instance, the occurrence of pelvic inflammatory disease might be enhanced by the decreased presence of CD4+ lymphocytes in the endometrium of HIV-infected women [41].

Candida

The most frequent gynecological complaint in HIV-infected women is not an STD, however, but pruritus vulvae caused by a vulvo-vaginal *Candida* infection (Figure 24.1). The first large observational study on gynecological manifestations of HIV-infected women came from Rhode Island in the USA and comprised 200 women [40]. Of these women, 63% were infected by sharing needles for drug use. In 117 women (59%), clinical manifestations were present before they had an AIDS-defining condition (in the old CDC classification). Recurrent vulvo-vaginal *Candida* infections were most frequently (37%) the first of these clinical manifestations. At follow-up, 76% of these 117 women had recurrent (>3 episodes per year) vaginal *Candida* infections. In HIV-infected women, the symptoms of vulvo-vaginal *Candida* infections are sometimes more severe and react less well to local antifungal treatment than those in HIV-uninfected women [40,42]. In most cases, vaginal candidiasis precedes oral thrush [43]. Recurrent vaginal candidiasis may occur already at relatively normal CD4+ cell counts and CD4+/CD8+ ratios. It is common experience of HIV-infected women that they suffer less from vaginal candidiasis

when their CD4+ cell counts have fallen below 200 cells/mm³. This may be explained by the increased probability that they have or have had systemic antifungal treatment for oral or esophageal candidiasis. As a side effect, not only the vulvo-vaginal candidiasis is treated, but also an existing intestinal reservoir is eradicated. Another explanation could be that the awareness of the vaginal candidiasis is increased at a relatively normal CD4+ count owing to the allergic type of immune response often found in this phase of the HIV disease.

Local antifungal treatment is still the treatment of choice in sporadic vaginal candidiasis. A total of 17.5% of the isolates of HIV-infected persons were found to be resistant to fluconazole, particularly those of AIDS patients [44]. *Torulopsis glabrata*, which has been found in nearly 10% of HIV-seropositive women [44,45], is more likely to be resistant than *Candida albicans*. If vaginal candidiasis recurs, fluconazole can be given as one dose of 150 mg. However, one should not only treat because of clinical symptoms like pruritus vulvae,

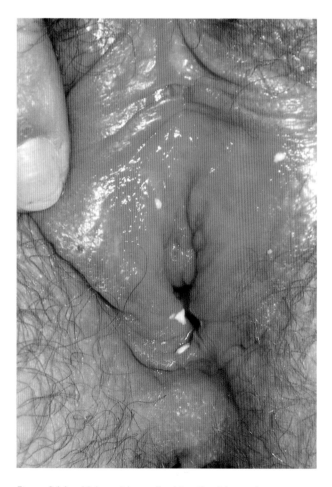

Figure 24.1. Vulva with small white *Candida* patches.

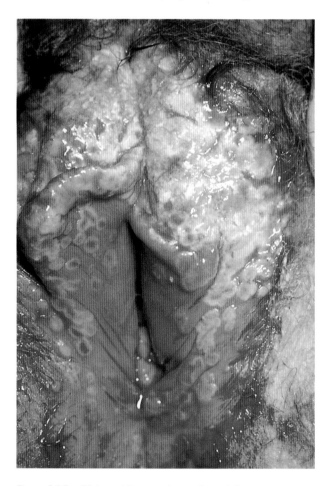

Figure 24.2. Vulva with many herpetic vesicles.

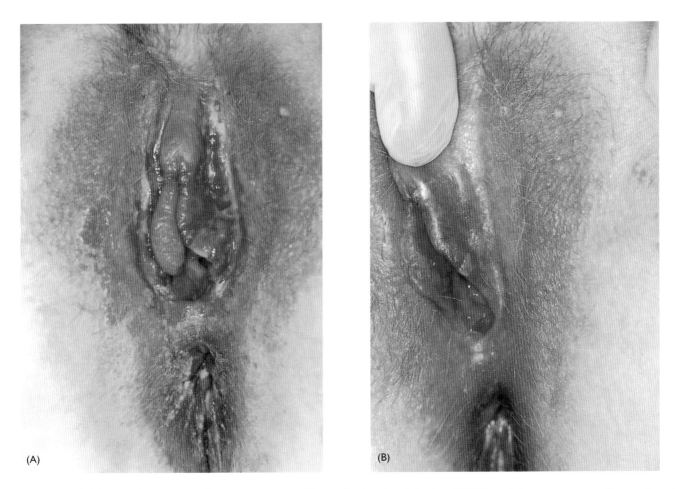

(A)　　　　　　　　　　　　　　　　　　　　　　(B)

Figure 24.3. (A) Vulva of a woman with severe recurrent *Herpes simplex* virus infection. (B) Vulva of the same woman after treatment, leaving behind an idiopathic HIV ulcer, which was cured by thalidomide.

but after or concurrently with proper laboratory diagnosis of the infection, including culture with susceptibility tests. Other causes of pruritus vulvae, like *Herpes simplex* infection, are sometimes alleviated by local treatment. However, they are not cured and so lead to a seemingly recurrent vaginal candidiasis and vice versa.

Herpes simplex virus

In the Rhode Island study, recurrent HSV infections were found in 10% of women [40]. In HIV-infected women, recurrent HSV infections are sometimes difficult to cure and can be persistent and ulcerative as in primary HSV infection (Figure 24.2). High oral or intravenous doses of aciclovir or famciclovir are needed in these cases. Frequently recurring HSV infections can be treated prophylactically by long-term low-dosage acyclovir (400 mg daily) [46].

In HIV-infected persons idiopathic ulcera are also found. In our department, an HIV-infected woman had extensive genital HSV ulcera that were treated adequately with high doses of acyclovir. One ulcus persisted, however (Figure 24.3). Histopathological examination, including immunohistochemistry, of a biopsy specimen showed no signs of any common bacterial or viral infection. Subsequent treatment with thalidomide 100 mg daily led to healing of the ulcer within 10 days [47].

Human papilloma virus infections

HPV infections of the lower genital tract appear to occur more frequently in HIV-seropositive women than in HIV-seronegative women. HPV infections of the female lower genital tract are strongly associated with genital squamous lesions, including condylomata acuminata and intraepithelial neoplasia or invasive

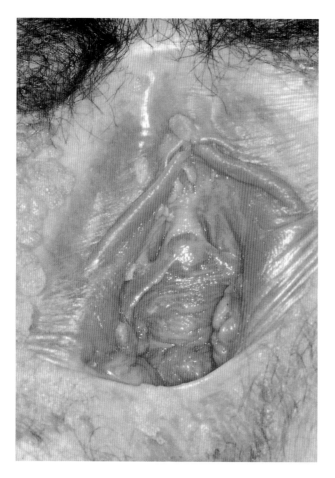

Figure 24.4. Vulva and vagina with condylomata acuminata.

carcinoma. In 1993, cervical carcinoma in HIV-seropositive women became an AIDS-defining diagnosis, and cervical dysplasia, squamous intraepithelial lesion (SIL) or cervical intraepithelial neoplasia (CIN) an AIDS-related event [48].

Condyloma accuminata

In the Rhode Island study condyloma acuminata constituted the second most frequent gynecological disease in HIV-infected women (16%) [40]. In a large cohort from New York, HIV-infected women had a tenfold higher incidence (8.2/100 person-years) of venereal warts than HIV-uninfected women, and the risk was highest with the lowest CD4+ cell counts [49]. These verrucous manifestations of the vulva, vagina and also cervix (Figure 24.4) are mainly caused by the HPV subtypes 6 and 11. In HIV-infected patients, however, clinically diagnosed condyloma acuminata can be caused by HSV [50]. Transmission of HPV is sexual or from mother to child during birth.

Like with cervical dysplasia in HIV-infected women (see below) condylomata acuminata are more likely to recur and are less well curable than in HIV-uninfected women [38].

Cervical dysplasia and cervical cancer

In relatively large cross-sectional studies, the prevalence of CIN or invasive squamous cervical carcinoma in HIV-seropositive women was reported to be as high as 20–41% compared with 4–9% in HIV-uninfected/unknown women belonging to HIV risk groups [51–55]. Only in a group of Nairobi prostitutes were the prevalences equal (26% v. 24%) [56]. More recently Korn analysed 19 studies including 728 HIV-infected women [57]. Of these women 38% had abnormal Papanicolaou (PAP) smears and 42% had cervical dysplasia, more than half of which were high grade. A much lower incidence (9.8%) of SIL was found in commercial sex workers in Senegal despite polymerase chain reaction (PCR)-detectable HPV in 56% of these women with a mean age above 30 years [58]. In this study, no difference was found between HIV-1- and HIV-2-infected women despite less immunosuppression in HIV-2-infected women. Within most groups of HIV-seropositive women, however, the prevalence of CIN appeared to be related to the level of immunosuppression as indicated by CD4+ cell counts [51–53,55,59–64]. Although the prevalence of oncogenic HPV types appeared to be higher in HIV-seropositive women than in those without (known) HIV infection [54,56,65–68], statistical analysis showed that HIV infection or HIV-induced immunosuppression were independent risk factors for the development of CIN in addition to the strongest factor, (oncogenic) HPV infection [51,52,62]. On the one hand, HIV infection may only be associated with an increased risk of CIN when immunosuppression is present [63]. On the other, at all levels of immunosuppression, HIV-infected women with HPV infection had an increased risk of CIN [60]. The importance of immunosuppression, either caused by HIV or by iatrogenic immunosuppression, on the development of CIN or cervical cancer became apparent from the longitudinal study of Petry [61]. In patients with (renal) allografts, the prevalence of CIN was found to be high (49% v. 10% in controls) [69], stressing the importance of immunosuppression.

In addition to the high prevalence of CIN in HIV-seropositive women, the recurrence rate (or persistence) of CIN after treatment is much higher than in HIV-uninfected/unknown women (56% v. 13% [70], 39% v. 9% [71]). In general, in immuno-suppressed women, whether or not due to HIV infection, the recurrence rate was higher [61], and in HIV-infected women, the recurrence was related to increasing immunosuppression: up to 61% when CD4+ cell counts were below 500 cells/μL [70,71].

Papanicolaou smear and colposcopy

Because of the increased risk of cervical dysplasia, the CDC advises that a PAP smear of the cervix should be performed every year [72]. Because of initial studies, there has been some concern about the reliability of the PAP smear for the detection of cervical dysplasia in HIV-infected women [73].

Subsequent studies in much larger groups showed that PAP smears in HIV-infected women are of similar reliability as in the general population [74,75].

There is one major concern, however. In HIV-infected women, lower tract genital dysplasia may be multifocal and involves not only the cervix, but also the vulva [76]. It manifests itself as vulvar intraepithelial neoplasia (VIN) (Figure 24.5). Like cervical dysplasia, VIN in young women is caused by HPV. When VIN is found in women in the fertile period, the risk of a concomitant HIV infection in a group of 28 women was 29% [76]. The recurrence rate in HIV-infected women after treatment of VIN was high compared with the HIV-uninfected women.

HIV and obstetrics

Influence of natural course

The first study in which HIV-seropositive women were followed after full pregnancy suggested an acceleration of disease progression by pregnancy [77]. A selection bias existed, however, towards women with advanced disease, since they were traced via their child after these developed a symptomatic HIV infection. Later studies indeed showed that disease progression of the child is related to disease stage of the mother at delivery [78]. Subsequent prospective studies on disease progression after pregnancy did not show clinical deterioration by pregnancy, at least in asymptomatic women [79]. During normal pregnancy, cell-mediated immune response is depressed [80]. The decline in CD4+ cells seems to be faster in HIV-

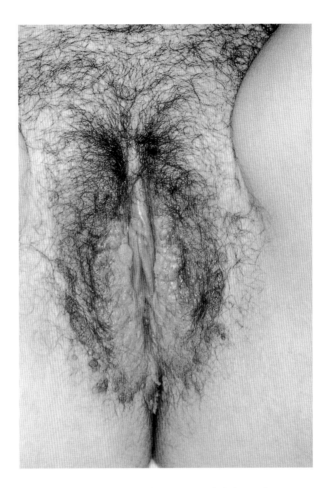

Figure 24.5.   A vulva with vulvar intraepithelial neoplasm.

seropositive pregnant women with less rebound in the last trimester of pregnancy and post partum than in HIV-seronegative pregnant women [81]. However, this phenomenon may also be explained by the natural course of HIV infection and has not been confirmed by another study [82]. Finally, transient p24 antigenemia can sometimes be observed, which is rare outside pregnancy in untreated persons except during acute HIV infection [83]. This may be due to either increased virus replication or a temporary decrease in HIV-antibody production, since only free circulating p24 antigen can be detected and not the immune complexed antigen.

Influence of HIV infection on pregnancy outcome

HIV infection is not a major problem with respect to the course of pregnancy and pregnancy outcome. Some studies show that the rate of abortion in HIV-infected women is increased [84]. It is not known whether the underlying reason must be looked for in immunological deficits of the mother, failure to protect the trophoblast against cytotoxic lymphocytes, or in an increased rate of genital infections or HIV transmission to the fetus in early pregnancy. The latter is suggested by the high rate (50%) of HIV-infections found in spontaneously aborted fetuses of HIV-infected women [85].

Preterm delivery is another complication of pregnancy that might be increased in HIV-infected women because of the concomitant risk of genital infections and low CD4+ cell counts. In the European collaborative study, the latter was found to be related to preterm labour in HIV-seropositive women [86]. In the same prospective study, the percentage of preterm labor was only 5% and thus not more than in a general population [87].

At the onset of the HIV epidemic, lower birthweights of babies born to HIV-infected women were mainly due to drug use. Only from studies linking infection status of the infant to birthweight did it become apparent that a moderate decrease in birthweight is due to HIV infection of the fetus [88,89]. On the one hand, this effect could be the result of bias, as HIV-infected symptomatic women are more likely both to infect their child and to have lighter children due to their physical condition. On the other hand, most infected infants are only infected during labor (see below), and the effect of intrauterine infection might be more pronounced if this were analysed separately.

Mother to child transmission of HIV

In non-selected populations having an HIV-1 infection, the mother to child transmission rate is usually between 15% and 30%, but in some groups, particularly among Africans, higher transmission rates up to over 40% are reported [87,90–92]. This is probably due to transmission by breastfeeding, which accounts for 14% [93]. HIV-2 infections, that are predominantly seen in West African people, are transmitted from mother to child in 0–3% of cases [94].

Transmission in pregnancy varies with HIV disease progression of the pregnant woman: a high CDC classification, a low CD4+ cell count, a low CD4+/CD8+ ratio, and the presence of p24 antigenemia during pregnancy are related to a 2–3 times increased transmission rate [87,95]. All these variables are an

expression of viral load in women without antiretroviral therapy. The large American–French intervention trial (ACTG-076 study) clearly showed the amount of replicated viruses (HIV-RNA load) in blood to be positively related to mother to child transmission: 41.7% in the highest quartile (>15 700 copies/ml) and 7.1% in the lowest quartile (<1730 copies/ml) [96]. Viral load is highest during acute infections and in symptomatic individuals. However, HIV viral load can also be high in individuals with a normal resistance and appears to be more or less steady in a given person until cellular resistance decreases (CD4+ cell counts less than 200 cells/mm^3) and viral load increases [97].

Transmission during pregnancy

The exact rates of transmission at different stages of pregnancy and delivery are still not known. Transmission during early pregnancy has been demonstrated convincingly [98,99]. It also appeared that spontaneously aborted fetuses from HIV-seropositive women were often infected with HIV [85]. In two small studies using PCR techniques, viral DNA could be detected in 30% and 57% of these fetuses [100,101]. Therefore, intrauterine infection with HIV seems likely. The high proportion of infections in spontaneous abortions (50%) seems to be biased, however, by the increased risk of abortion in HIV-infected women. [84]. Intrauterine infection is also supported by the finding that, in the first week of neonatal life, viral markers, such as p24 antigen, anti-HIV IgM, and viral DNA are detectable in 30–50% of HIV-infected children [102–104]. Neither p24 antigen nor IgM antibodies cross the placenta. The detection of DNA by means of PCR in neonatal blood is the most sensitive early proof of infection, but it may not distinguish between intrauterine infection and transmission of appreciable quantities of HIV during delivery. Recently, it appeared that transmission before late gestation or delivery is probably not a common occurrence. A carefully designed study on 100 fetuses from HIV-seropositive women, who nearly all aborted electively beyond 15 weeks of gestation (mean: 22.4 weeks) showed only 2 infections (CI: 0.2–7) [105].

There seem to be two distinct patterns of AIDS development in congenitally HIV-infected children. A total of 25–30% will develop AIDS very rapidly, usually during the first year of life. The remainder follow a more adult pattern of disease progression

[106,107]. This can be explained in two ways. One explanation is that children who develop AIDS during the first year of life might be infected by large quantities of HIV. In support of this explanation is the finding that advanced disease progression of the mother is not only reflected in a high rate of mother to child transmission, but also in the severity of disease in the infected children [108]. A second explanation might be that children who are infected during pregnancy are at high risk to develop AIDS in their first year of life. In support of this explanation is the finding that in the fetus HIV infects thymic cells and so affects the immune apparatus in its origin [85,109]. The results of the twin registration study corroborate this latter explanation (see below).

The mode of HIV transmission during pregnancy is still not fully established. It is clear from the transmission rates that HIV fortunately does not cross the placenta freely. This was confirmed in our laboratory by quantitative HIV-RNA determinations in maternal blood at labor and umbilical cord blood (unpublished data). However, if during pregnancy a syphilis infection occurs, transmission of HIV is high [110], which can be explained by placentitis and 'leaking' of the placenta. In general, chorioamnionitis is more often found in HIV-seropositive than HIV-uninfected women and is associated with an increased transmission rate [111]. It may be that HIV spreads to the fetal circulation after infection of the placenta (just as the rubella virus does). It is unclear whether the fetal macrophagic Hofbauer cells in the stroma of the placenta, which sometimes contain HIV [112,113], protect against HIV infection of the fetus or mediate it. Further, HIV-infected lymphocytes crossing the placental barrier might also induce a fetal infection. Transfer of maternal lymphocytes across the placenta to the fetus appears to occur in 30% [114]. This could be the result of microlesions in most of these women or partial placental abruption in some. It seems prudent not to perform invasive diagnostics (amniocentesis) or version of breech infants in order to avoid maternofetal blood contamination [115].

Transmission during delivery

Delivery is a process during which HIV-contaminated fluids, such as cervical secretions and maternal blood surround the fetus and are sometimes present in the neonatal oropharynx or stomach [116]. HIV was cultured from the cervicovaginal secretion of 4 (21%) out of 19 pregnant women and from the gastric aspirates of 2 out of 16 children, both of which were infected, whereas none of the 12 uninfected children had a positive culture [116]. Genital shedding of HIV-DNA during pregnancy was found in 32% of 212 cervical and 10% of 215 vaginal specimens [117]. Shedding appeared related to low CD4+ counts and to severe vitamin A deficiency. The latter was found to be related to HIV transmission in a Malawi cohort of mother child pairs [118].

The duration of ruptured membranes appears to be an important determinant of HIV transmission from mother to child, in particular in women with a low CD4+ cell count [115,119]. Vaginal delivery thus appears to be a hazardous period for the fetus of an HIV-infected woman. The question is to what extent does delivery contribute to the mother to child transmission rate and which (other) factors are related to the risk of infection.

The European Collaborative Study (ECS) showed that one of the clear risk factors for mother to child transmission is preterm delivery below 34 weeks, with an odds ratio of 3.8 [87]. The percentage of deliveries before 34 weeks was only 5%, which is not higher than expected, arguing against intrauterine HIV infection as the cause of preterm labor. Since later analyses of the ECS showed that low maternal CD4+ counts were related to preterm delivery [86], it cannot be excluded, however, that the increased risk of HIV transmission in preterm infants occurred intrauterine. Another explanation for the increased risk of HIV transmission in preterm infants is that they are less protected against HIV-infection during the process of birth by (maternal) anti-HIV antibodies, as passive antibody transfer across the placenta largely occurs during the last 2 months of pregnancy [120].

The international twin registration study showed most elegantly that at least 50% of infected children are infected during birth [121]. It established that second twins are infected much less frequently than first twins (15% v. 35%). This difference is still apparent in twins born via caesarean section, since in these twins the infection rate is less frequent than in twins born vaginally (8% v. 16%). For twins, most risk factors are equal and the second twin endures even more contractions. The only difference is that the passage through the birth canal and the duration of ruptured membranes is usually (much) longer for the first-born than for the second-born twin. These factors thus clearly enhance mother to child transmission of HIV.

It seems likely that second-born twins who are infected are predominantly infected *in utero*, and first-born twins have mixed *in utero* and *intrapartum* infection. This is supported by the shorter median time interval to AIDS in second-born compared with first-born twins (17 months v. 42 months). The twin study also showed a difference between the transmission rate after vaginal delivery (25%) and after a caesarean section (12%). It attributed 76% of the transmission risk to vaginal exposure (lower confidence limit 48%).

A multicenter evaluation of the sensitivity of HIV-1 DNA PCR in neonatal blood taken during the first 2 days of life showed DNA to be detectable in 38% of the infected children and in 93% by 14 days of age [122]. This suggests that intrauterine infection occurs in 40% of the infected infants and at birth in 60%. This is corroborated by a metaanalysis of published and unpublished data of prospective studies, showing that caesarean section halves the risk of infection [123]. The effect was largely explained, however, by the data of the large ECS [124]. Surprisingly, no effect at all was found in the large French collaborative study and in a large cohort from the USA [115,119]. It was seen, however, in other studies that were not included in the metaanalysis, such as a prospective study in South Africa [125].

Summarizing, circumstantial evidence exists, that at least 50% and possibly 70% of infected infants are infected during birth by ingestion of HIV-containing maternal fluids. Knowledge of the timing and mode of transmission is of course very important for preventive strategies.

Transmission during lactation

Transmission of HIV through breast feeding has been well documented from the onset of the AIDS epidemic following acute HIV infections caused by blood transfusions in the puerperium [126,127]. Acute HIV infections are more likely to result in transmission than chronic infections because of the absence of antibodies in the baby and the high viral load and infectivity of the mother. Transmission rates are 26% (CI 13–39%) for acute infections [128] and 14% (CI 7–22%) for women that were already infected before pregnancy [93]. HIV has been shown to result into a productive infection of mammary epithelial cells in culture [129] and cell-free HIV has been detected in milk [130]. The presence of HIV-infected cells in milk of the mother predicts the mother to child transmission rate

[128,131]. Since colostrum and early breast milk contain many more cells than later milk, the risk of infection might be highest in the early phase of lactation. The risk of infection was also shown to be high in the presence of a breast abscess even during late lactation [132]. A matter of special concern is that a study in rhesus monkeys showed, that susceptibility to SIV infection is enhanced during progesterone dominancy [30]. This suggests that during pregnancy, and also during breastfeeding, the risk of a primary HIV infection of the woman and so of her child is relatively high in case of an HIV-infected partner.

Among the many favorable aspects of breast milk and breastfeeding is the fact that human milk contains immunoglobulins against agents causing diarrhea and respiratory diseases. Immunoglobulins against HIV are also present in milk. The secretion of both anti-HIV IgA and IgM takes place into the mammary gland, probably as a local reaction to HIV, and does not reflect serum levels [133]. The presence of anti-HIV secretory IgA in early milk samples appeared to be associated with absence of mother to-child transmission [128]. Likewise, as shown by multivariate analysis, the presence anti-HIV IgM during the entire period of lactation was inversely related to HIV-1 mother to child transmission [128].

In order to prevent infant mortality from other diseases than HIV infection and from malnutrition, the World Health Organization and UNICEF still recommend for developing countries to advise breastfeeding [134].

Prevention of mother to child transmission

Table 24.1. summarizes potential methods to reduce mother to child transmission. To date the only proven and most effective strategy is the use of antiretroviral medication, hitherto zidovudine, during pregnancy and delivery. The French–American multicenter placebo-controlled, ACTG 076 study showed a 76% reduction of transmission from 22.6% (95% CI 17.0–29.0%) to 7.6% (CI 4.3–12.3%) in a selected group of women who did not need zidovudine for themselves and who started between 14 and 34 weeks (median 26 weeks) of pregnancy [96,135]. They used 500 mg zidovudine per day orally in five doses. During delivery, an infusion was given yielding a double dose and the children received zidovudine via the bottle for 6 weeks after birth.

Table 24.1. Possible methods of reducing mother to child transmission of HIV.

Reducing transmission to women, especially during pregnancy and lactation
Termination of pregnancy
Prevention of placental leakage by syphilis
Prevention of genital ulcers
Vitamin A supplementation
Antiretroviral therapy
Prevention of preterm delivery
No invasive diagnostics during pregnancy or labor
Caesarean section
Vaginal lavage
Immunization/vaccination
Artificial bottle feeding

The absolute reduction in HIV transmission was highest in women with the heaviest viral RNA load before therapy. Reduction was also encountered, however, in women with low viral load. The reduction of mother to child transmission could not be fully explained by viral RNA load reduction in plasma [96]. Viral load in cervical secretions was not measured. It has been found that plasma does not reflect HIV load in cervical secretion [116], whereas HIV load in cervical shedding might be clinically more important for contamination and thus infection during birth. Moreover, accidents during pregnancy, like partial placental abruption and maternofetal transfusion, may be conditions that cannot be avoided, but have a high risk of infection even in women with low viral load.

Another possibility, for which purpose the children are treated after birth, is postexposure prophylaxis. Whether this principle is of much importance is not certain. In some centers, women who already used zidovudine before pregnancy (and who usually had a lower resistance and were thus at higher risk to infect their child) were also analyzed. They were excluded from the ACTG076 trial and their children did not receive zidovudine during the first weeks of life. They too appeared to have a decreased transmission rates compared with untreated women (14% v. 23%) [136].

In clinical practice, zidovudine treatment fortunately appears as effective as in the context of the ACTG076 trial [137]. Teratogenetic and short-term side effects are absent or low when zidovudine is given during the whole course of pregnancy [135,138].

Early onset of treatment as in the ACTG076 trial might be less effective than a later start, since probably very few fetuses are infected in the first two trimesters of pregnancy (as discussed earlier), whereas zidovudine resistance can develop within 12 weeks of treatment [139,140]. In these cases, the most risk-bearing period would not be covered. In practice, this means that it is quite possible to postpone treatment beyond 20 weeks if the woman and her partner need time to cope with a recent knowledge of HIV infection.

Combination therapy is much more effective than zidovudine to reduce viral load, whereas the risk of developing resistance is much lower. It thus seems logical to advise combination therapy also for preventing mother to child transmission. However, the dilemma is that we are uncertain about long-term drug side effects on the offspring [141]. This is increasingly important, when the potential extra benefit gets smaller. In the case of zidovudine, long-term carcinogenic side effects in mice were found [142]. The least we have to do is to inform the pregnant women of these still unknown possibilities.

When women do not want to use zidovudine during pregnancy, it seems justified to advise an elective caesarean section (as discussed above). When women receive zidovudine during pregnancy, the additional benefit of a ceasarean section is not yet proven. In view of the fact that the highest risk of mother to child transmission is at birth, short-term aggressive combination treatment starting a few days before elective term delivery may be the least harmful way of prevention in the future. The results of randomized trials considering this treatment are awaited.

Acknowledgment

We wish to thank Professor F.B. Lammes for providing some of the figures.

References

1 World Health Organisation. HIV/AIDS: The global epidemic. *Week Epidemiol Rec* 1997; **72**: 17–21.

2 Centers for Disease Control. First 500,000 AIDS cases – United States, 1995. *MMWR* 1995; **44**: 849-8-53.

3 Centers for Disease Control. Update: AIDS among women – United States, 1994. *MMWR* 1995; **44**: 81–84.

4 Cotton DJ. AIDS in women. In: *Textbook of AIDS Medicine* Broder S, Merigan TC, Bolognesi D (eds) Baltimore: Williams & Wilkins, 1994: 161–168.

5 Hankins CA, Handley MA. HIV disease and AIDS in women: current knowledge and a research agenda. *J Acquir Immune Defic Syndr* 1992; **5**: 957–971.

6 Brettle RP, Leen CLS. The natural history of HIV and AIDS in women. *AIDS* 1991; **5**: 1283–1292.

7 Rothenberg R, Woelfel M, Stoneburner R, Milberg J, Parker R, Truman B. Survival with the acquired immunodeficiency syndrome. *N Engl J Med* 1987; **317**: 1297–1302.

8 The Italian Seroconversion Study. Disease progression and early predictors of AIDS in HIV-seroconverted injecting drug users. *AIDS* 1992; **6**: 421–426.

9 Gardner LI, Brundage JF, McNeil JG et al. Predictors of HIV-1 disease progression in early- and late-stage patients: the US army natural history cohort. *J Acquir Immune Defic Syndr* 1992; **5**: 782–793.

10 Anzala OA, Nagelkerke NJD, Bwayo JJ et al. Rapid progression to disease in African sex workers with human immunodeficiency virus type 1 infection. *J Infect Dis* 1995; **171**: 686–689.

11 Phillips AN, Antunes F, Stergious G et al. A sex comparison of rates of new AIDS-defining disease and death in 2554 AIDS cases. *AIDS* 1994; **8**: 831–835.

12 Melnick SL, Sherer R, Louis TA et al.Survival and disease progression according to gender of patients with HIV infection. *JAMA* 1994; **272**: 1915–1921.

13 Sha BE, Benson CA, Pottage JC, Urbanski PA, Daugherty SR, Kessler HA. HIV infection in women: an observational study of clinical characteristics, disease progression, and survival for a cohort of women in Chicago. *J Acquir Immune Defi Syndr* 1995; **8**: 486–495.

14 Fleming PL, Ciesielski CA, Byers RH, Castro KG, Berkelman RL. Gender differences in reported AIDS-indicative diagnoses. *J Infect Dis* 1993; **168**: 61–67.

15 Vlahov D, Munoz A, Solomon et al. Comparison of clinical manifestations of HIV infection between male and female injecting drug users. AIDS 1994; **8**: 819–823.

16 Cooley TP, Hirschhorn LR, O'Keane JC. Kaposi's sarcoma in women with AIDS. *AIDS* 1996; **10**: 1221–1225.

17 Clark RA, Blakley SA, Rice J, Brandon W. Predictors of HIV disease progression in women. *J Acquir Immune Defic Syndr* 1995; **9**: 43–50.

18 Bacchetti P, Moss AR. Incubation time of AIDS in San Francisco. *Nature* 1989; **388**: 251–253.

19 Katzenstein DA, Hammer SM, Hughes MD et al. The relation of virologic and immunologic markers to clinical outcomes after nucleoside therapy in HIV-infected adults with 200 to 500 CD4 cells per cubic millimeter. *N Engl J Med* 1996; **335**: 1091–1098.

20 Bush CE, Donovan RM, Markowitz N, Baxa D, Kvale P, Saravolatz LD. Gender is not a factor in serum human immunodeficiency virus type 1 RNA levels in patients with viremia. *J Clin Microbiol* 1996; **34**: 970–972.

21 Stewart GJ, Cunningham AL, Driscoll GL et al. Transmission of human T-cell. Lymphotropic virus type III (HTLV-III) by artificial insemination by donor. *Lancet* 1985; **ii**: 581–584.

22 Araneta MR, Mascola L, Eller A et al. HIV transmission through donor artificial insemination. *JAMA* 1995; **273**: 854–858.

23 Anonymous. Comparison of female to male and male to female transmission of HIV in 563 stable couples. European Study Group on Heterosexual Transmission of HIV. *MJ* 1992 **304**: 809–813.

24 Nicolosi A, Correa Leite ML, Musicco M, Arici C, Gavazzeni G, Lazzarin A. The efficiency of male-to-female and female-to-male sexual transmission of the human immunodeficiency virus: a study of 730 stable couples. Italian Study Group on HIV Heterosexual Transmission. *Epidemiology* 1994; **5**: 570–575.

25 de Vincenzi I. A longitudinal study of human immunodeficiency virus transmission by heterosexual partners. European Study Group on Heterosexual Transmission of HIV. *N Engl J Med* **331**: 341–346.

26 Padian N, Shiboski S, Jewel N. Female-to-male transmission of human immunodeficiency virus. *JAMA* 1991; **266**: 1664–1667.

27 Renzullo P, McNeil J, Levin L et al. Risk factors for prevalent human immunodeficiency virus (HIV) infection in active duty army men who initially report no identified risk: a case-control study. *J Acquir Immune Defic Syndr* 1990; **2**: 266–271.

28 Padian N, Abrams J, Shurnick JH, Van Devanter NL, O'Brien TR. Risk factors for postcoital bleeding among women with or at risk for infection with human immunodeficiency virus. *J Infect Dis* 1995; **172**: 1084–1087.

29 Halsey N, Coberley J, Holt E et al. Sexual behavior, smoking, and HIV-1 infection in Haitian women. *JAMA* 1992; **267**: 2062–2066.

30 Marx PA, Spira AI, Gettie A et al. Progesterone implants enhance SIV vaginal transmission and early virus load. *Nat Med* 1996; **2**: 1084–1089.

31 Spira AI, Marx PA, Patterson BK et al. Cellular targets of infection and route of viral dissemination after an intravaginal inoculation of simian immunodeficiency virus into rhesus macaques. *J Exp Med* 1996; **183**: 215–225.

32 Satten GA, Mastro TD, Longini IM Jr. Modelling the female-to-male per-act HIV transmission probability in an emerging epidemic in Asia. *Stat Med* 1994; **13**: 2097–2106.

33 Mastro TD, Satten GA, Nopkesorn T, Sangkharomya S. Longini IM Jr. Probability of female-to-male transmission of HIV-1 in Thailand. *Lancet* 1994; **343**: 204–207.

34 Celentano DD, Nelson KE, Suprasert S et al. Risk factors for HIV-1 seroconversion among young men in northern Thailand *JAMA* 1996; **275**(2): 122–127.

35 Forrest BD. Women, HIV, and mucosal immunity. *Lancet* 1991; **337**: 835–836.

36 Kreiss J, Willerford DM, Hensel M et al. Association between cervical inflammation and cervical shedding of human immunodeficiency virus. *J Infect Dis* 1994; **170**: 1597–1601.

37 Wald A, Corey L, Handsfield HH, Holmes KK. Influence of HIV infection on manifestations and natural history of other sexually transmitted diseases. *Annu Rev Public Health* 1993; **14**: 19–42.

38 Wasserheit JN. Epidemiological synergy. Interrelationships between human immunodeficiency virus infection and other sexually transmitted diseases. *Sex Transm Dis* 1992; **19**: 61–77.

39 Korn AP, Landers DV. Gynecologic disease in women infected with human immunodeficiency virus type 1. *J Acquir Immune Defic Syndr Hum Retrovirol* 1995; **9**: 361–370.

40 Carpenter CCJ, Mayer KH, Stein MD. Human immunodeficiency virus infection in North American women: experience with 200 cases and a review of the literature. *Medicine* 1991; **70**: 307–325.

41 Johnstone FD, Williams AR, Bird GA, Bjornsson S. Immunohistochemical characterization of endometrial lymphoid cell populations in women infected with human immunodeficiency virus. *Obstet Gynecol* 1994; **83**: 586–593.

42 Rhoads J, Wright D, Redfield R et al. Chronic vaginal candidiasis in women with human immunodeficiency virus infection. *JAMA* 1987; **257**: 3105-3107.

43 Imam N, Carpenter CCJ, Mayer KH et al. Hierarchical pattern of mucosal candida infections in HIV-Seropositive Women. *Am J Med* 1990; **89**: 142–146.

44 Law D, Moore CB, Wardle HM, Ganguli LA, Keany MGL, Denning DW. High prevalence of antifungal resistance in *Candida* spp. From patients with AIDS. *J Antimicrob Chemother* 1994; **34**: 659–668.

45 Spinillo A, Michelone G, Cavanna C, Colonna L, Capuzzo E, Nicola S. Clinical and microbiological characteristics of sumptomatic vulvovaginal candidiasis in HIV-seropositive women. *Genitourin Med* 1994; **70**: 268–272.

46 Kaplowitz LG, Baker D, Gelb D et al. Prolonged continuous acyclovir treatment of normal adults with frequently recurring genital herpes simplex virus infection. *JAMA* 1991; **265**: 747–751.

47 Verberkmoes A, Boer K, Wertheim PME, Bronkhorst CM, Lange JMA. Thalidomide for genital ulcer in HIV-positive woman. *Lancet*, 1996; **347**: 974.

48 1993 revised classification for HIV infection and expanded surveillance case definition for AIDS among adolescents and adults. *MMWR* 1992; **41**: 1–19.

49 Chirgwin KDm Feldman J, Augenbraun M, Landesman S, Minkoff H. Incidence of venereal warts in human immunodeficiency virus-infected and uninfected women. *J Infect Dis* 1995; **172**: 235-238.

50 Tong P, Mutasim DF. Herpes simplex virus infection masquerading as condyloma acuminata in a patient with HIV disease. *Br J Dermat* 1996; **134**: 797–800.

51 Wright TC Jr, Ellerbrock TV, Chiasson MA, Van Devanter N, Sun XW. Cervical intraepithelial neoplasia in women infected with human immunodeficiency virus: prevalence, risk factors, and validity of Papanicolaou smears. New York Cervical Disease Study. *Obstet Gynecol* 1994; **84**: 591–597.

52 Klein RS, Ho GY, Vermund SH, Fleming I, Burk RD. Risk factors for squamous intraepithelial lesions on Pap smear in women at risk for human immunodeficiency virus infection. *J Infect Dis* 1994; **170**: 1404–1409.

53 Conti M, Agarossi A, Parazzini F et al. HPV, HIV infection, and risk of cervical intraepithelial neoplasia in former intravenous drug abusers. *Gynecol Oncol* 1993; **49**: 344-348.

54 Laga M, Icenogle JP. Marsella R et al. Genital papillomavirus infection and cervical dysplasia–opportunistic complications of HIV infection. *Int J Cancer* 1992; **50**: 45–48.

55 Schafer A, Friedmann W, Mielke M, Schwartlander B, Koch MA. The increased frequency of cervical dysplasia-neoplasia in women infected with the human immunodeficiency virus is related to the degree of immunosuppression. *Am J Obstet Gynecol* 1991; **164**: 593–639.

56 Kreiss JK, Kiviat NB, Plummer FA et al. Human immunodeficiency virus, human papillomavirus, and cervical intraepithelial neoplasia in Nairobi prostitutes. *Sex Transm Dis* 1992; **19**: 54–59.

57 Korn AP, Landers DV. Gynecologic disease in women infected with human immunodeficiency virus type 1. *J Acquir Immune Defic Syndr Hum Retrovirol* 1995; **9**: 361–370.

58 Langley CL, Benga-De E, Critchlow CW et al. HIV-1, HIV-2, human papillomavirus infection and cervical neoplasia in high-risk African women. *AIDS* 1996; **10**: 413-417.

59 Maiman M, Tarricone N, Vieira J, Suarez J, Serur E, Boyce JG. Colposcopic evaluation of human immunodeficiency virus-seropositive women. *Obstet Gynecol* 1991; **78**: 84–88.

60 Sun XW, Ellerbrock TV, Lungu O, Chiasson MA, Bush TJ, Wright TC Jr. Human papillomavirus infection in human immunodeficiency virus-seropositive women. *Obstet Gynecol* 1995; **85**: 680–686.

61 Petry KU, Scheffel D, Bode U et al. Cellular immunodeficiency enhances the progression of human papillomavirus-associated cervical lesions. *Int J Cancer* 1994; **57**: 836–840.

62 Williams AB, Darragh TM, Vranizan K, Ochia C, Moss AR, Palefsky JM. Anal and cervical human papillomavirus infection and risk of anal and cervical epithelial abnormalities in human immunodeficiency virus-infected women. *Obstet Gynecol* 1994; **83**: 205–211.

63 Smith JR, Kitchen VS, Botcherby M et al. Is HIV infection associated with an increase in the prevalence of cervical neoplasia? *Br J Obstet Gynaecol* 1993; **100**: 149–153.

64 Spinillo A, Tenti P, Zappatore R et al. Prevalence, diagnosis and treatment of lower genital neoplasia in women with human immunodeficiency virus infection. *Eur J Obstet Gynecol Reprod Biol* 1992; **43**: 235–241.

65 Kuhler-Obbarius C, Milde-Langosch K, Helling-Giese G, Salfelder A, Peimann C, Loning T. Polymerase chain reaction-assisted papillomavirus detection in cervicovaginal smears: stratification by clinical risk and cytology reports. *Virchows Arch* 1994; **425**: 157–163.

66 Seck AC Faye MA, Critchlow CW et al. Cervical intraepithelial neoplasia and human papillomavirus infection

among Senegalese women seropositive for HIV-1 or HIV-2 or seronegative for HIV. *Int J STD AIDS* 1994; **5**: 189–193.

67 Van Doornum GJ, Van den Hoek JA, Van Ameijden EJ et al. Cervical HPV infection among HIV-infected prostitutes addicted to hard drugs. *J Med Virol* 1993; **41**: 185–190.

68 ter Meulen J, Eberhardt HC, Luande J et al. Human papillomavirus (HPV) infection, HIV infection and cervical cancer in Tanzania, east Africa. *Int J Cancer* 1992; **51**: 515–521.

69 Alloub MI, Barr BBB, McLaren KM, Smith IW, Bunney MH, Smart GE. Human papillomavirus infection and cervical intrepithelial neoplasia in women with renal allografts. *Br Med J* 1989; **298**: 153–156.

70 Wright TC Jr, Koulos J, Schnoll F et al. Cervical intraepithelial neoplasia in women infected with the human immunodeficiency virus: outcome after loop electrosurgical excision. *Gynecol Oncol* 1994; **55**: 253–258.

71 Maiman M, Fruchter RG, Serur E, Levine PA, Arrastia CD, Sedlis A. Recurrent cervical intraepithelial neoplasia in human immunodeficiency virus-seropositive women. *Obstet Gynecol* 1993; **82**: 170–174.

72 Centers for Disease Control. Risk for cervical disease in HIV-infected women – New York City. *MMWR* 1990; **39**: 846–849.

73 Maiman M, Tarricone N, Vieira J et al. Colposcopic evaluation of human immunodeficiency virus-seropositive women. *Obstet Gynecol* 1991; **78**: 84–88.

74 Adachi A, Fleming I, Burk RD et al. Women with human immunodeficiency virus infection and abnormal papanicolaou smears: a prospective study of colposcopy and clinical outcome. *Obstet·Gynecol* 1993; **81**: 372–377.

75 Korn AP, Autry M, DeRemer PA, Tan W. Sensitivity of the Papanicolaou smear in human immunodeficiency virus-infected women. Obstet Gynecol 1994; **83**: 401–404.

76 Korn AP, Abercrombie PD, Foster A. Vulvar intraepithelial neoplasia in women infected with human immunodeficiency. *Gynecol Oncol* 1996; **61**: 384–386.

77 Scott GB, Fischl MA, Klimas N et al. Mothers of infants with the acquired immunodeficiency syndrome. Evidence for both symptomatic and asymptomatic carriers. *JAMA* 1985; **253**: 363–366.

78 Blanche S, Mayaux M-J, Rouzioux C et al. Relation of the course of HIV infection in children to the severity of the disease in their mothers at delivery. *N Engl J Med* 1994; **330**: 308–312.

79 Brettle, P. Pregnancy and its effects on HIV/AIDS. In: Johnstone FD (ed.) *HIV Infection in Obstetrics and Gynaecology.* London: Bailliere Tindall, 1992: 125–136.

80 Sridama V, Pacini F, Yang S-L, Moawad A, Reilly M, DeGroot LJ. Decreased levels of helper T cells: a possible cause of immunodeficiency in pregnancy. *N Engl J Med* 1982; **307**: 352–356.

81 Biggar RJ, Pahwa S, Minkhoff H et al. Immunosupression in pregnant women infected with human immunodeficiency virus. *Am J Obstet Gynecol* 1989; **161**: 1239–1244.

82 Miotti PG, Liomba G, Dallabetta GA, Hoover DR, Chiphangwi JD, Saah AJ. T lymphocyte subsets during and after pregnancy: analysis in human immunodeficiency virus type 1 infected and uninfected Malawian mothers. *J Infect Dis* 1992; **165**: 1116–1119.

83 Puel J, Gayet-Mengelle C, Berrebi A, Tricoire J, Rousseau A, Castelin M. Protocoles d'exploration et de surveillance de l'infection a virus de l'immunodeficience humaine chez la mère et l'infant. In: Berrebi A, Puel J, Tricoire J, Pontonnier G (eds) *HIV Infection in Mother and Child.* Toulouse: Privat, 1988: 63–84.

84 Temmerman M, Chomba EN, Ndinya-Achola J et al. Maternal human immunodeficiency virus-1 infection and pregnancy outcome. *Obstet Gynecol* 1994; **83**: 495–501.

85 Langston C, Lewis DE, Hammill HA et al. Excess intrauterine fetal demise associated with maternal human immunodeficiency virus infection. *J Infect Dis* 1995; **172**: 1451–1460.

86 Thorne C, Newell ML, Dunn D, Peckham C. The European Collaborative Study: clinical and immunological characteristics of HIV 1-infected pregnant women. *Br J Obstet Gynaecol* 1995; **102**: 869–875.

87 European Collaborative Study. Risk factors for mother-to-child transmission of HIV-1. *Lancet* 1992; **339**: 1007–1012.

88 Abrams EJ, Matheson PB, Thomas PA et al. Neonatal predictors of infection status and early death among 332 infants at risk of HIV-1 infection monitored prospectively from birth. *Pediatrics* 1995; **96**: 451–458.

89 Moye J, Rich KC, Kalish LA et al. For the Women and Infants Transmission Study Group. Natural history of somatic growth in infants born to women infected by human immunodeficiency virus. *J Pediatr* 1996; **128**: 58–69.

90 Blanche S, Rouzioux C, Moscato M-LG et al. A prospective study of infants born to women seropositive for human immunodeficiency virus type 1. *N Engl J Med* 1989; **320**: 1643–1648.

91 Gabiano C, Tovo P-A, de Martino M et al. Mother-to-child transmission of human immundeficiency virus type 1: risk of infection and correlates of transmission. *Pediatrics* 1992; **90**: 369–374.

92 Lallemant M, Le Coeur S, Samba L et al. and the Congolese Research Group on Mother-to-Child Transmission of HIV. Mother-to-child transmission of HIV-1 in Congo, central Africa. *AIDS* 1994; **8**: 1451–1497.

93 Dunn DT, Newell ML, Ades AE, Peckham CS. Risk of human immunodeficiency virus type 1 transmission through breastfeeding. *Lancet* 1992; **340**: 585–588.

94 Andreasson P-A, Dias F, Naucler A, Andersson S, Biberfeld G. A prospective study of vertical transmission of HIV-2 in Bissau, Guinea-Bissau. *AIDS* 1993; **7**: 989–993.

95 Report of a Consensus Workshop Sienna, Italy, 1992. Maternal factors involved in mother-to-child transmission of HIV-1. *J AIDS* 1992; **5**: 1019–1029.

96 Sperling RS, Shapiro DE, Coombs RW et al. Maternal viral load, zidovudine treatment, and the risk of transmission of human immunodeficiency virus type 1 from mother to infant. *N Engl J Med* 1996; **335**: 1621-1629.

97 Weverling GJ, Keet IPM, De Jong MD et al. HIV-rna level is set early in the HIV infection and predicts clinical outcome. *XI International Conference on AIDS.* Vancouver, July 1996 [abstract Th.B. 4330].

98 Jauniaux E, Nessmann C, Imbert MC, Meuris S, Puissant F, Hustin J. Morphological aspects of the placenta in HIV pregnancies. *Placenta* 1988; **9**: 633–642.

99 Mauray W, Potts BJ, Rabson AB. HIV-1 infection of first-trimester and term placental tissue: a possible mode of maternal-fetal transmission. *J Infect Dis* 1989; **160**: 583–588.

100 Seiro R, Rubinstein A, Rashbaum WK, Lyman WD. Maternofetal transmission of AIDS: frequency of human immunodeficiency virus type 1 nucleic acid sequences in human fetal DNA. *J Infect Dis* 1992; **166**: 699–703.

101 Mano H, Chermann J-C. Fetal human immunodeficiency virus type 1 infection of different organs in the second trimester. *AIDS Res Human Retrovirol* 1991; **7**: 83–88.

102 Krivine A, Firtion G, Cao L, Francoual C, Henrion R, Lebon P. HIV replication during the first weeks of life. *Lancet* 1992; **339**: 1187–1189.

103 Borkowsky W, Krasinski K, Pollack H, Hoover W, Kaul A, Ilmet-Moore T. Early diagnosis of human immunodeficiency virus infection in children <6 months of age: comparison of polymerase chain reaction, culture, and plasma antigen capture techniques. *J Infect Dis* 1992; **166**: 616–619.

104 Burgard M, Mayaux M-J, Blanche S et al. The use of viral culture and p24 antigen testing to diagnose human immunodeficiency virus infection in neonates. *N Engl J Med* 1992; **327**: 1192–1197.

105 Brossard Y, Aubin JT, Mandelbrot L et al. Frequency of early in utero HIV-1 infection: a blind DNA polymerase chain reaction study on 100 fetal thymuses. *AIDS* 1995; **9**: 359–366.

106 European Collaborative Study. Children born to women with HIV-1 infection: natural history and risk of transmission. *Lancet* 1991; **337**: 253–260.

107 Auger I, Thomas P, Gruttola de V et al. Incubation periods for paediatric AIDS patients. Nature 1988; **336**: 575–577.

108 Blanche S, Mayaux M-J, Rouzioux C, et al. Relation of the course of infection in children to the severity of the disease in their mothers at delivery. *N Engl J Med* 1994; **330**: 308–312.

109 Papiernik M, Brossard Y, Mulliez N et al. Thymic abnormalities in fetuses aborted from human immunodeficiency virus type 1 seropositive women. *Pediatrics* 1992; **89**: 297–301.

110 Pollack H, Borkowsky W, Krasinski K. Maternal syphilis is associated with enhanced perinatal transmission. *30th Interscience Conference on Antimicrobial Agents and Chemotherapy* (IcAAC), Atlanta, 1990, p. 1274A (Abstract).

111 St Louis ME, Kamenga M, Brown C et al. Risk for perinatal HIV-1 transmission according to maternal immunologic, virologic, and placental factors. *JAMA* 1993; **269**: 2853–2859.

112 Lewis SH, Reynolds-Kohler C, Fox HE, Nelson JA. HIV-1 in trophoblastic and villous Hofbauer cells, and haematological precursors in eight-week fetuses. *Lancet* 1990; **335**: 565–568.

113 Backé E, Jimenez E, Unger M, Schäfer, Jauniaux E, Vogel M. Demonstration of HIV-1 infected cells in human placenta by in situ hybridisation and immunostaining. *J Clin Pathol* 1992; **45**: 871–874.

114 Pollack MS, Kirkpatrick D, Kapoor N, Dupont B, O'Reilly RJ. Identification by HLA typing of intrauterine-derived maternal T cells in four patients with severe combined immunodeficiency. *N Engl J Med* 1982; **307**: 662–666.

115 Mandelbrot L, Mayaux MJ, Bongain A et al. and the French Pediatric HIV Infection Study Group. Obstetric factors and mother-to-child transmission of human immunodeficiency virus type 1: the French perinatal cohorts. *Am J Obstet Gynecol* 1996; **175**: 661–667.

116 Nielsen K, Boyer P, Dillon M et al. Presence of human immunodeficiency virus (HIV) type 1 and HIV-1-specific antibodies in cervicovaginal secretions of infected mothers and in the gastric aspirates of their infants. *J Infect Dis* 1996; **173**: 1001–1004.

117 John GC, Nduati RW, Mbori-Ngacha D et al. Genital shedding of human deficiency virus type 1 DNA during pregnancy: association with immunosuppression, abnormal cervical or vaginal discharge, and severe vitamin A deficiency. *J Infect Dis* 1997; **175**: 57–62.

118 Semba RD, Miotti JD, Saah AJ, Canner JK, Dallabetta GA, Hoover DR. Maternal vitamin A deficiency and mother-to-child transmission of HIV-1. *Lancet* 1994; **343**: 1593–1597.

119 Landesman SH, Kalish LA, Burns DN et al. Obstetrical factors and the transmission of human immunodeficiency virus type 1 from mother to child. The Women and Infants Transmission Study. *N Engl J Med* 1996; **334**: 1617–1623.

120 Regelman WE, Mills EL, Quie PG. Immunology of the newborn. In: Feigin RD, Cherry JD (eds) *Textbook of Pediatric Infectious Diseases*. Philadelphia: Saunders WB, 1987: 927–931.

121 Duliege AM, Amos CI, Felton S et al. Birth order, delivery route, and concordance in the transmission of human immunodeficiency virus type 1 from mothers to twins. International Registry of HIV-Exposed Twins. *J Pediatr* 1995; **126**: 625-632.

122 Dunn DT, Brandt CD, Krivine A et al. The sensitivity of HIV-1 DNA polymerase chain reaction in the neonatal period and the relative contribution of intra-uterine and intra-partum transmission. *AIDS* 1995; **9**: F7–F11.

123 Dunn DT, Newell ML, Mayaux MJ et al. Mode of delivery and vertical transmission of HIV-1: a review of prospective studies. Perinatal AIDS Collaborative Transmission Studies. *J Acquir Immune Defic Syndr* 7: 1064–1066.

124 The European Collaborative Study . Caesarean section and risk of vertical transmission of HIV-1 infection. *Lancet* 1994; **343**: 1464–1467.

125 Kuhn L, Bobat R, Coutsoudis A et al. Cesarean deliveries and maternal–infant HIV transmission: results from a prospective study in South Africa. *J Acquir Immune Defic Syndr* 1996; **11**: 478–483.

126 Ziegler JB, Johnson RO, Cooper DA, Gold G. Postnatal transmission of AIDS-associated retrovirus from mother to infant. Lancet 1985; **i**: 896–897.

127 Van de Perre P, Simonon A, Msellati P et al. Postnatal transmission of human immunodeficiency virus type 1 from mother to infant. *N Engl J Med* 1991; **325**: 593–598.

128 Van de Perre P. Postnatal transmission of human immunodeficiency virus type 1: the breast feeding dilemma. *Am J Obstet Gynecol* 1995; **173**: 483–487.

129 Toniolo A, Serra C, Conaldi PG, Basolo F, Falcone V, Dolei A. Productive HIV-1 infection of normal human mammary epithelial cells. *AIDS* 1995 **9**: 859–866.

130 Thiry L, Sprecher-Goldberg S, Jonckheer T et al. Isolation of AIDS virus from cell-free breast milk of three healthy virus carriers. *Lancet* 1985; **ii**: 891–892.

131 Van de Perre P, Simonon A, Hitimana DG et al. Infective and anti-infective properties of breast milk from HIV-1 infected women. *Lancet* 1993; **341**: 914-918.

132 van de Perre P, Hitimana D-G, Simonon A, Msellati P, Karita E, Lepage P. Postnatal transmission of HIV-1 associated with breast abscess. *Lancet* 1992; **327**: 1490–1491.

133 van de Perre P, Hitimana D-G, Lepage P. Human deficiency virus antibodies of IgG, IgA, and IgM subclasses in milk of seropositive mothers. *J Pediatr* 1988; **113**: 1039–1041.

134 World Health Organization. Global Programme on AIDS. Consensus statement from the WHO/UNICEF consultation on HIV transmission and breast-feeding. *Week Epidemiol Rec* 1992; **24**: 177–179.

135 Connor EM, Sperling RS, Gelber R et al. Reduction of maternal–infant transmission of human immunodeficiency virus type 1 with zidovudine treatment. *N Engl J Med* 1994; **331**: 1173–1180.

136 Matheson PB, Abrams EJ, Thomas PA et al. Efficacy of antenatal zidovudine in reducing perinatal transmission of human immunodeficiency virus type 1. *J Infect Dis* 1995; **172**: 353-358.

137 Fiscus SA, Adimora AA, Schoenbach VJ et al. Perinatal HIV infection and the effect of zidovudine therapy on transmission in rural and urban counties. *JAMA* **275**: 1483–1488.

138 Kumar RM, Hughes PF, Khurranna A. Zidovudine use in pregnancy: a report on 104 cases and the occurrence of birth defects. *J Acquir Defic Syndr* 1993; **7**: 1034–1039.

139 Larder BA, Darby G, Richman DD. HIV with reduced sensitivity to zidovudine (AZT) isolated during prolonged therapy. *Science* 1989; **243**: 1731–1734.

140 Medina DJ, Tung PP, Lerner-Tung MB, Nelson CJ. Mellors JW, Strair RK. Sanctuary growth of human immunodeficiency virus in the presence of 3′-azido-3′-deoxythymidine. *J Virol* 1995; **69**: 1606–1611.

141 Johnstone FD. HIV and pregnancy. *Br J Obstet Gynaecol* 1996; **103**: 1184–1190.

142 Anonymous. US expert panel reaffirms benefit of perinatal zidovudine. *Lancet* 1997; 349: 258.

Part III

Jacques W.A.J. Reeders
John R. Mathieson

Quick Reference Tables

Radiological abnormalities in AIDS-related disease of the Central Nervous System, Cardiovascular System, Chest, Lumenal Gastrointestinal Tract, and Liver, Spleen, and Biliary Tract according to the organ involved (Tables A–E).

A Central Nervous System (CNS)

Organism/disease	Organ involved	Radiological abnormality	Extent of disease	Differential diagnosis
Toxoplasmosis (*Toxoplasma gondii*)	CNS	*CT:* hypodense (82%) contrast enhancement; well-defined, annular, nodular (rare), subependymal (rare) lesions; calcifications	• cerebral hemispheres more frequently affected than cerebellum/ brainstem; • cortico-medullary junction with basal ganglia	AIDS-related lymphoma
		MR: increased signal foci on long TR-images with iso/hypointense centers. Short TR-images: hypointense/contrast enhancement	Other organs involved: • Lymph nodes • GI tract • Respiratory tract	
AIDS-related lymphoma	CNS	*CT:* multiple isodense masses (less common), hyperdense enhancement (80%): round, oval, nodular lesions with ringlike enhancement. Linear/nodular subpial and subependymal enhancement is characteristic!	(Multi)focal lesions: • Striatum • Hemispheric • White matter • Periventricular • Supratentorial brain	Toxoplasmosis
		MR: hypointense on T_1-weighted images; isointense less common; after contrast center remains hypointense; margins enhance in smooth/ringlike appearance. T_2-weighted images: variable appearances – increased, isointense and decreased signal intensity	Other organs involved: • GI tract • Bone marrow	
Cryptococcus (*Cryptococcus neoformans*)	CNS	*CT:* spherical, well-defined iso or/hypodense lesion(s); cryptococcoma, gelatinous pseudocysts	• Meninges • Basal ganglia • Thalami • Midbrain • Corpus callosum • Cerebral cortex • Posterior fossa	Other lesions with CNS mass effect
		MR: high signal on long TR-images, decreased signal on short TR-images; peri-vascular space dilatation	Other organs involved: • Chest • Lymph nodes • Liver/spleen • Bone marrow	

Organism/disease	Organ involved	Radiological abnormality	Extent of disease	Differential diagnosis
Herpes (Herpes simplex virus (HSV), Varizella zoster virus (VZV)	CNS	CT/MR: encephalitis; ventriculitis; necrotizing vasculitis of entire cord/spinal roots; generalized swelling, abnormal density or signal changes in white matter; cortical enhancement (rare)	Diffuse involvement Other organs involved (mucocutaneous): • Perianal region • Oropharynx • Esophagus	Cytomegalovirus (CMV)
Mycobacteria [Mycobacterium tuberculosis, M. avium-intracellulare (MAI)]	CNS	CT/MR: Hydrocephalus Meningeal enhancement Parenchymal involvement (less common): ring-like, nodular lesions	• At site of the perforating end-arteries at the base of the brain Other organs involved: • Lymph nodes • Liver/spleen • Peritoneum • Bone marrow • GI tract • Chest • GU tract • Skin (rare) • Heart (rare)	Toxoplasmosis AIDS-related lymphoma
Brain atrophy	CNS	CT/MR: supratentorial (100%) and infratentorial (70%) atrophy; caudate head atrophy cortical atrophy; widened sulci	Generalized; Supratentorial or infratentorial	
Progressive multifocal leucencephalopathy (PML) (JC-virus)	CNS	CT: Demyelination: areas of diminished density MR: Demyelination: zones of increased signal on long TR images; decreased signal on short TR images. Lesions against cortico-medullary junction, in (deep) gray matter posterior fossa (common), cervical cord (uncommon)	• Cortico-medullary junction, • Gray matter • Posterior fossa • Cervical cord • Kidneys	
Focal white matter hyperintensities (FWMH)	CNS	MR: zones of perivascular demyelination or dilated perivascular spaces secondary to atrophy: white matter hyperintensity	• Perivascular spaces	

Organism/disease	Organ involved	Radiological abnormality	Extent of disease	Differential diagnosis
HIV encephalitis	CNS	Non-specific atrophy with deep white matter changes; microglial nodules undetectable by CT, but rarely seen on MR. Symmetrically diffuse or periventricular white matter disease without mass effect. *CT*: areas of low attenuation *MR*: high signal intensity on long TR images; combined lobal atrophy and diffuse symmetrical white matter hyperintensity on T_2-weighted images	Diffuse	PML
Cytomegalovirus (CMV)	CNS	Ependymitis; ependymal necrosis; calcifications in neonates; encephalitis; microglial nodules predominantly in cortex *CT*: usually normal, progressive ventriculomegaly; smooth periventricular enhancement with compression of ventricular margins *MR*: non-specific appearances; ventriculo-ependymitis; abnormal high signal changes in periventricular brain	Generalized/diffuse Other organs involved: ● Oropharynx ● Adrenals ● Chest ● GI tract ● Retina ● Biliary tract ● Liver/gallbladder	AIDS-related lymphoma

CT, computed tomography; MR, magnetic resonance; GU, genitourinary; GI, gastrointestinal.

B   Cardiovascular System (CVS)

Organism/disease	Organ involved	Radiological abnormality	Extent of disease	Differential diagnosis
Pericardial effusion (*Mycobacterium tuberculosis*, MAI, CMV, Coxsackie virus, *Herpes simplex*, *Cryptococcus neoformans*, *Salmonella typhimurium*, *Nocardia asteroides*, *Listeria monocytogenes*, *Toxoplasma gondii*, Kaposi's sarcoma, non-Hodgkin lymphoma)	CVS	*Echocardiography*: echo-free/echo-poor space between parietal pericardium and epicardium	Pericardium/epicardium	
Ventricular dysfunction (*Mycobacterium tuberculosis*, MAI, CMV, Coxsackie virus, *Herpes simplex*, *Toxoplasma gondii*, *Pneumocystis carinii*(?), *Candida albicans*, *Cryptococcus neoformans*, *Aspergillus fumigatus*, *Staphylococcus aureus*, *Nocardia asteroides*, *Streptococcus pneumoniae*, Kaposi's sarcoma, Hodgkin/non-Hodgkin lymphoma)	CVS	Myocarditis (50%) and dilated myocardiopathy (20%) Endocarditis Pericarditis/pericardial effusion Left ventricular enlargement *Echocardiography*: enlarged right/left ventricle, abnormal septum position/motion; marked pulmonary hypertension: both diastolic/systolic flattening of ventricular septum in response to markedly abnormal transeptal pressure gradient	Myocardium Endocardium Pericardium	

C Chest

Organism/disease	Organ involved	Radiological abnormality	Extent of disease	Differential diagnosis
Pneumocystis carinii (PCP)	Chest	Normal chest X-ray: 10% *Chest X-ray:* *Early disease:* bilateral perihilar/or basal fine interstitial pattern without pleural effusion; diffuse symmetric to medium reticular or reticulo-nodular pattern and ground glass opacification. *Advanced disease:* homogeneous scattered alveolar consolidation; peripheral reticular pattern. *Late disease:* asymmetrically scattered alveolar consolidation (mosaic pattern); reticular pattern: thickening of interlobular/interlobar interstitial tissue *Final stage:* ARDS-like appearance Less common: miliary/coarse interstitial pattern Thin-walled cystic lesions (multiple, confluent) in upper lobes (pneumatoceles): (0–13%) pneumothorax (1–6%) Atypical pattern: air space disease; cavitary nodules, hilar/mediastinal lymphadenopathy; pleural effusions (0–2%). *High-resolution CT:* symmetrical ground-glass appearance; interstitial pattern; sparing of lung periphery	Diffuse; upper or lower zone predominance Bilateral Other organs involved: ● Liver/spleen ● Lymph nodes	Other opportunistic infections: tuberculosis, cryptococcosis, fungal infection, toxoplasmosis. HSV, Kaposi's sarcoma, CMV

Organism/disease	Organ involved	Radiological abnormality	Extent of disease	Differential diagnosis
Toxoplasmosis (*Toxoplasma gondii*)	Chest	Uncommon *Chest X-ray*: bilateral, predominantly coarse, nodular pattern	Bilateral Other organs involved: ● CNS ● GI tract (rare)	PCP, tuberculosis, cryptococcosis, fungal infection.
Cytomegalovirus (CMV)	Chest	*Chest X-ray*: pneumonia: bilateral interstitial infiltrates; nodular pattern or asymmetrically scattered alveolar opacities with a preference for central/lower regions. Pneumothorax; pneumomediastinum	Bilateral Other organs involved: ● Oropharynx ● Adrenals ● GI tract ● CNS ● Retina ● Biliary tract Liver/gallbladder	PCP fibrosis
Herpes simplex virus (HSV)	Chest	*Chest X-ray*: bilateral interstitial pattern; scattered focal alveolar abnormalities; pleural effusions: rare; lymphadenopathy: rare		PCP CMV
Varicella zoster virus (VZV)	Chest	*Chest X-ray*: bilateral, scattered, round, nodular alveolar opacities with tendency to coalesce; pleural effusions: rare; lymphadenopathy: rare		PCP CMV
Pyogenic infections (*Hemophilus influenzae*, *Streptococcus pneumoniae*, *Nocardia asteroides*, *Legionella pneumoniae*, *Corynebacterium equi* (*Rhodococcus*)	Chest	*Chest X-ray*: diffuse, unilateral or bilateral, patchy or lobar consolidation; pleural effusions/empyema; peripheral nodules/ nodular infiltrates with a basal predominance; cavitation does occur (Staphylococci and anaerobes); multiple lung abscesses may occur; intrathoracic lymphadenopathy: very uncommon *CT*: feeding vessels leading to the nodules; pleural effusions; pleural empyema	Diffuse Unilateral/bilateral	

Organism/disease	Organ involved	Radiological abnormality	Extent of disease	Differential diagnosis
Tuberculosis (*M. tuberculosis*)	Chest	Normal chest X-ray: 5% *Primary form (60%)* *Early disease:* cavitary infiltrates predominantly in the posterior segments of the upper lobes or superior segments of lower lobes; not usually accompanied by lymphadenopathy. *Advanced disease:* dissiminated extra-pulmonary sites; diffuse coarse, nodular, reticulo/nodular pattern. *Third form (15%):* miliary pattern: diffuse fine nodular pattern; focal alveolar infiltrates in mid/lower lung zones; hilar and/or mediastinal lymphadenopathy. *CT:* enlarged nodes with central low attenuation (necrosis) and peripheral ring enhancement; widening mediastinum; pleural effusion	Other organs involved: ● GI tract (esophagus) ● Liver/spleen ● Lymph nodes ● GU tract (kidneys) ● Bone marrow ● Adrenals	PCP Atypical mycobacterial infection Fungal infection AIDS-related lymphoma
Mycobacterium avium complex	Chest	Normal chest X-ray: 20% *Chest X-ray:* diffuse, bilateral, reticulo-nodular or patchy infiltrates or nodules, with a tendency to form cavities and a preference for the superior lobes; focal or diffuse alveolar disease; miliary pattern: less common; hilar and/or mediastinal lymphadenopathy; pleural effusions.	Dissiminated, focal, or diffuse Other organs involved: ● Lymph nodes ● Liver/spleen ● Peritoneum ● Bone marrow ● GI tract ● GU tract ● CNS (rare) ● Skin (rare) ● Heart (rare)	Tuberculosis

Organism/disease	Organ involved	Radiological abnormality	Extent of disease	Differential diagnosis
Fungal infections: cryptococcosis (*Cryptococcus neoformans*)	Chest	*Chest X-ray:* diffuse, bilateral, scattered, patchy, nodular or alveolar infiltrates and/or intrathoracic lymphadenopathy (80%). Less frequent: single nodule/mass with/without cavitation or focal segmental consolidation; pleural effusion; miliary pattern	Solitary/multiple lesions Other organs involved: ● CNS ● Lymph nodes ● Liver/spleen ● Bone marrow	*Toxoplasma* PCP Tuberculosis
Nocardiosis (*Nocardia asteroides*)	Chest	*Chest X-ray:* unilateral segmental or lobar consolidation often with cavity formation	Unilateral/focal	Other opportunistic infection
Histoplasmosis (*Histoplasma capsulatum*)	Chest	Normal chest X-ray: 40% *Chest X-ray:* diffuse interstitial infiltrates. Less common: miliary pattern; focal infiltrates; hilar/mediastinal lymphadenopathy	Disseminated More diffuse than focal Other organs involved: ● Bone marrow	Other opportunistic infections
Coccidioidomycosis (*Coccidioides immitis*)	Chest	Normal chest X-ray: 70% *Chest X-ray:* diffuse nodular infiltrates; focal opacities; cavities; lymphadenopathy; solitary or multiple cavity-forming lesions (thin-walled)	Diffuse	Other opportunistic infections
Aspergillosis (*Aspergillus fumigatus*)	Chest	*Chest X-ray:* upper lobe thick-walled cavities (multiple); intracavitary masses; pleural-based nodules; consolidation; pleural effusions	Diffuse	Other opportunistic infections
Kaposi's sarcoma (KS)	Chest	*Chest X-ray:* diffuse, bilateral, poorly defined, reticulonodular opacities (1–2 cm) in a perihilar distribution; bilaterally scattered mostly round opacities, whose delineation varies in definition; interstitial abnormalities coarser in nature than those in PCP; lobar/sublobar patchy consolidations/atelectasis; pleural effusions, mostly	Bilateral Unilateral (<10%) Other organs involved: ● Mucocutaneous ● Sternum ● Ribs ● Thoracic spine ● GI tract ● Liver/spleen ● Lymph nodes	PCP CMV

Organism/disease	Organ involved	Radiological abnormality	Extent of disease	Differential diagnosis
		bilateral, often in large amounts (<40%); intrathoracic lymphadenopathy (30%) *CT*: nodules with irregular margins; areas of consolidation along a predominantly bronchovascular distribution: peribronchovascular interstitial thickening, radiating from the perihilar region; subpleural nodules; ground-glass attenuation adjacent to nodules/masses (hemorrhage); interlobular septal thickening (38%)	Pulmonary KS is preceded in 95% with KS-mucous membrane/skin lesions	
AIDS-related lymphoma	Chest	Intrathoracic involvement: <10% *Chest X-ray*: Pleural effusions: 50%; unilateral or bilateral; solitary or multiple, smooth-contoured nodules which rapidly enlarge; masses with central cavitation; air broncho-gram; chest wall invasion; axillary/hilar/mediastinal lymphadenopathy (25%) Less frequent: interstitial infiltrates; alveolar opacities; pericardial effusion/masses; myocardial involvement.	Unilateral or bilateral; solitary or multiple lesions Other organs involved: ● CNS ● Lumenal GI tract ● Liver, spleen, pancreas ● Retroperitoneum	Typical/atypical mycobacterial infection. PCP. Fungal infection.
Lymphocytic interstitial pneumonia (LIP)	Chest	Normal chest X-ray: 50% *Chest X-ray*: non-specific findings: fine to coarse reticular/reticulo-nodular pattern; patchy alveolar/ground-glass opacities; pleural effusion: unusual; no intrathoracic lymphadenopathy	Diffuse Bilateral Most frequently in children with AIDS	Other opportunistic infections PCP

CT, computed tomography

D Lumenal Gastrointestinal Tract

Organism/disease	Organ involved	Radiological abnormality	Extent of disease	Differential diagnosis
Candida (*Monilia*) (*Candida albicans*)	Oropharynx/ esophagus	*DC-esophagogram:* Oral thrush *Mild disease:* edematous folds; minimal mucosal plaques, covering a friable erythematous mucosa, coarse filling defects, oriented along the long axis of the esophagus; ulcerations. *Moderate disease:* diffuse mucosal plaques, fine longitudinal ulcerations. *Severe/advanced disease:* fold thickening; abnormal motility; diffuse deep ulceration (longitudinal); 'cobblestone' appearance; extensive diffuse or focally clustered plaques ('shaggy esophagus'); pseudomembranes. *Endstage of disease:* polypoid lesions; strictures; mucosal 'bridging'	Diffuse Other organs involved: ● Skin ● Chest ● CNS	*Herpes simplex* virus (HSV)
Herpes simplex virus (HSV1,HSV2)	Oropharynx/ esophagus	*DC-esophagogram:* *Mild disease:* multiple, scattered, diamond/stellate-shaped shallow ulcers, separated by normal mucosa; lucent halo of edema. *Advanced disease:* diffuse nodularity/ulcerations with 'cobblestoning'; inflammatory exudates; Irregular esophageal contour similar to CMV	Focal or diffuse Other organs involved: ● Mucocutaneous ● Perianal region Focal or diffuse	*Candida* CMV

Organism/disease	Organ involved	Radiological abnormality	Extent of disease	Differential diagnosis
Cytomegalovirus (CMV)	Esophagus/ Stomach	*DC-esophagogram:* Diffuse granular mucosa due to clustered superficial erosions and/or aphthous ulcers; irregular thickening of mucosal folds; shallow, poorly defined, diamond-shaped ulcers; irregular thickening of mucosal folds; nodular wall thickening; tiny ulcers; granularity of mucosa; narrowing of lumen with limited distensibility with attenuation;	Distal esophagus with extension into esophago-gastric junction Other organs involved: ● Adrenals ● Chest ● CNS ● Retina ● Biliary tract ● Liver/gallbladder Predilection: antrum Focal or diffuse; common	Idiopathic HIV
	Small intestine	*Enteroclysis:* Mild dilatation: edematous submucosal nodules (0.25–0.75 cm); separation of loops; shallow or deep, round or serpiginous ulceration of various size/depths. *Late stage:* narrowing of lumen; fistula	Segmental or diffuse Predilection: terminal ileum	
	Colon/ano-rectum	*Mild disease:* DC barium enema; diffuse mild or coarse mucosal granularity; cecal spasm; irregular thickening of mucosal folds (edema); superficial or deep punctate or linear ulcerations; aphthous ulcers. *CT:* low-density edematous bowel wall; marked mucosal/ serosal enhancement. *Severe/advanced disease:* DC barium enema: large ulcers; skip lesions; areas of mass effect (granulation tissue/submucosal hemorrhage); nodular filling defects (pseudomembranes) *CT:* increased density in bowel wall (hemorrhage); thickening of bowel wall.	Common predilection: ascending colon/cecum/terminal ileum Sometimes entire colon	

Organism/disease	Organ involved	Radiological abnormality	Extent of disease	Differential diagnosis
		Late stage disease: DC barium enema/ CT: narrowing of lumen		
Idiopathic HIV	Esophagus/ ano-rectum	*DC barium studies:* Giant (≥2 cm) well-defined shallow ulceration with surrounding normal mucosa	Usually solitary; multiple may occur	CMV HSV Mycobacterial infection
Cryptosporidiosis (*Cryptosporidium*)	Small bowel	*Enteroclysis:* Mild small bowel dilatation; hypersecretion; 'sprue-like appearance' *CT:* small bowel wall thickening/dilatation small bowel/increased intra-lumenal fluids; non-specific mesenteric lymphadenopathy	Diffuse Other organs involved: ● Duodenum ● Colon ● Biliary tract ● Gallbladder ● Chest	Other opportunistic infections: Giardiasis *Isospora belli*
Mycobacterium (*M. avium-intra cellulare* (MAI), *M. tuberculosis*)	Esophagus	*DC-esophagogram:* Focal extrinsic mass impression; longitudinal deep ulcerations; sinus tracts to the mediastinum/esopha-gotrachial fistulae; traction diverticula; strictures in chronic disease	Focal Other organs involved: ● Lymph nodes ● Liver/spleen ● Peritoneum ● Bone marrow ● Chest ● GU tract ● CNS (rare) ● Skin (rare) ● Heart (rare)	Idiopathic HIV CMV
	Stomach/ Duodenal bulb	*DC-stomach examination* Ulceration; hypertrophic fibrotic encasement; bulky gastric mass extending into mesentery. Thickening of mucosal folds; aphthous ulcers	Segmental hepatosplenomegaly, common	Crohn's disease
	Small intestine	*Enteroclysis:* Mild dilatation with irregular fold thickening; separation/displacement of bowel loops due to lymphadenopathy; spasm, irregularity; fine nodularity; mild hypertension with segmental/ flocculation of barium; appendical mass ?; 'pseudo-Whipple's' disease.	Segmental Predilection: proximal jejunum	Other opportunistic infections: PCP Giardiasis *Isospora belli* CMV

Organism/disease	Organ involved	Radiological abnormality	Extent of disease	Differential diagnosis
	Small intestine	*CT*: moderate-sized mesenteric/retroperitoneal lymphadenopathy: low density (necrosis)		
	Colon	*DC barium enema*: circumferential thickening of cecal wall and terminal ileum; fistula formation. *CT*: regional low-attenuation necrotic lymphadenopathy	ileo-cecal region Segmental	
Kaposi's sarcoma	Oropharynx/ esophagus/ Stomach/ duodenum Small bowel/ Colon/ano-rectum	*DC barium studies*: *Early disease:* flat lesions, not demonstrated on barium studies; granularity of mucosa; *Advanced disease:* irregular thickening of mucosal folds; discrete sharp submucosal nodules (6 mm–3 cm) with or without central umbilication (bull's eye/target appearance); normal intervening mucosa; nodular wall thickening or small bowel; sometimes large, bulky, polypoid, segmental masses; narrowing of lumen *CT*: high-attenuation lymphadenopathy	Diffuse Other organs involved: ● Skin ● Chest ● Lymphnodes ● Liver/spleen ● Heart ● GU tract (kidneys)	Opportunistic infections Crohn's disease, AIDS-related lymphoma Multiple polyps, hematogenous metastasis
AIDS-related lymphoma	Stomach/ Small intestine/ Colon/ano-rectum	*DC barium studies*: Diffuse wall thickening; mesenteric polypoid lesions simulating adenocarcinoma; loss of mucosal pattern; irregular fold thickening; discrete penetrating ulcers; narrowing of lumen *CT*: extraluminal extent of enteric lymphomas	Other organs involved: ● CNS ● Bone marrow ● Abdominal viscera: kidney (hydronephrosis due to obstructing lymph nodes) ● Ano-rectum/colon	Kaposi's sarcoma

CT, computed tomography

E　Liver/Spleen/Biliary tract

Organism/disease	Organ involved	Radiological abnormality	Extent of disease	Differential diagnosis
Pneumocystis [*Pneumocystis carinii* (PCP)]	Liver/spleen	*US:* numerous nodules (liver/spleen/kidneys) usually hyperechoic >2 cm *CT:* calcifications (liver/spleen) usually hypodensity nodules, <2 cm in both liver and spleen	Focal Other organs involved: ● CNS ● Bone marrow ● Chest	*Candida Aspergillus* MAI Cytomegalovirus Tuberculosis Bacillary peliosis Fungal infection Kaposi's sarcoma AIDS-related lymphoma Smooth-muscle tumor
Bacillary peliosis	Liver/spleen	*US/CT:* hypoechoic/hypodense nodules <2 cm (liver/spleen/lymph nodes)	Rare; associated with chronic diseases (malignancies, tuberculosis, etc.)	Tuberculosis MAI PCP Fungal infection Kaposi's sarcoma AIDS-related lymphoma Smooth-muscle tumor
Fungal infections (*Histoplasma capsulatum, Coccidioides immites, Cryptococcus neoformans, Candida albicans*)	Liver/spleen	*US/CT:* hypoechoic hypodense nodules <2 cm (liver/spleen); hepatosplenomegaly	Diffuse Other organs involved: ● Chest ● Bone marrow ● GI tract ● CNS ● Lymphnodes ● Liver/spleen	Tuberculosis MAI Bacillary peliosis PCP Kaposi's sarcoma AIDS-related lymphoma
CMV	Liver/spleen	*US/CT:* multiple focal small, hyper- or hypoechoic/low density lesions	Focal or diffuse Other organs involved: ● Lumenal GI tract ● Adrenals ● Chest ● CNS ● Retina	Other opportunistic infections
	Biliary tract	*ERCP:* mimicking sclerosing cholangitis; irregular dilatation CBD; decreased arborization of intrahepatic ducts; irregular/'brush border' of biliary mucosa; multiple vesicular filling defects; thickened duct wall of intra/extrahepatic bile ducts; papillary stenosis; strictures; pruning; acalculous cholecystitis	Segmental/diffuse	*Cryptosporidium*

Organism/disease	Organ involved	Radiological abnormality	Extent of disease	Differential diagnosis
Mycobacterium avium-intracellulare (MAI)	Liver/spleen	*US/CT:* hypoechoic/hypodense nodules <2 cm (liver/spleen); more hepatosplenomegaly than MTb	Diffuse Other organs involved: ● Lymph nodes ● Peritoneum ● Bone marrow ● Lumenal GI tract ● Chest ● GU tract ● CNS (rare) ● Skin (rare) ● Heart (rare)	Tuberculosis Bacillary peliosis PCP Fungal infections Kaposi's sarcoma AIDS-related lymphoma
Mycobacterium tuberculosis (MTb)	Liver/spleen	*US/CT:* hypoechoic/hypodense nodules <2 cm; less hepatosplenomegaly than MAI lymph node necrosis	Diffuse Other organs involved: ● Chest ● Lymph nodes ● GU tract (kidneys) ● Adrenals ● Bone marrow ● Lumenal GI tract	MAI Bacillary peliosis PCP Fungal infections Kaposi's sarcoma AIDS-related lymphoma
Kaposi's sarcoma	Liver/spleen	*US:* small (5–12 mm) hyperechoic nodules in liver/spleen *CT:* hypodense periportal bands ('prominent portal triads') (liver); hypodense nodules <2 cm (liver/spleen); hepatosplenomegaly	Other organs involved: ● Skin ● Chest ● Lumenal GI tract ● Lymph nodes ● Liver/spleen ● Heart ● GU tract (kidneys)	Tuberculosis MAI Bacillary peliosis PCP Fungal infections AIDS-related lymphoma Metastatic disease Hemangiomas
AIDS-related lymphoma	Liver/spleen/pancreas	Three patterns: 1. Large infiltrating masses: US: hypoechoic; CT: hypodense with homogenous attenuation 2. Multiple focal nodules: US: hypoechoic; CT: low-density; variable size 1–5 cm or larger; liver/spleen, pancreas, lymph nodes 3. Diffuse infiltrating 'peritoneal lymphomatosis': US: hypoechoic; *CT:* hypodense; mimics fluid, also with ascites	Other organs involved: ● Chest ● CNS ● Retroperitoneum ● Lumenal GI tract	Tuberculosis, MAI Bacillary peliosis PCP Fungal infections Kaposi's sarcoma Smooth-muscle tumor

CT, computed tomography; US, ultrasound

F   Observations of Different Radiological Patterns on Chest X-ray in AIDS

Observations	Incidence	Differential diagnosis
Bronchial or bronchiolar wall thickening	Common	PCP, pyogenic infections Mycobacterial infections (TB, MAC) Kaposi's sarcoma
	Uncommon/absent	ARL Viral infections Fungal infections LIP
Bronchial or bronchiolar impaction	Common	Mycobacterial infections (TB, MAC) Pyogenic infections, PCP
	Uncommon/absent	Kaposi's sarcoma LIP ARL Viral infections Fungal infections
Bronchiectasis	Common	Mycobacterial infections (TB, MAC) Pyogenic infections, PCP
	Uncommon/absent	Fungal infections Kaposi's sarcoma ARL Viral infections LIP
Endoluminal polyp/mass	Uncommon	Mycobacterial infections (TB, MAC) Fungal infections Kaposi's sarcoma ARL (rare)
	Absent	Pyogenic infections, PCP Viral infections LIP
Intrathoracic (mediastinal/hilar) lymphadenopathy	Common	Mycobacterial infections (TB, MAC) Fungal infections Kaposi's sarcoma ARL
	Uncommon/absent	PCP Viral infections Bacterial infections
Pleural effusions(isolated)	Common	Kaposi's sarcoma ARL Bacterial infections
	Uncommon/absent	PCP Viral infections Mycobacterial infections (TB, MAC) Fungal infections LIP

Observations	Incidence	Differential diagnosis
Thick-walled cavities	Common	Fungal infections Mycobacterial infections (TB, MAC)
	Uncommon/absent	PCP Viral infections Kaposi's sarcoma LIP ARL
Thin-walled cavities	Common	PCP Fungal infections
Solitary (parenchymal) nodules	Common	Kaposi's sarcoma (peribronchovascular and subpleural) ARL Fungal infections Mycobacterial infections (TB, MAC) Septic emboli (perivascular (±cavitation)
	Uncommon/absent	PCP Viral infections (CMV) Bacterial infections (cryptococcosis)
Multiple (miliary) nodules	Common	Kaposi's sarcoma Viral infections Mycobacterial infections (TB, MAC) Fungal infections
	Uncommon/absent	PCP Bacterial infections
Consolidation	Common	Bacterial infections (cryptococcosis) Fungal infections
	Uncommon/absent	PCP (lobar/segmental) Viral infections (diffuse) Mycobacterial infections (TB, MAC) Kaposi's sarcoma ARL
Ground glass attenuation	Common	PCP Pyogenic infections Viral infections (CMV) Bacterial infections LIP
Reticular/reticulonodular pattern	Common	PCP Viral infections (CMV) Kaposi's sarcoma ARL LIP
Interstitial infiltrates plus lymphadenopathy	Common	Kaposi's sarcoma Mycobacterial infections (TB, MAC) Bacterial infections (cryptococcosis) ARL

Abbreviations:
PCP = pneumocystis carinii pneumonia
TB = mycobacterium tuberculosis
MAC = mycobacterium avium complex
ARL = AIDS-related lymphoma
CMV = cytomegalovirus
LIP = lymphocytic interstitial pneumonia

Refs: − Chapter 14,
− McGuinness G., Gruden J.F., Bhalla M., Harkin T.J., Jagirdar J.S., Naidich D.P.
  AIDS-Related Airway Disease; Review Article; AJR: 168, 67–77, 1997

G   Pathogens and Neoplasms in AIDS: Cytological Methods

Infections	Diagnostic method	Cytogenic staining	PA characteristics
Viruses			
Cytomegalovirus	Broncho-alveolar lavage (BAL) smears FNA biopsies Transbronchial biopsies Open lung biopsies	PAP, HE, Giemsa Immunoperoxidase Monoclonal antibodies for immunochemistry *In situ* hybridization	Dark red, intranuclear, inclusion bodies with thin halo
Herpes simplex virus (HSV)	Sputum BAL Smears FNA biopsies	PAP, HE, Giemsa Monoclonal antibodies for immunochemistry *In situ* hybridization	Vesicles/ulceration: small, eosinophyllic, intranuclear, inclusion bodies
Bacteria			
Mycobacterium avium-intracellulare	Smears	Ziehl–Nielson stain Kynynuon stain Rhodamine-Aaramine stain DNA probes PAS/GMS HE stain Metenamine stain Diff quick Polymerase chain reaction (PCR) techniques	Acid fast microorganisms in cytoplasm of macrophages
Parasites			
Cryptosporidium *Microsporidium* *Isospora belli*		Cytology plays no significant role	
Fungi			
Candida albicans	Endoscopy specimen Bronchoscopy specimen	PAP, PAS GMS stain Culture	
Histoplasmosis (*Histoplasma capsulatum*)	FNA biopsy of mass BAL	PAP, PAS Giemsa stain GMS stain Bone marrow culture	
Cryptococcosis (*Cryptococcus neoformans*)	Lumbar puncture (CSF) FNA specimen Skin biopsy	PAP PAS GMS or mucicarmine stain India ink stain (CSF)	Multi-nucleated giant cells with organisms in their cytoplasm
Coccidioidomycosis	BAL Transbronchial biopsy	PAP PAS GMS or mucicarmine stain India ink stain (CSF)	

Infections	Diagnostic method	Cytogenic staining	PA characteristics
Neoplasms			
Kaposi's sarcoma	Deep endoscopy Biopsy	Cytology plays no role in diagnosis	
AIDS-related lymphoma	FNA biopsy	HE Diff quick Giemsa stain Gram stain AFB	

FNA, fine-needle aspiration; PAP, Papanicolaou stain; HE, hematoxylin and eosin stain; GMS, Grocott's methenamine silver stain; PAS, periodic acid–Schiff stain; CSF, cerebrospinal fluid; AFB, Acid Fast Bacilli; BAL, bronchoalveolar lavage; PA, Pathology.

INDEX

Numbers in italics refer to illustrations or tables

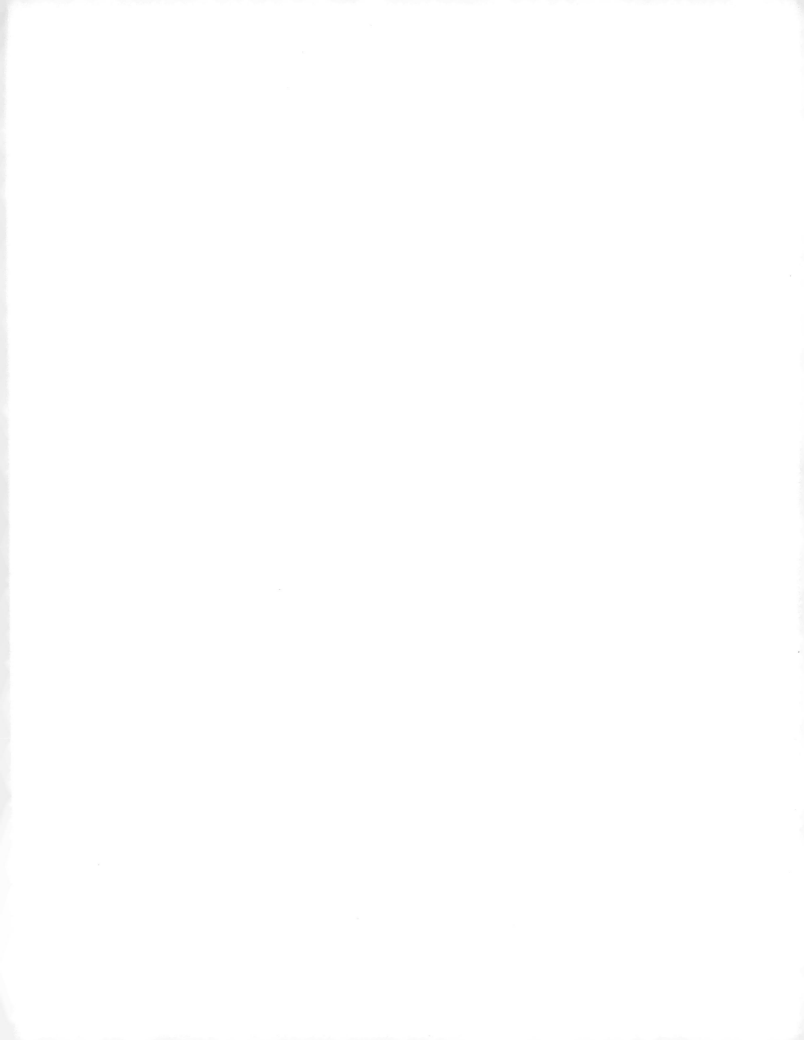